Umbilicus and Umbilical Cord

Mohamed Fahmy

Umbilicus and Umbilical Cord

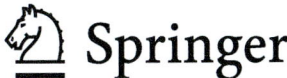 Springer

Mohamed Fahmy
Pediatric Surgery
Al Azher University Pediatric Surgery
Cairo
Egypt

Additional material to this book can be downloaded from http://extras.springer.com

ISBN 978-3-319-87306-0   ISBN 978-3-319-62383-2   (eBook)
https://doi.org/10.1007/978-3-319-62383-2

Printed on acid-free paper

This Springer imprint is published by the registered company Springer International Publishing AG part of Springer Nature.
The registered company address is: Gewerbestrasse 11, 6330 Cham, Switzerland

It is my honor to dedicate this illustrative textbook to our diseased and disabled children, and their mothers, who tolerate their illness with a bitter smile and at the same time give us the data to investigate and elaborate on their diseases, while also giving us a sense of satisfaction to see our procedures succeeding and our publication spreading.

The original version of this book was revised: Acknowledgment has been added in the Frontmatter. An erratum can be found at https://doi. org/10.1007/978-3-319-62383-2_37

Acknowledgements

I am grateful to all my colleagues who permitted me to use some of their patients' photos in this illustrative textbook.

For additional information and references on the umbilical cord see Silent Risk Issues about the human umbilical cord 2nd Edition Copyright © 2014 by Jason H. Collins, MD, MSCR.

Contents

Part II   Umbilical Cord

Part I
Introduction

Nomenclature and Synonyms of the Umbilicus

Nomenclature: Umbilicus, belly button, navel, omphalos, outie, innie, centrepiece of the human body, and sole button

Umbilical cord known as: Lifeline, thread of life, funis and funiculus, which is derived from the Latin word used for rope or cord

Umbilicus is the common scientific and medical name, but in the common language, it is called belly button; it represents the rounded, knotty depression in the centre of the abdomen caused by the detachment of the umbilical cord.

Navel: The term omphalos in Greek or umbilicus in Latin means a 'navel' which is a conical stone that was deemed in antiquity to have marked a 'Centre of the Earth'.

Omphalos: This is the scientific and medical term used to represent the umbilicus; the origin of this name will be explained later.

Outie and innie: In humans, the umbilical scar can appear as a depression (often referred to as an *innie*) or as a protrusion (*outie*), although umbilicus could be classified into these two categories.

M. Fahmy, *Umbilicus and Umbilical Cord*, https://doi.org/10.1007/978-3-319-62383-2_1

The navel clinically known as the umbilicus, colloquially known as the belly button or tummy button, is a hollowed or sometimes raised area on the abdomen at the attachment site of the umbilical cord. All placental mammals have a navel. The umbilicus is used to visually separate the abdomen into quadrants.

The umbilicus itself has been described as a round dermal projection or depressed scar on the centre of anterior abdominal wall surrounded by a natural skin fold that measures 1.5–2 cm in diameter and lies anatomically within the midline at the level of the superior iliac crests [1].

Reference

1. Craig SB, et al. In search of the ideal female umbilicus. Plast Reconstr Surg. 2000;105:389.

Origin of the Name of Umbilicus

The mythical story is telling us that the rocks married the Earth and the Earth became pregnant. *Salevao*, the god of the rocks, observed motion in the moa or the centre of the Earth. The child was born and named Moa (Moa or *Dinornis* is an extinct animal known through fossil records; it is an extinct flightless bird of New Zealand). Depending on species, they ranged in height from 3 to about 4 m; Moas were the largest birds that ever lived (Fig. 3.1), from the place where it was seen moving. Salevao ordered the umbilicus to be laid on a club and cut with a stone; and hence the custom ever after on the birth of a man-child. Salevao then provided water for washing the child and made it sa or sacred to *Moa*. The rocks and the Earth said they wished to get some of that water to drink. Salevao replied that if they got a bamboo, he would send them a streamlet through it and hence the origin of springs. Salevao said he would become loose stones and that everything which grew would be sa ia Moa, or sacred to Moa, till his hair was cut. After a time his hair was cut, and the restriction has taken off, and hence also the rocks and the Earth were called sa ia Moa, or as it is abbreviated, SAMOA. It is a visible testimony to the fact that one was a product of a natural birth.

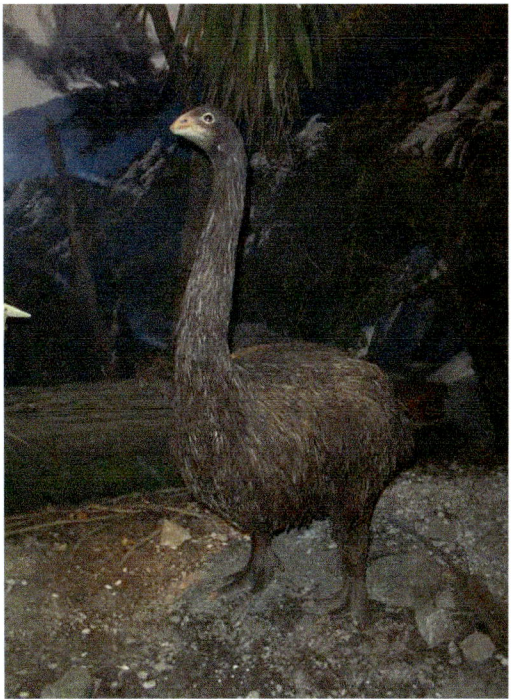

Fig. 3.1 Moa or *Dinornis* is an extinct animal known through fossil records

© Springer International Publishing AG 2018
M. Fahmy, *Umbilicus and Umbilical Cord*, https://doi.org/10.1007/978-3-319-62383-2_3

3.1 Origin of Omphalos

Greeks had placed a 'holy stone' in the Temple of Apollo at Delphi on the slope of Mt. Parnassus (near the Gulf of Corinth), and they called this rounded stone the 'Omphalos', since they believed this site marked the exact centre of the universe, just as the navel is supposed to mark the centre of the human body (Fig. 3.2).

An omphalos is an ancient religious stone artefact or baetylus; baetylus or bethel is a Semitic word denoting a sacred stone, which was supposedly endowed with life (Fig. 3.3). These objects of worship were meteorites and were dedicated to the gods or revered as symbols of the gods themselves [1].

In Greek, the word omphalos means 'navel' (compare the name of Queen Omphale). According to the ancient Greeks, Zeus sent out two eagles to fly across the world to meet at its centre, the 'navel' of the world. Omphalos stones used to denote this point were erected in several areas surrounding the Mediterranean Sea; the most famous of those was at the oracle in Delphi [2].

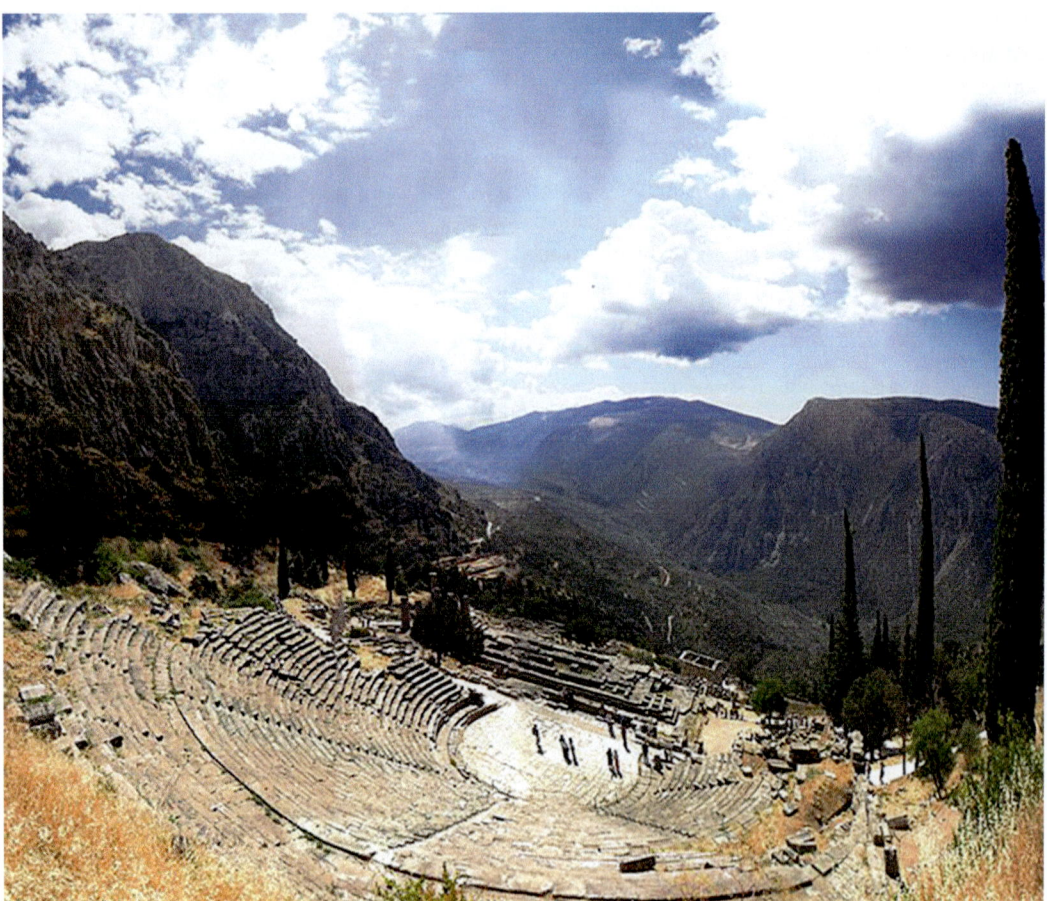

Fig. 3.2 Temple of Apollo at Delphi

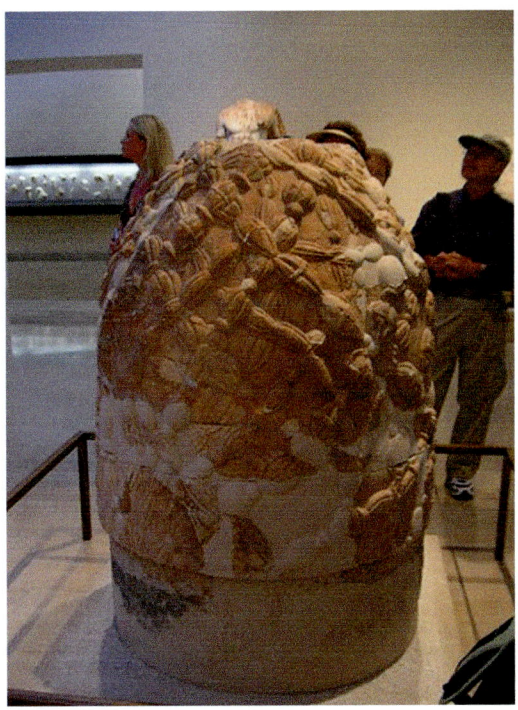

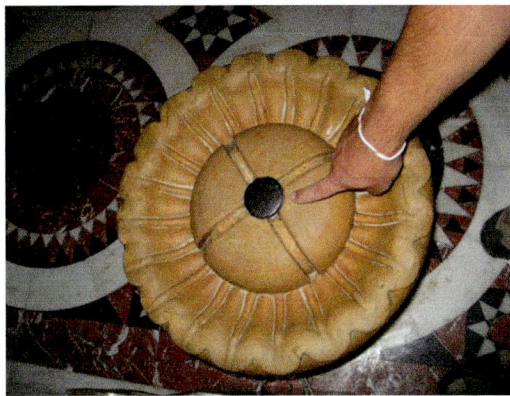

Fig. 3.4 Omphalos stone has a carving of a knotted net covering its surface

Fig. 3.3 Omphalos the holy stone in the Temple of Apollo at Delphi

3.2 The Omphalos in Delphi

Most accounts locate the Omphalos in the temple adyton. 'Adton in Greek means inaccessible or don't enter, and usually used to refer to a spaces reserved for oracles, priests or acolytes, and not for the general public near the "Pythia". The Pythia (Gr. Πυθία) was the priestess presiding over the Oracle of Apollo at Delphi, located on the slopes of Mount Parnassus.

The stone itself (which may have been a copy) has a carving of a knotted net covering its surface and has a hollow centre, which widens towards its base (Fig. 3.4).

Origin of umbilicus in Ancient Egypt: In the late Egyptian period, all dead women were called Hathors. The goddess Hathor is one of the oldest known deities of Egypt, and it is certain that in the form of a cow she was worshipped in the early part of the archaic period. She was also regarded as the great mother of the world, as the personification of the great power of nature which was perpetually conceiving, creating, rearing and maintaining all things great and small. It was Hathor, in the form of a cow, who received the dead when they entered the underworld; she gave them new life and celestial food wherewith to maintain it [3] (Fig. 3.5). In the person of Hathor, we thus have the complete circle from the cradle to the grave. Various peoples have held the belief that human life is determined (sometimes at birth) by maternal goddesses or supernatural beings, and that life ends when a cord, or thread, is severed. The Assyrian mother goddess Ishtar spins the thread of life and cuts it. Alcinous promises Odysseus that he will take care of him till he touches 'the soil of his beloved home', and he will have to face then 'whatever hard fate has in store for him and what the Moirai have spun on his thread of life when he was born'. A thread has been spun at birth for each mortal by Moira or Aisa, and the texture of this thread determines whatever will happen to him, both good and bad. Moiragenes was anyone who might be regarded as favoured

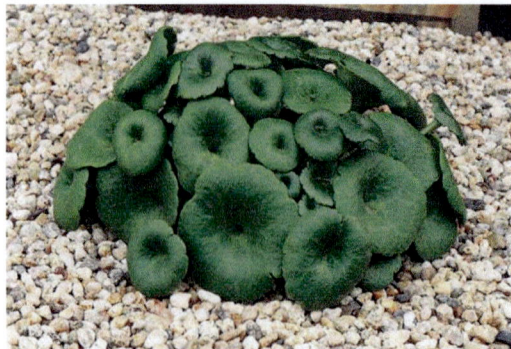

Fig. 3.6 Wild flowers, *Umbilicus rupestris* (navelwort)

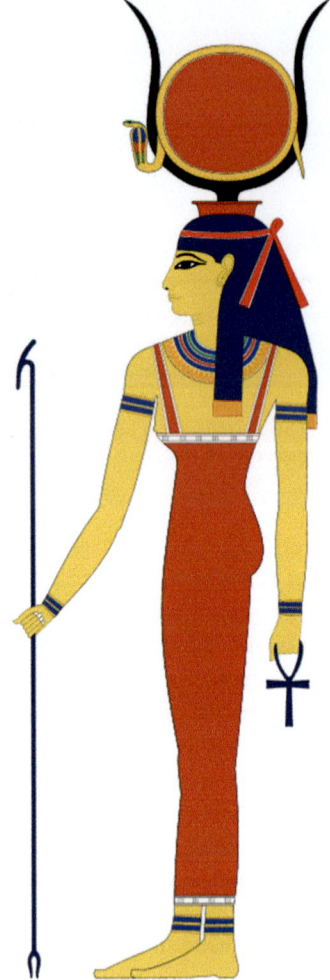

Fig. 3.5 The Goddess Hathor wearing her headdress

by these goddesses; they would care for him like good mothers and spin all the luck they could into his thread. The Moirai are closely related to the Erinyes (Furies); their altar in Sikyon was in the forest devote [4, 5].

3.3 Agricultural Origin of the Name of Umbilicus

Balsamo Umbilicus schmidtii plant: The term umbilicus also originated after the name of plants and flowers; a lot of roses which is ancient in origin are called umbilicus.

Umbilicus rupestris flowers: Wall pennywort (or navelwort) is a wild flower, rather fleshy species with almost circular leaves found on old stone walls or on natural rock outcrops. It is frequent in many areas but rare on basaltic rock. This succulent plant, a member of the stonecrop family, has its leaves joined into a tube. Navelwort is commonly found on walls and steep banks, especially in permanently damp, shaded areas; its English name is navelwort, and its scientific name is *Umbilicus rupestris* (Fig. 3.6).

Umbilicus chrysanthus: *Umbilicus* is a genus of over 90 species of flowering plants in the family Crassulaceae. Many of its species have been given synonyms under different genera such as *Rosularia, Cotyledon* and *Chiastophyllum*.

Also the term umbilicus is often used in descriptions of gastropod shells, i.e. it is a feature present on the ventral (or under) side of many (but not all) snail shells, including some species of sea snails, land snails and freshwater snails.

The umbilicus of a shell is the axially aligned, hollow cone-shaped space within the whorls of a coiled mollusc shell.

The word 'umbilicus' is also applied to the depressed central area on the planispiral coiled shells of Nautilus species and fossil ammonites. (These are not gastropods, but shelled cephalopods (Fig. 3.7)).

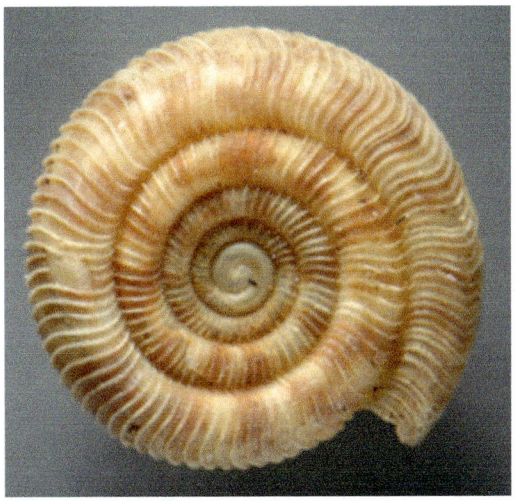

Fig. 3.7 Planispiral gastropod coiled shell with a central umbilicus

References

1. Pliny's natural history xvii. 9; Patriarch photios I of constantinople, Myriobiblon, Codex 242.
2. Holland O, Leicester B. The mantic mechanism at Delphi. Am J Archaeol. 1933;37:201–14.
3. Erman A. Die ägyptishe religion. Berlin: G. Reimer; 1909. p. 95–6.
4. Budge EAW. The gods of the Egyptians, vol. I. London: Methuen & Co.; 1904. p. 428.
5. Opler ME. Childhood and youth in Jicarilla apache society. Los Angeles: Publications of the Frederick Webb Hodge Anniversary Publication Fund; 1945. p. 5.

In English umbilicus is a common name which is Latin in origin, but the less common name which is German in origin is navel, (adj navel).

But the common term for ordinary people to call is "belly button"

- In Greek langue: *omphalos*
- In France: ombilical
- In Netherlands: navel, navelstreng, verbinding (figuurlijk)
- In Germany: nabelpunkt
- In Greece: Ελληνική
- In Italy: ombelicale
- Portugal: umbilical
- Russian: Русский пупочный, прочно соединенный, неотъемлемый, фала для связи астронавта или водолаза с кораблем, трубопровод наземного топливного питания ракеты
- Spanish: cordón
- Swedish: svenska
- Simplified Chinese: 中国话
  - adj.: 脐带的, 脐状的, 脐的
  - non: 脐带
- Traditional Chinese:
- 中國話
  - adj.: 臍帶的, 臍狀的, 臍的
  - n.: 臍帶
- Japanese: 日本語
  - adj.: 臍の, へその近くの, へその
  - n.: へその緒, つなぐもの
- Hebrew: נירובט, החפשממה תוישנ - .adj
- Turkish: göbek bağı (funicle, navel cord, umbilical)
- Farsi: فان هاگدنوویپ ,دننام فان یگتفرفرورف
- Arabic: سره

© Springer International Publishing AG 2018
M. Fahmy, *Umbilicus and Umbilical Cord*, https://doi.org/10.1007/978-3-319-62383-2_4

Names Related to Umbilicus

5

Many terms will be used in this book related to the original root of the words umbilicus, omphalos and navel:

- Omphalopsychite: A name of the Hesychasts, from their habit of gazing upon the navel
- Omphaloskepsis
- Omphaloscopy (Chap. 25)
- *Omphalos argument* (Chap. 9)
- Navel gazing (Chap. 25)
- Omphalitis (Chap. 26)
- Omphalocele (Chap. 34)
- Examophalous
- Gastroschisis (Chap. 33)
- *Caput Medusa*: which is a pathological distension of the veins on the anterior abdominal wall, seen to radiate from the umbilicus like the snakes that formed the hair of the mythical gorgon (Fig. 5.1). Caput is a Latin word which means head. Medusa originally is a beautiful young woman whose crowning glory was her magnificent long hair and was desired and courted by many suitors. Yet before she could be betrothed to a husband, Poseidon (Neptune) found her worshipping in the temple of Athena (Minerva) and ravished her. Athena was outraged at her sacred temple being violated and punished Medusa by turning her beautiful tresses into snakes and giving her the destructive power to turn anyone who looked directly at her into stone (Fig. 5.2).

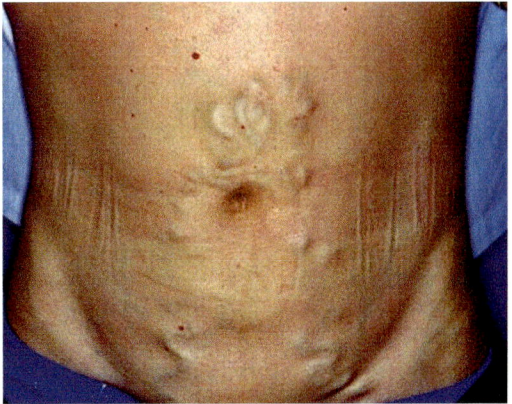

Fig. 5.1 A case of portal hypertension with prominent veins around the umbilicus, looks like Medusa's head (caput medusa)

© Springer International Publishing AG 2018
M. Fahmy, *Umbilicus and Umbilical Cord*, https://doi.org/10.1007/978-3-319-62383-2_5

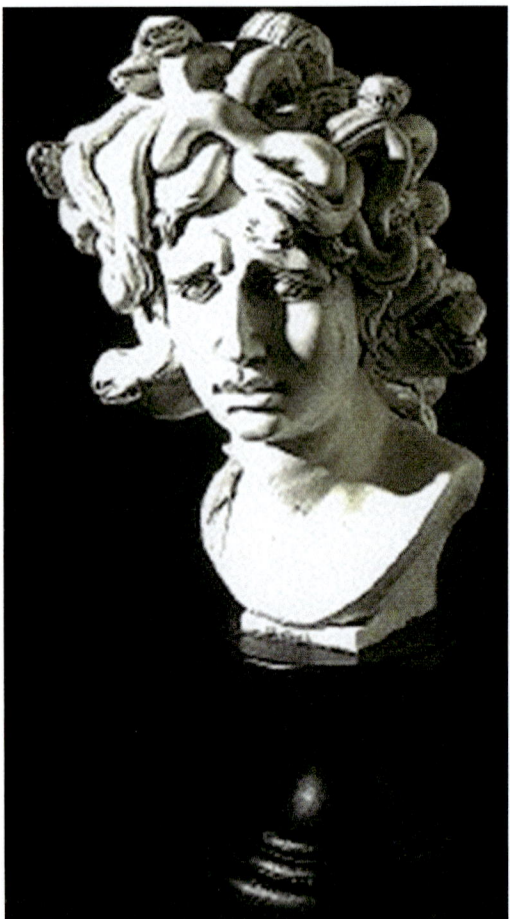

Fig. 5.2 Medusa

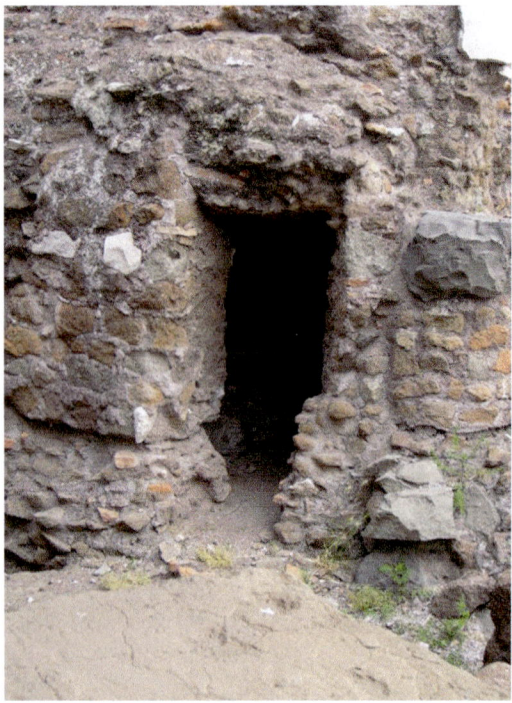

Fig. 5.3 The Umbilicus Urbis

- *The Umbilicus Urbis*: The Umbilicus Urbis of the City of Rome, it is the designated centre of the city from which and to which all distances in Rome and the Roman Empire were measured, is situated in the Roman Forum. It was built between the Basilica Aemilia, which predates it, and the Basilica Julia, which does not, in the late Republican period.

The Rostra, the platform from which orators addressed the Roman citizens, was built overlooking it. Originally covered in marble, the umbilicus is now a forlorn-looking brick structure some 2 m high and 2 m in diameter (Fig. 5.3).

- *Hercules and Omphale*: When Heracles and Deianira were parted, he was sold as a slave in Lydia; the one who bought him was a woman, a widow named Omphale. To her house Heracles went, carrying his armour and wearing his lion's skin. And Omphale laughed to see this tall man dressed in a lion's skin coming to her house to do a servant's tasks for her.

Other Uses of the Name of Umbilicus

The word 'navel', or its equivalent in other languages, has been used sometimes for the centre for something, e.g. 'nave' for the hub of a wheel. Tortellini might represent the belly button of Venus.

In recent years the cell phone was called the world's longest umbilical cord. The term 'umbilical cord' or just 'umbilical' has also come to be used for other cords with similar functions, such as the hose connecting a surface-supplied diver to his surface supply of air and/or heating or a space-suited astronaut to his spacecraft.

The phrase 'cutting the umbilical cord' is used symbolically to describe a child's breaking away from the parental home.

In Siberian the midwife is called 'navel mother' and the child 'navel son' or 'navel daughter'.

Alexandria city itself is called as 'the umbilicus of the ancient world'.

The Umbilicus Urbis in Rome was a special monument in the Forum Romanum, indicating the symbolic centre of the city: the 'Navel of the City of Rome'. The remains of the monument are located beside the Arch of Septimius Severus, behind the Rostra and near the Temple of Concord and the Temple of Saturn.

© Springer International Publishing AG 2018
M. Fahmy, *Umbilicus and Umbilical Cord*, https://doi.org/10.1007/978-3-319-62383-2_6

Umbilicus of Plants

Almost most of the whole creatures and every being had an umbilicus, as a reminder of its past or as a centrepiece of its architecture; the fruit has a stem that connects it to its branch, when it is ripe, and when it falls, it leaves a scar, as a navel, with very few exceptions; this is true for vegetables, fruits, fungi and mushrooms.

Some plants are named after its characteristic navel or umbilicus, and given the name of umbilicus or omphalos, the most obvious example is navel or umbilicated orange (Fig. 7.1).

Other plants are scientifically named and classified with specific terms including the word navel- or umbilicus-like:

Umbilicus botryoides: Small, pendulent flower spikes about 10 cm and pinkish in colour (Fig. 7.2).

Umbilicus chrysanthus: A genus of over 90 species of flowering plants in the family Crassulaceae. Many of its species have been given synonyms under different genera such as *Rosularia*, *Cotyledon* and *Chiastophyllum* which had a wide umbilicus at its dome with variable depths (Fig. 7.3).

Umbilicus rupestris: A flower wall pennywort (or Navelwort) is a wild flower, rather fleshy species with almost circular leaves, and a central depression looks like navel, found on old stone walls or on natural rock outcrops in Western Europe (Fig. 7.4) [1].

Omphacomeria: Its name originally from Greek "omphax," which means unripe fruit, sour or bitter and "meris" which means portion or part referring to the very sour fruits *Omphacomeria acerba* (Fig. 7.5) [2].

Omphalandria: From Greek word, omphalos; umbilicus and andros mean male or man parts, is a plant genus of the family Euphorbiaceae first described as a genus in 1759. It is native to tropical parts of the Americas, the West Indies, Asia, Australia and Africa [3].

Navel orange: A sweet orange that is usually seedless and has at its apex a navel-like depression enclosing an underdeveloped secondary fruit. The varieties of orange are called Navelina, Navel Caracara, Navelate, Navel Lane Late and Navel Ricalate in relation to the characteristic navel it had.

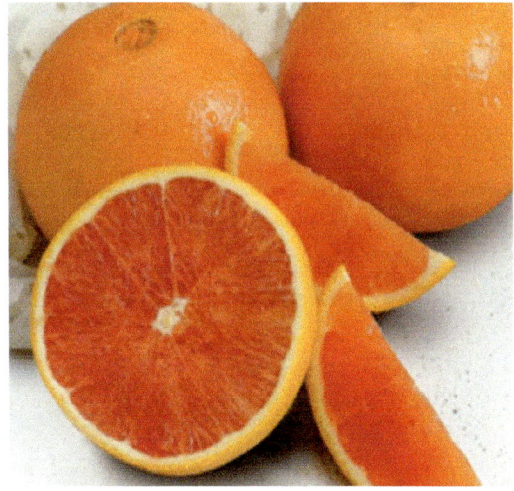

Fig. 7.1 Scarlet navel orange

© Springer International Publishing AG 2018
M. Fahmy, *Umbilicus and Umbilical Cord*, https://doi.org/10.1007/978-3-319-62383-2_7

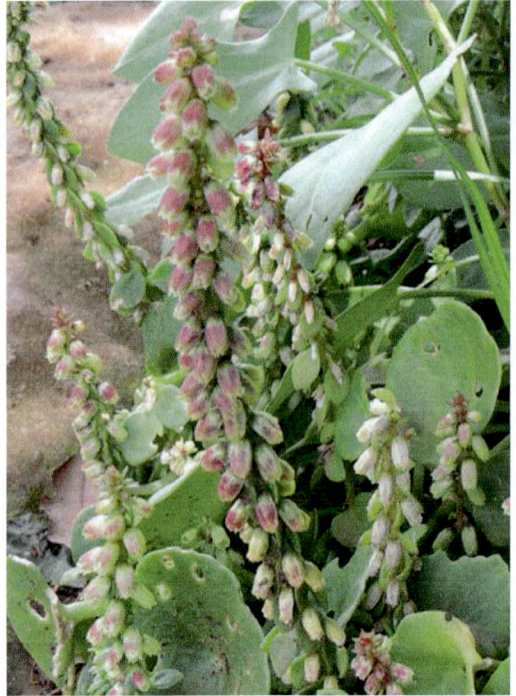

Fig. 7.2 *Umbilicus botryoides*

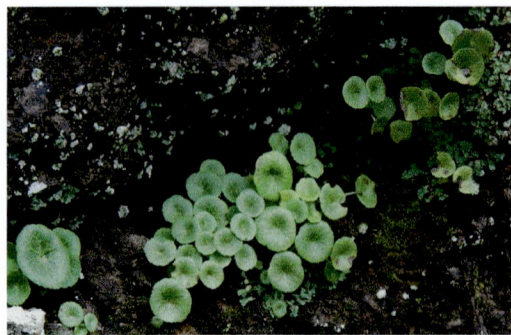

Fig. 7.4 *Umbilicus rupestris*

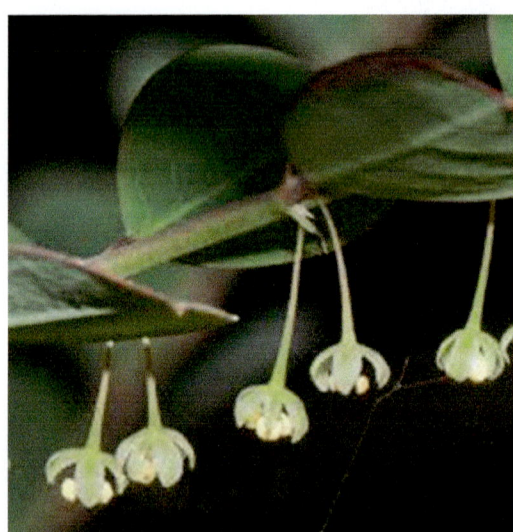

Fig. 7.5 *Omphacomeria*

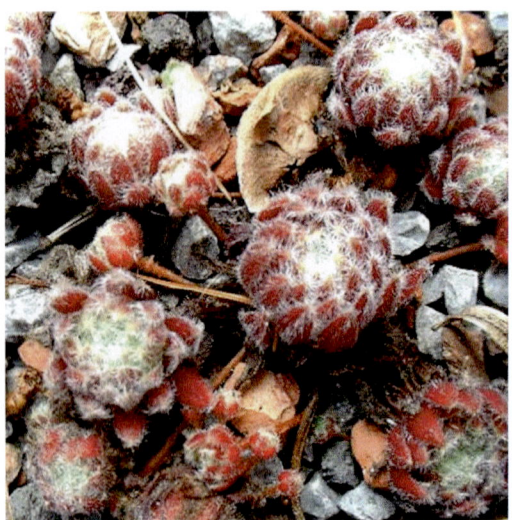

Fig. 7.3 *Umbilicus chrysanthus*

Basidiomycota: Filamentous large fungi; *Agaricales* is the common specie, with a characteristic head and a hyphen attached to its centre, and it looks like the placenta, with the umbilical cord attached to it (Fig. 7.6) [4].

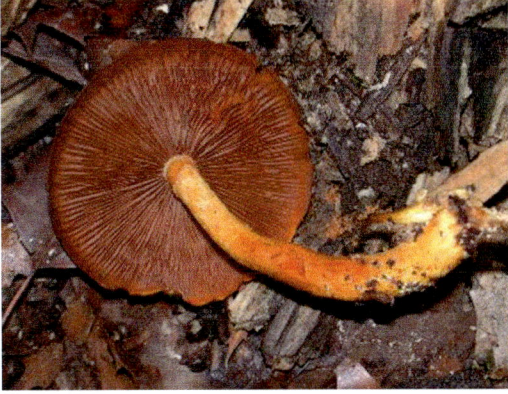

Fig. 7.6 *Agaricales basidiomycota* a giant mushroom; looks like umbilical cord and placenta

References

1. Everett TH. The New York botanical garden illustrated encyclopedia, vol. 10. New York: Taylor & Francis. https://books.google.com.eg/books?id=KeGzp-YXrPYC&lpg=PA3446&ots=MuINjC9EEk&dq=Umbilicus%20of%20fruits&pg=PA3446#v=onepage&q=Umbilicus%20of%20fruits&f=false
2. Quattrocchi U. CRC world dictionary of plant. Boca Raton: CRC Press; 1999. p. 1873.
3. Millspaugh CF. Omphalandria linearibracteata Millsp. Publ Field Columb Mus Bot Ser. 1900;2(1):59–60.
4. Gillespie LJ. Omphalea (Euphorbiaceae) in Madagascar: a new species and a new combination. Novon. 1997;7(2):127–36. doi:10.2307/3392184.

Animal's Navel

8

Most mammals had an umbilical cord and eventually umbilicus, but sea shellfish, the whole animal, looks like an umbilicus (Figs. 8.1 and 8.2).

Some animals are delivered with the umbilical cord attached to the placenta, and after a not completely understood process, the cord is atrophied and detached from the newly born animal's abdominal wall; other animals are delivered after the cord detachment, and all will have the umbilical scar naturally.

Two arteries and two veins are found in the nine-banded armadillo, with many subtle variations and other animals may have an admixture of yolk sac (vitelline) vessels (Fig. 8.3). Cats may have four vessels of each type.

The umbilical cord in some mammals, including cows and sheep, contains two distinct umbilical veins. Goats and other mammals umbilical cords are relatively shorter than the human cord [1].

Animals that lay eggs seem to have a false umbilical cord that attaches the embryo and yolk sac together in much the same way.

In most of domestic animals like sheep, cows, cattle etc., the mother eats the cord of its kids, and sometimes the ram or ibex help in eating the cord remnants.

In other mammals, the mother animal generally will gnaw the cord off separating the placenta from the baby. It is often consumed by the mother which nourishes her, recycles the protein, and reduces tissue that would attract scavengers or predators (Fig. 8.4). In chimpanzees, the mother focuses no attention on umbilical severance, instead staying still and nursing and holding her baby (with cord, placenta) until the cord dries and separates within a day of birth, at which time she leaves the cord and placenta on the forest floor where it is recycled by scavengers. This was first documented by zoologists in the wild at 1974 [2].

8.1 Fate of Animal Cord and How They Are Cut

Normally at birth, when the umbilical cord ruptures, the internal parts of the umbilical cord retract into the abdomen. Those parts are the two

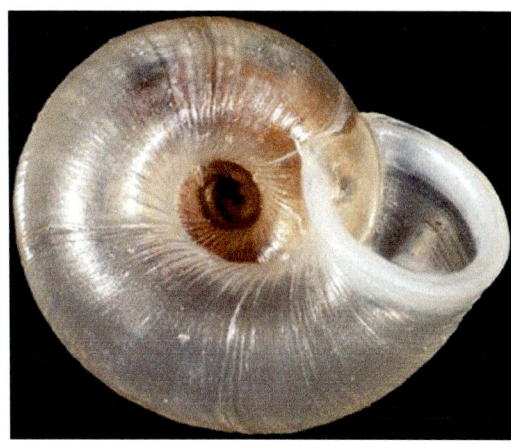

Fig. 8.1 Sea shellfish

© Springer International Publishing AG 2018
M. Fahmy, *Umbilicus and Umbilical Cord*, https://doi.org/10.1007/978-3-319-62383-2_8

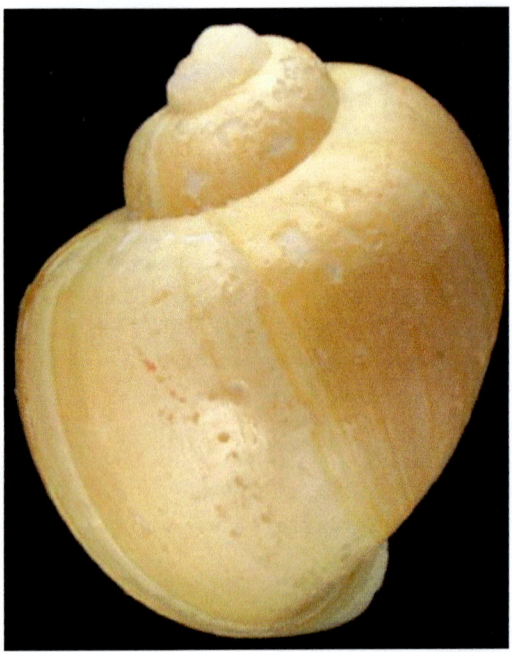

Fig. 8.2 Golden apple snail

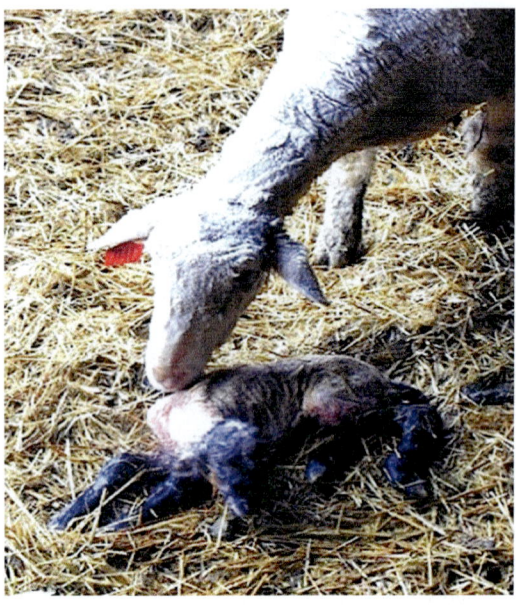

Fig. 8.4 Sheep mother eating the cord of its kids

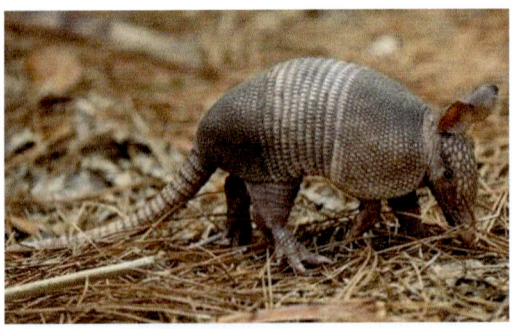

Fig. 8.3 Nine-banded armadillo

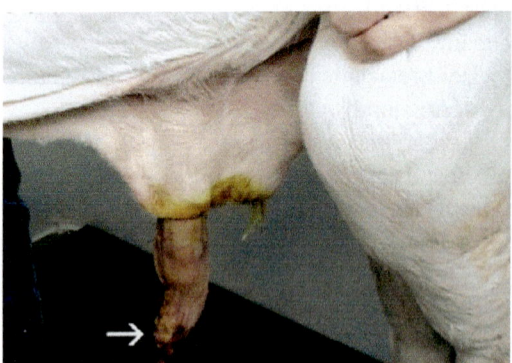

Fig. 8.5 Umbilical cord is often left hanging from the calf's belly

umbilical arteries, the umbilical vein and the tube leading from the bladder (urachus). Inside the abdomen they are better protected from the environment. In only a few days, these arteries, vein and urachus will all shrink. In a normal calf, the blood vessels are just a thread by a couple of weeks. The urachus shrinks to a very small ligament.

The hole through which these pass in the abdominal wall is the navel. It will gradually close during the first 2 months of life. The ruptured umbilical cord, what we normally see outside the calf's body, extends at birth through the navel. It should be essentially an empty tube.

Two to 6 inches of umbilical cord are often left hanging from the calf's belly. It will shrivel and dry up during the 7–10 days of life as long as it is neither infected nor repeatedly sucked on by another calf. At that point the navel opening is no longer needed, and it continues to close (Fig. 8.5).

Kangaroo: Among the world's most curious creatures is Australia's amazing kangaroo. He appears standing proud and tall on the Australian coat of arms and has been a rallying symbol for national sporting teams.

Born a mere 1–1.5 cm (half-inch) long and weighing less than a gram, kangaroos can grow taller than a man (Fig. 8.6). As with most other

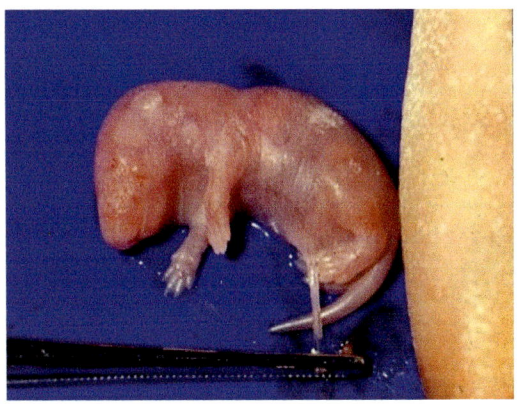

Fig. 8.6   A tiny newborn kangaroo

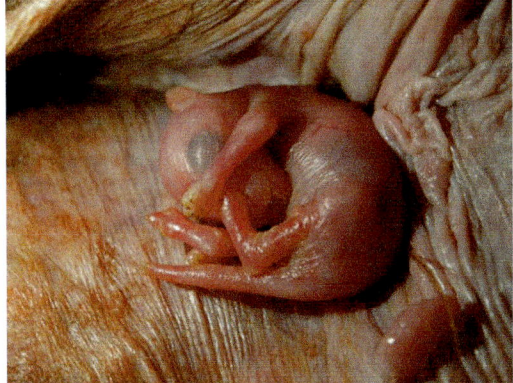

Fig. 8.7   Kangaroo in the pouch

marsupials, one of the three orders of mammals, they raise their young in body pouches. But kangaroos have another advantage—an expectant female can retain an embryo in ready reserve for months, until the conditions are right for its continued development (Fig. 8.7).

When it comes to marsupials, no place on earth can count a greater variety than the island continent of Australia. Of 250 existing species, some 170 of them—including wombats, bandicoots and kangaroos—live only in Australia or its immediate surroundings. All the rest, except the opossum found in the United States and Canada, are limited to Latin America.

Fertility cycle: The young is born 33 days after mating, and mating can occur again a day or two after this. The embryo resulting from the mating remains in a quiescent state until the previous young is about to vacate the pouch. During this period the suckling stimulus prevents the recurrence of fertility cycles. If the young is lost prematurely from the pouch, the quiescent embryo resumes development (as is normal at the end-of-pouch life), and cyclic reproductive activity is resumed.

There are no external signs that the kangaroo is pregnant, and the first indication that birth is imminent is when the mother begins to clean her pouch. About 24 h or more before birth, the pregnant female begins to lean forward and puts her head inside the pouch, which is usually held open by the forepaws, and licks, and perhaps bites, the inside of her pouch. This pouch licking continues as the female assumes a birth position, the tail passing between her hindlegs, hindquarters resting on the ground and back supported against a tree or other object. The pouch licking becomes more intense as birth approaches.

At the point of birth, the young appears head first enclosed in the amniotic sac and either the continued vigorous licking by the mother or may be the sharp claws of the young (or a combination of both factors) causes the sac to rupture. In any case, the hairless newborn almost immediately breaks free and begins its journey to the pouch [3].

Up to the Pouch: The newborn young crawls over the mother's fur by grasping the fur with alternate movements of the forelegs and claws. The hindlimbs play no part and are mere buds at this stage. Simultaneously with the movements of the forelimbs, the head is moved from side to side, and the young appears to move in a sinuous manner over the fur. For part of the journey, the umbilical cord is attached to the yolk sac inside the mother, but it is finally broken, probably by the licking of the mother or perhaps occasionally by the pulling of the young. The young reaches the pouch and disappears inside. Crawling behaviour and head movement continue until it finds a nipple and attaches. The journey is accomplished in a remarkably short time—on average in less than 3 min. It is not known how long the young takes to attach to a nipple, but it is certainly shorter than 15 min.

The pouch contains four teats. The mother offers no resistance to the young and, indeed, appears to be quite oblivious of its existence.

While the young is crawling to the pouch, the mother is vigorously licking up the blood and birth fluids, carefully cleaning all traces from her fur. This licking is done after the young has gone, although she occasionally licks over or ahead of the young while it is crawling to the pouch, thus giving rise in some people's minds to the idea that the mother prepares a well licked track for the young to follow.

There is, in fact, no necessity to postulate that the young needs assistance to get to the pouch and attach to a teat, for it is endowed with all the necessary equipment at birth. It has well-developed and active forelimbs, jaw muscles and tongue. Although it has no functional eyes or ears, it has large nostrils and presumably a well-developed sense of smell which probably plays a major part in its location of the pouch. It has often been stated that the newborn young is incapable of sucking, and the mother therefore forces milk into its mouth by means of certain abdominal muscles, but this is incorrect [4].

References

1. Reeves TB. A double umbilicus. Anat Rec 10:15–18 Jane Goodall: in the shadow of man, textbook published April 21st 2000 by Mariner Books (first published January 1st 1971); 1916.
2. Oldest live-birth fossil found; fish had umbilical cord. National Geographic News. 28 May 2008.
3. Flannery TF. Kangaroos: 15 million years of Australian bounders. In: Archer M, Clayton G, editors. Vertebrate zoogeography and evolution in Australasia. Carlisle: Hesperian Press; 1984. p. 817–35.
4. Frith HJ, Coleby JH. Kangaroos. Melbourne: F.W. Cheshire Publishing Pty Ltd; 1969. p. 110–9.

Umbilicus in History and Its Religious Background

9.1 Adam and Eve Umbilicus

Did Adam and Eve have belly buttons?

Did God create Adam and Eve with navels?

In 1944, a subcommittee of the United States House of Representatives Military Committee refused to authorize a little 30-page booklet titled Races of Man, which was to be handed out to soldiers and airmen fighting in World War II, because this little booklet had a drawing that depicted Adam and Eve with belly buttons. The members of this subcommittee ruled that showing Adam and Eve with navels 'would be misleading to gullible American soldiers' [1].

In 1646, Sir Thomas Browne, a doctor and philosopher from Norwich, published a work titled 'Pseudodoxia Epidemica' and he devoted an entire chapter to 'Pictures of Adam and Eve with Navels'. He points out that even such notables as Raphael and Michelangelo were guilty of such 'vulgar errors'. He declared that to paint Adam and Eve with belly buttons would be to suggest that 'the Creator affected superfluities, or ordained parts without use or office'. The Catholic Church, as a rule, seemed to be against artists depicting Adam and Eve with navels in their paintings, so this posed quite a problem for a number of these artists who didn't want to antagonize the church. A good many of them, therefore, chose to take the 'safe path' and simply painted the couple with strategically placed foliage, long hair or forearms blocking the abdomen [2] (Fig. 9.1).

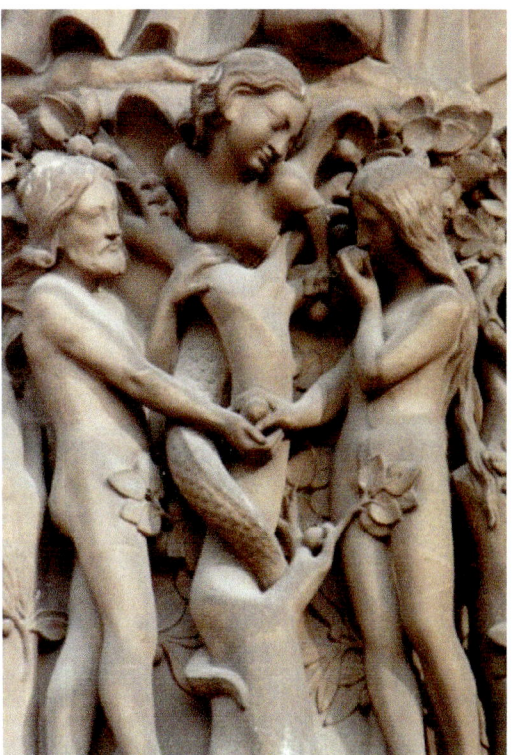

Fig. 9.1 Adam and Eve, serpent at the entrance to Notre Dame Cathedral in Paris

The original version of this article was revised: Acknowledgment had been missing in the original version. Reference [4] was added in Chapter 9 and the references following thereafter were renumbered in the reference list. An erratum to this chapter is available at https://doi.org/10.1007/978-3-319-62383-2_37

M. Fahmy, *Umbilicus and Umbilical Cord*, https://doi.org/10.1007/978-3-319-62383-2_9

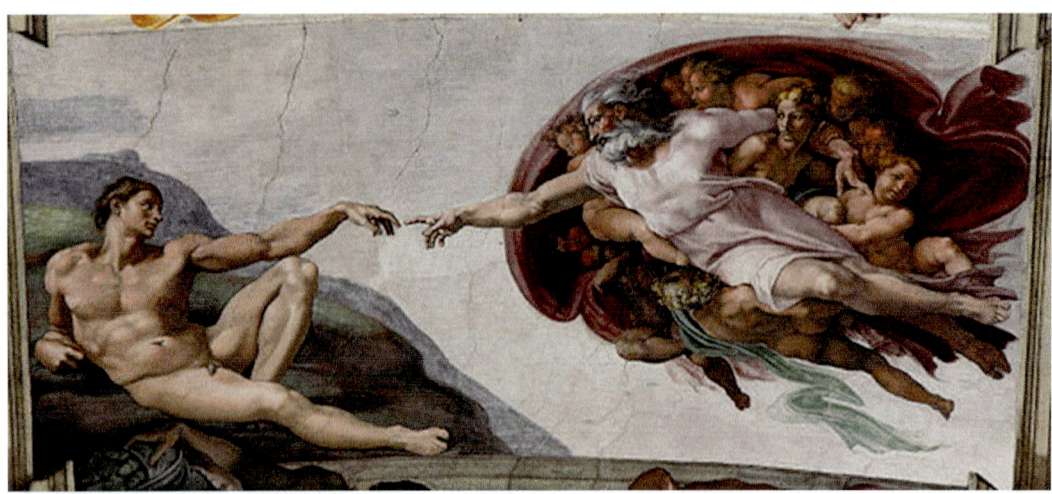

Fig. 9.2 Michelangelo, public domain, https://commons.wikimedia.org/w/index.php?curid=15461165

And yet Michelangelo dared to paint Adam with a navel and to place it right there on the ceiling of the Sistine Chapel, for which he was accused of heresy by some theologians of his day (Fig. 9.2).

The Omphalos argument: There were some who maintained that God did create Adam and Eve with navels, although there was considerable debate as to exactly when this mark was placed upon them. This is known as the Omphalos argument. The man who is most often credited with being the primary promoter of this theory was the British naturalist and experimental zoologist, Philip Henry Gosse (1810–1888) [3]. He formulated what has come to be known as 'the Omphalos argument' in which he advocated the view that God created the universe, including man (Adam and Eve), with the appearance of prior history. Adam and Eve were given navels to present the appearance of natural childbirth, even though such never happened. This was all advocated in 1857 in his book: *Omphalos: An Attempt to Untie the Geological Knot.*

There are three primary theories regarding Adam and Eve navel as follows:

Pre-umbilicism: the view that Adam and Eve were given navels at the moment of their creation by God. Some of these theorists get pretty bizarre in their speculations. Since man is created in the image of God, and since they regard this to in some way refer to physical characteristics, they actually suggest Adam and Eve were in some manner connected to the Creator with a cosmic umbilical cord. They also suggest that since Adam and Eve had a navel, and since they are 'in the image of God', God Himself must have a navel, which leads to some absolutely heretical conjectures.

Mid-umbilicism: This particular view suggests that Adam's navel was created when the Lord God took the rib from him and created the woman Eve. God chose to pull the rib from the centre of Adam's blank abdomen, thus forming a puncture wound. Therefore, the navel on Adam, unlike all future navels, was not a visible sign that he had come from a woman, but actually a visible sign that a woman had come from him. Eve, according to these mid-umbilicists, never did have a navel, as there was no need for her to have one.

Post-umbilicism: This last theory places the umbilicus on both Adam and Eve after their sin and at the point of being driven from the garden. This 'scar' in their midsection would forever be a reminder to this couple, and to all mankind, that they had, by their sin, been 'severed from' their God, just as a baby is severed from its mother when the umbilical cord is cut, with the navel being a constant visible reminder of that previous connection now forever severed by Garry Wills in the New York Review (November 22, 1990, pp. 6–10).

An originary myth from Turkey, for instance, relates that on seeing the first man created by Allah, the Devil spat at his stomach. Allah then made a grab at and removed the polluted spot, the resultant scar thus explaining why humans have a belly button. The absence of navels on this first human couple would be a powerful, long-lasting witness to the creation itself and to the power of our Creator God.

For Jesus nobody records any minute details of his birth, however according to the mythology of the middle ages, he didn't have a belly button (navel) so by association wouldn't have had an umbilical cord either, a couple different sagas (song of roland for one) tell of heroes fighting giants, with basically the same riddle, the opponent is invincible on every part of his body except one, a place found on every man that ever lived, save one, which they make to be the navel as Christ was divinely conceived rather than through the union of a man and woman.

9.2   Umbilicus and Umbilical Cord in Different Cultures

The umbilical cord considered as 'the thread of life' and the placenta are magical doubles of the child and they symbolize the dual union of infant and mother, the tie that unites mother and child.

Umbilical cord in history: One has to wonder what thoughts prehistoric humans had when confronted with the stillbirth of a baby entangled in its umbilical cord. Some insights from more recent times suggest the umbilical cord represented an omen, a sacred talisman, predictor of future fertility. In some popular classes in Europe, Australia, Africa and Hawaii, the umbilical cord was dried and soaked in water for consumption to ensure future fertility. It was eaten, hung from tree branches and stuffed in volcanic rock crevices at sites such as the Birthing Stones in Kukahiioko, Oahu [4]. Chinese literature suggests the cord had many medicinal properties.

The new European insights for umbilical cord began with Galen (129–200 A.D.), who suggested that the umbilical cord served to nurture the fetus through arteries and veins. Leonardo da Vinci (1452–1519) observed that the cord was as long as the fetus at a given gestational age (Fig. 9.3). Spiglius (1631) determined blood flow direction, and Harvey (1657) suggested that interruption of this blood flow could be the cause of fetal death if the cord was compressed.

Umbilical cord in Ancient Egypt: Hiqit is the frog-headed goddess called *'l'un des premiers berceaux d'Abydos'*. The goddesses arrive and Isis gives the child its name of Ousirhaf (the one whose double is powerful). The goddesses wash the infant, cut its umbilical cord and put it on a bed. Similar proceedings follow with the other two infants of the triplets. We suspect that in all these fantasies, the end of life is modelled on the beginning: the thread of life is the umbilical cord [5] (Fig. 9.4).

The goddesses of Egypt who correspond to the Moirai of the Greeks are the Hathors. The Hathors appear as seven or more beautiful young girls foretelling the future of the newborn infant. They are represented attending the infant as midwives. Whenever a child is born, the seven Hathors appear and proclaim the fate that has been allotted to the infant by its god. Death is called 'that which has been fated' (*das Verhdngte*) in an official document. Some of them attend the young mother to protect her with their incantations; others receive the newborn baby and pass it from one to the other. The sun god Ra sends the goddesses Isis, Nephtys, Mashkonouit and Hiqit to act as midwives to Rounditdit, a mother pregnant with triplets. The first two goddesses are well known; the latter two may require introduction [6] (Fig. 9.5).

All Egyptian goddesses are in a sense mothers, midwives and fates (Hathors). Hathor is the divine representative of women, the goddess of love and pleasure. She is both the goddess of sunrise and sunset and, therefore, also of the hereafter. In the late Egyptian period, all dead women were called Hathors. 'The goddess Hathor is one of the oldest known deities of Egypt and it is certain that in the form of a cow,

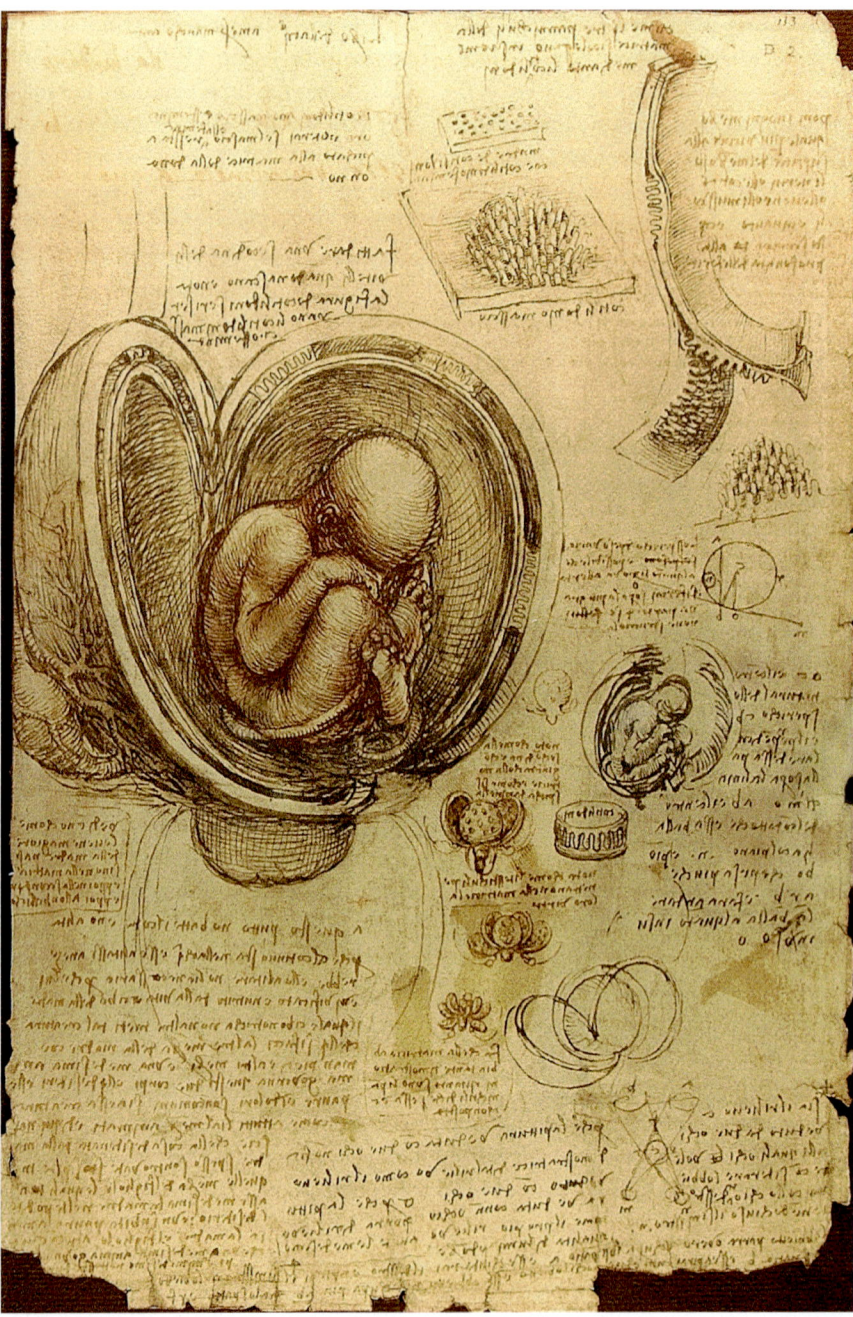

Fig. 9.3 Drawing of the human fetus in utero from Da Vinci's anatomical notebooks

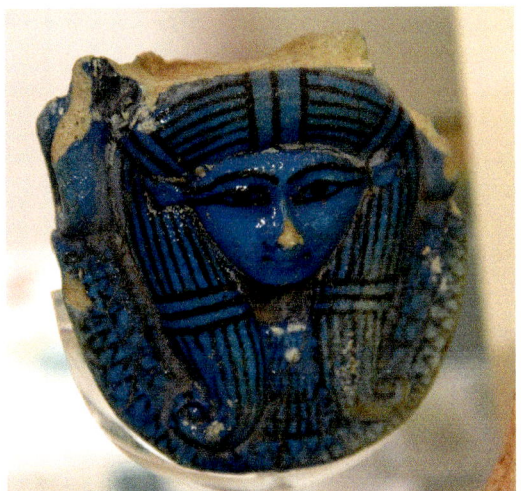

Fig. 9.4 Hathor's head. Faience, from a sistrum's handle. Eighteenth Dynasty. From Thebes, Egypt. The Petrie Museum of Egyptian Archaeology, London

she was worshipped in the early part of the archaic period'. She was also regarded as the great mother of the world, as the personification of the great power of nature which was perpetually conceiving, creating, rearing and maintaining all things great and small. It was Hathor who received the dead when they entered the underworld; she gave them new life and celestial food wherewith to maintain it. In the person of Hathor, we thus have the complete circle from the cradle to the grave, but she also represents an annually recurring periodicity for she is the star Sothis and is thereby connected with the rise of the Nile before the inundation. Sothis rose helically on the first day of the Egyptian New Year, and when the sun god Ra entered his boat, Hathor, the goddess of the star Sothis, went with him [7].

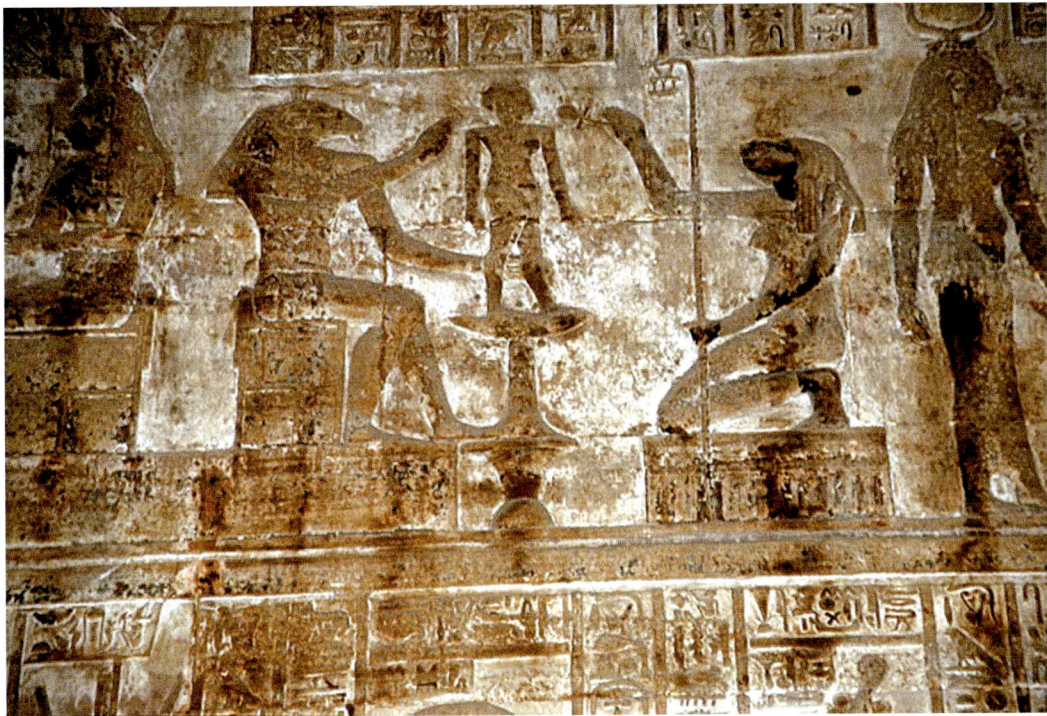

Fig. 9.5 The god Khnum, accompanied by Hiqit, moulds Ihy in a relief from the mammisi (birth temple) at Dendera Temple complex

9.3 Umbilical Cord and Tradition [8–10]

The thread of life is the umbilical cord and the final separation from the world is a repetition of the first separation when the physical unity of mother and child is disrupted. That the 'thread' is the umbilical cord symbolism is unmistakable. In Europe, the umbilical cord appears frequently in the life of a child. All over Europe, the stump is preserved as an amulet and frequently buried with its original owner.

Among the *Jicarilla Apache* (New Mexico), when a couple knows that the woman is pregnant, they cease tying their moccasin laces, tucking them instead inside. Were they to tie them, the umbilical cord would be wound around the child's neck with the risk of choking it during delivery, the moccasin string is the symbolic equivalent of the umbilical cord. In numerous instances, the placenta or the cord is regarded as magically identical with the child. At *Torda Aranyosszek,* the placenta is called the child's double.

In *Bavaria,* they keep the placenta for 3 days in a parcel under the mother's bed, and then they throw it into running water to prevent witches from getting hold of it and substituting a changeling for the child.

In *eastern England,* the stump of the umbilical cord must not fall on the ground when it separates.

In *Saxonia*, some people eat the placenta, which was regarded as a safeguard against epilepsy.

In *Russia* (*Orenburg*), the placenta is buried with great reverence. If it is wished to prevent the mother from having more children, the placenta is dug out and reburied upside down.

In the area of *Obolensk,* the placenta is put on the head of the newborn infant who is then washed in its mother's urine. This is to prevent it from being afflicted with chorea.

In *Hungary,* the umbilical cord is kept to fumigate the child when it gets sick. If witches get hold of the cord, they can use it to suck milk out of cows from a great distance. In southern Hungary, as soon as the child can walk, a powder is made of the umbilical cord and mixed with the child's food to make it strong. The same remedy is used for stomach ache or sleeplessness.

Gypsies in Hungary resort to the following rite to exorcize the spirits of sickness from the child. The oldest man present, the sorceress and the child's mother throw the cord (which has been concealed up to that moment) into a brazier. When the smoke ascends, all three say the following prayer:

Dear God give us luck and protect us all the time.
Rescue us everywhere.
We give you the heavy chain
To chain the spirit of evil
And make it flee this place.

The chain is the umbilical cord, an amulet against all evil. They call it *devleskero lancos-*god's chain- or *devleshero shelo-*god's rope.

The *Aranda* cut the umbilical cord with a stone knife at a distance of some inches from the child's body. It is never bitten off, as is the custom in many primitive tribes. After a few days, the remaining part of the cord is cut off by the mother who, by swathing it in strips of fur, makes it into a string which is kept by the father's mother for a few days and then wound around the child's neck. This necklace facilitates the growth of the child and keeps it quiet and contented. It averts illness and prevents the child from hearing the noise made by dogs in the camp.

On the *Pennyfather* River (East England), the placenta is buried at birth. It contains the vital principle. When the portion of cord falls off the infant, it is carried in the mother's dilly bag. The mother does not bury it before the little one begins to walk, because if she were to do so, the baby would die.

Siberian customs are especially interesting. Among the Tungus and Jakut, the father and his friends eat the placenta. According to Pallas, the Ostiaks put the placenta in a little box, and after adding a piece of meat or fish to it, they hang it on the tree. The midwife is called 'navel mother' and the child 'navel son' or 'navel daughter'.

In the *Tremjugan district,* they pretend to see human features in the expelled placenta. They personify it and call it 'the child nourishing woman'; it is also the object of a cult. They make a little shirt, a belt and a shawl for it and put all this in the 'navel basket'. Before carrying the 'navel basket' into the forest, they arrange a little festival called 'navel meal', and they place whatever food they have, and tea, on a plate for 'the child nourishing woman', the placenta. The 'navel mother', the midwife, tells the women to bow to this spirit and say: 'Child nourishing woman eat! Mother of the fire eat and drink. Then we shall have luck and blessing'.

In *Czechoslovakia*, the mother keeps the umbilical cord in a knot. Before the child begins going to school, they give it to him; if he can untie the knot, all will be well. It is the Graeco–Walach custom to show the child the cord to bring him luck. The Székelys in Transylvania make the child look through the umbilical cord to see his future. Usually a boy gets the knotted umbilical cord at the age of 7; if he can untie it, he will be a real man.

In *Baden and Franconia* (Germany), the cord is kept 6 years, and then it is chopped into scrambled eggs fed to the child. It is believed this will make him smart, or the cord is sewn into his clothes to prevent him from losing his mind. In Bavaria, it is burnt after 7 years.

In *Oldenburg* (Lower Saxony, Germany), they form a circle out of the umbilical cord; if the child looks through it and sees the alphabet, it will learn to read quickly.

The *Graeco–Walachs* keep the cord (called *asalos*, the equivalent of the Greek *omphalos*) dry because if it gets wet, the child feels pain in its body. When the child has grown a little, they show him the umbilical cord to make him successful in everything. 'He has seen his *asalos*' means 'he is very successful'. The mother must never show a child's umbilical cord to other children.

In *France*, the umbilical cord is cut short for girls, but for boys 'selon la longeur au moment de la naissance, du petit membre viril'; also it is almost exclusive for the male sex that the cord is preserved.

The *Polish* custom of calling out to the man who cuts the last handful of corn, 'you have cut the umbilical cord', is a conscious or allegorical representation of separation.

According to the Saxons in *Transylvania*, a pregnant woman must be careful not to get her neck entwined in anything or wear a string of pearls on her neck because the umbilical cord might get twisted around the child's neck when it is born. The Wends say if a pregnant woman passes under a rope, the cord will get twisted around the child's neck and kill it.

The *Mularatara* (*South Australian border*), they cut a long umbilical cord and then let it break when it is dry. They tie it with a string and put it on the boy's neck to make him grow big and fat. It also prevents the child from crying.

Among the tribes of the *Nullarbor* (semiarid country of southern Australia) plains, the string made from the umbilical cord and worn around the infant's neck is supposed to contain part of the child's spirit. When it withers and falls off, the baby has finally completed absorption of the spirit.

At *Cape Bedford* (town in the centre of the Eastern Cape province of South Africa), the cord is tied in a coil and hung around the child's neck. The child wears it for some time, and it is finally presented to the father's father if the child is a boy and to the mother's father if a girl.

Among the *Somali*, when a male child is born, they take pains to cut the umbilical cord in such a way as to leave as much as possible and then they try to stretch it, for the longer it is, the longer will be the penis. They tie the part that has been cut off into a knot which the mother keeps in her bag. If a delivery is not going smoothly, this piece of the cord is held over a fire and a woman sniffs the steam.

In *Vietnam*, the tradition is to bury the remnants of the umbilical cord in the gardens in special jars, believing that this will make the man retain back, whatever happens to him to the place where his cord remnants were buried.

In the Philippines, some of the traditional health practices based on superstitious beliefs are the covering of the navel of the newborn baby with sand for the purpose of quick healing and the burying of the placenta and umbilical cord of a newborn baby together with a pencil and paper in the belief that the act will make the baby intelligent. Other practices are the use of indigenous objects like the 'buho' or bamboo in cutting the umbilical cord of a newborn baby instead of unnatural objects, like scissors, the use of which, it is believed, will influence the child to be disloyal to the family and the hanging of dried umbilical cord 'pusod' of a newborn baby beneath the doorway or window in the belief that this will keep the infant safe from accident or harm.

In Bangladesh, the cutting and tying of the cord generally takes place under unhygienic conditions. Many said a bamboo slip is used for cutting of umbilical cord, saying it is better than a metal blade. The thread used was not boiled. The TBAs also smear ash on the navel area of the baby. This is believed to help the area to heal after cutting the cord. Often, it is done by the birthing woman herself or by her mother or mother-in-law in order to avoid the large payment associated with this task.

In Turkey, giving a middle (umbilical) name to the child is also common. The name given to the child while the umbilical cord is being cut is called its 'umbilical name'.

The umbilical name is given to children in Anatolia because it is believed that the child will be called by his/her umbilical name in the grave. He/she will be called by his/her umbilical name as the imam reads the final repentance and forgiveness prayer for him/her as he/she is lowered into the grave.

These data presented show the relationship between the severed thread and the umbilical cord; but is this really the latent, repressed meaning of the myth? In other words, does the myth go back to the trauma of the severed umbilical cord? This is hardly likely. The symbolism is either conscious (allegory) or preconscious. The severance of the umbilical cord is a 'trauma' we have all mastered. In the rites and myths discussed, it is but a preconscious substitute for the sword of Damocles, the ever-threatening castration anxiety. The wish is the Oedipal desire charged with anxiety. But the myth represents this as merely the cutting of the umbilical cord; it transforms the end into a beginning.

Tradition of cord cut in Islam believing countries: The seventh day of the baby's birth, is crucial when both the umbilical cord fell off, and the foreskin removed by circumcision, there are no specific regulations or tradition for the cord cut or umbilical care.

The umbilical cord is only mentioned twice in documents: Once was when Isaac, Abraham's son from Sarah, was born, his umbilical cord fell off, but his foreskin did not. This happened on the seventh day of his birth. The same Hadith indicates Abraham was the first one commanded to perform circumcision. Second was when the prophet Muhammad explained that if a woman dies with a child in her womb, or she dies during childbirth or after childbirth but within the period of post-partum bleeding, she is considered to be a martyr. The Messenger of Allah said: 'And if a woman dies during the post partum period, her child will drag her to Paradise by his umbilical cord'. The umbilical cord is that which is cut when the child is born. Prophet Muhammad said in an authentic statement: 'Who is counted as a shaheed among you?' (*Bihar al-anwar*).

Traditional practices in developing countries: About two-thirds of births in developing countries take place outside health facilities and almost half of the women are delivered by untrained traditional birth attendants, family members or deliver on their own. A wide variety of traditional practices and beliefs are associated with care of the umbilical cord. Traditional beliefs must be taken into account when introducing clean cord care programmes in a community since these beliefs may conflict with programme recommendations. Some traditional practices such as applying unclean substances to the cord are dangerous and should be discouraged or replaced with safer alternatives. Practices will not change unless people are convinced that the new practice is indeed better. Some traditional practices are beneficial and should be promoted, while others may be ignored.

The following are examples of traditional cord care practices:

In many cultures, people believe that all life from the placenta must be transferred to the newborn for otherwise the baby may die. Therefore the cord is usually cut after cord pulsations stop or after the delivery of the placenta. This practice is harmless and may even be beneficial to the baby. In some areas, the cord is milked, especially

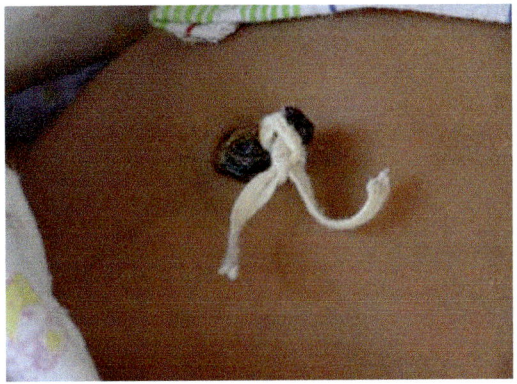

Fig. 9.6 UC tie by domestic thread

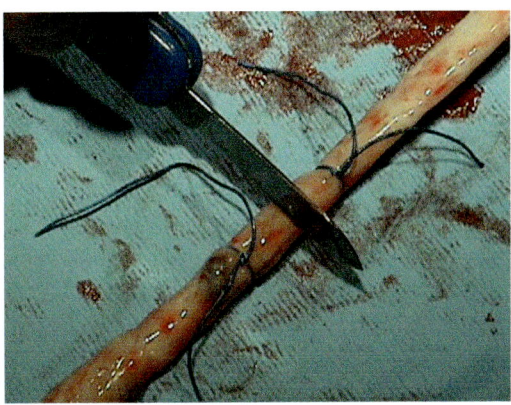

Fig. 9.7 Cord cut between two ties by a pocket knife

if the baby is not breathing, in order to bring the baby's soul back from the mother.

Materials used to tie the cord include strings, threads and strips of cloth (Fig. 9.6).

In Nepal, the custom is to use home-made cord ties of raw cotton in accordance with the saying, 'a new thread for the new baby'. Sometimes, blades of grass, bark fibres, reeds or fine roots are used: This is harmful because such materials often harbour tetanus spores from the soil and thus increase the risk of neonatal tetanus. In some areas, no tie is used or the cord is tied only if bleeding occurs. This practice increases the risk of bleeding from the stump. In traditional societies in India, the practice of waiting for placental expulsion and using a blunt instrument to cut the cord, which results in more vessel spasm than using a sharp one, ensures that cord bleeding is uncommon even if the cord is not tied very tightly.

A variety of tools are used to cut the cord. They are usually items that are available in the house or that relate to the father's trade, such as scissors, knives, broken glass, stones, sickles or used razor blades. These are rarely cleaned or boiled before use and are dangerous sources of infection. Some cultures have more beneficial customs such as heating the knife over a fire or candle before cutting the cord (Fig. 9.7).

The umbilical cord is left long in most traditional cultures. Exceptionally, it is cut very short, as in some communities in Uganda (this practice is associated with the danger of umbilical bleeding

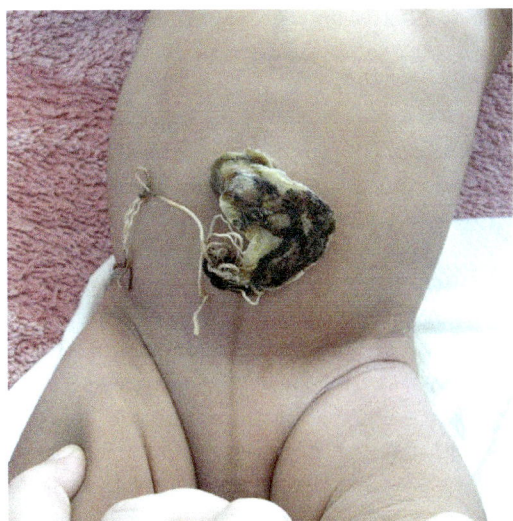

Fig. 9.8 Long umbilical cord stump (most of the cord left to dry)

as it makes the cord hard to tie). In Ecuador, the cord is left 12–15 cm long in girls because it is believed that anything shorter than that would cause a girl to have a small uterus and narrow hips later in life and therefore have difficulty in childbirth. The effect of leaving the cord long on cord infections has not been studied. It is, however, harder to keep the cord dry and clean if it is long, and it could more easily come into contact with urine and faeces (though this would not happen where the cord is tied loosely around the neck or arm, as is the custom in some African countries) (Fig. 9.8).

In most cultures, some kind of substance is applied to the cord stump. Ash, oil, butter, spice pastes, herbs and mud are substances that are commonly used. These substances are often contaminated with bacteria and spores and thus increase the risk of infection. One of the most dangerous practices is the application of cow, chicken or rat dung to the stump; this is associated with a high risk of neonatal tetanus. Ghee application has also been found to be a risk factor for tetanus. The most common reasons given for applying a substance to the cord are to prevent bleeding from the stump, to promote separation of the stump, and to keep spirits away. The effect of these practices on bleeding and separation has not been studied. Some Latin American cultures have beneficial customs regarding treatment of the cord, such as cauterizing the stump with a candle flame, hot coal or burning stick. In Kwa Zulu-Natal and in some communities in Kenya, some women apply expressed breast milk (colostrum) to the cord stump (this could in fact be beneficial in view of the antibacterial factors present in breast milk) (Fig. 9.9).

In many cultures, it is common to bind the newborn's abdomen with cloth or bandages. This practice keeps the stump moist, thus delaying healing and increasing the risk of infection, especially if the material used is unclean. Various reasons are given for the custom of binding, such as to prevent the umbilicus from bulging or protruding from the body, to secure the newborn's internal organs or to protect the stump from 'bad air'

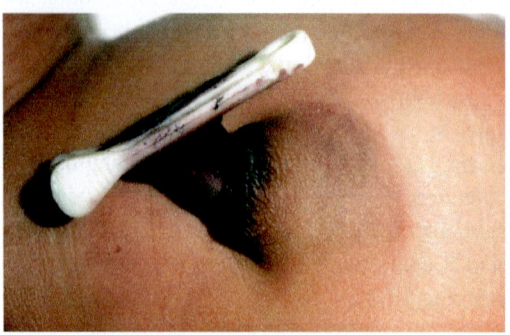

Fig. 9.9 Cord stump managed with (Khull) domestic eyeliner

which is considered in some cultures to be a cause of illness.

Placenta prints: Recently, some parents used paper towels to pat all the blood off the placenta and then painted the placenta and the cord with green washable, water-based liquid paint, then flipped it over onto a large piece of paper and made a print of it.

9.4 Spiritual Facts About Umbilicus and Umbilical Cord

The navel is the locus and the centrepiece of the human body. It's the communal scar of humanhood, the sole button on your birthday suit.

Japanese spiritualist Hogen Fukunaga writes, 'The navel is the core of everything about the person'. So it logically follows that the unlucky person who ends up with an abnormal version of this most central of body parts is doomed to a life of dubious distinction.

Notice that the Milky Way tree serves as an extension of Pacal's umbilicus. The umbilicus is a human being's entrance into life and entrance into death as well.

People consider the navel a vestigial nub and think nourishment only comes through the mouth not so. Tao is the great mother and vitality untold lies in the region of the umbilicus.

The old books call Tao (in Chinese philosophy the absolute principle underlying the universe) the great mother. Tao provides for us as a mother would. It shelters us, nourishes us and makes our life possible. We are literally tied to the vitality of Tao.

Lying dormant inside us are points of concentration. Most people are unaware that concentration on these points will yield specific forces, cure ailments, alter consciousness and still the mind. Like a treasure buried in the ruins of a sacred place, these spots only await discovery before they give their owner wondrous powers. One such spot is the area of the navel. When you concentrate there, you will find that great vitality comes your way. It will be as if you are still

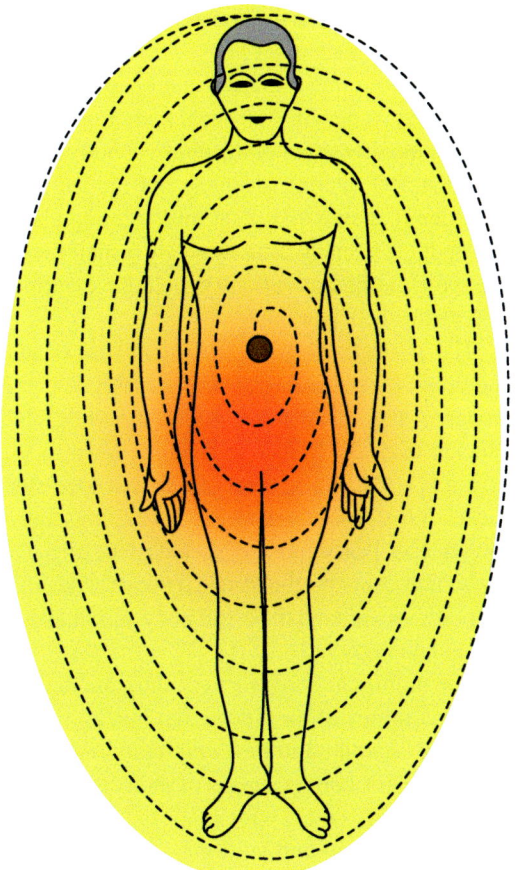

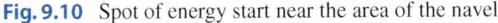

Fig. 9.10 Spot of energy start near the area of the navel

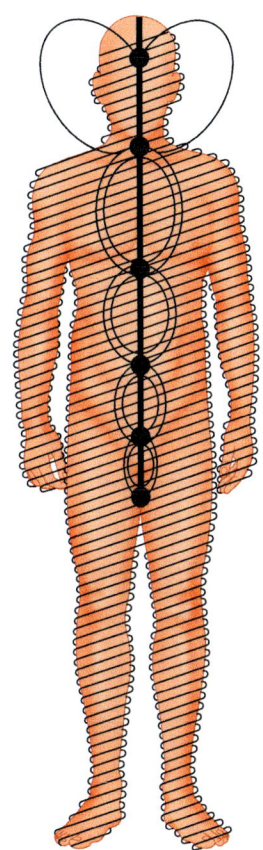

Fig. 9.11 Double helix pattern of energy starting from navel

connected to your mother through the umbilicus and power and tremendous physical well-being will come your way (Fig. 9.10).

Energy currents: The energy currents in the Caduceus flow in a double helix pattern (similar to the structure of DNA) creating a spiral of energy around the body known as the East–West current. Also a spiral of energy radiates out from the umbilicus (Fig. 9.11)

The Breath of Brahma: A spiral has the unique ability to move in two directions at the same time. All vibration is serpentine in motion, reflecting this dynamic. The gunas universally embody this ubiquitous force, the 'breath of Brahma'. Living vital fields are pulsating with life. The pulses undulate through the field in oval spirals from within to without and at the same time, from without to within.

Luminosity, heat and caloric energy are sustained by the vibrational frequency of fire. This electric pattern of energy predominates in the fields of force which manifest warmth and function, as in the vital organs and muscles. Fire is the yang, directed, working, passionate, vital energy in the body. Its radiant working energy rules the organs and the processes of metabolism and is the motive force of the musculature. Any stimulating or rajasic contact resonates with fire and promotes its attainment. Fire is centred in the solar plexus, two finger widths below the umbilicus (Fig. 9.12).

Describing the same phenomenon, Itzhak Bentov explains rhythm entrainment, the process where 'periodic events that are close in fre-

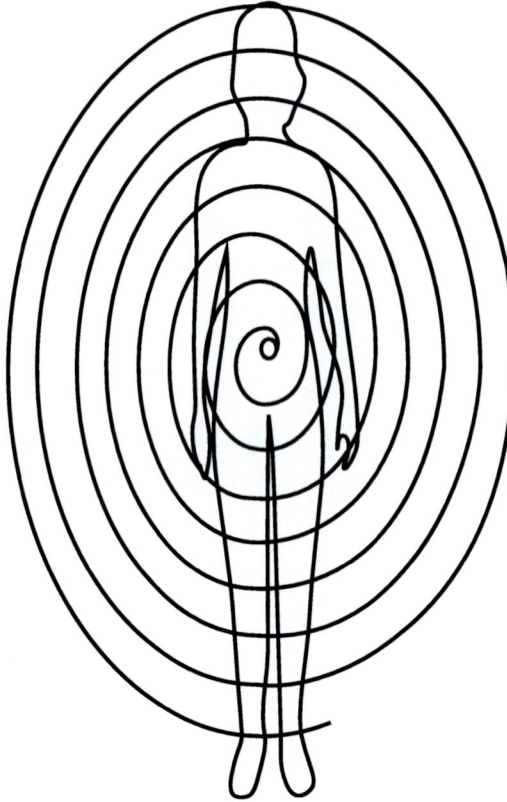

Fig. 9.12 Umbilicus is the centre of energy and polarity

quency occur in phase or in step with each other'. He goes on to write: 'Our biological rhythms are entrained by light and to a certain extent by gravity. Magnetic, electromagnetic, atmospheric, and subtle geophysical effects influence us in ways that are not presently well understood'. This process is significant in the macrocosm as well, where 'the big and mighty asteroids and planets are rhythm entrained and develop resonances in their orbits as they rotate about the sun [11]'.

The law of sympathetic vibration describes the tendency of vibrations of the same wavelength to resonate together. Sympathetic resonance may be the glue that holds creation together. Waveforms of the same frequency will entrain (synchronise their vibrations) to energize and influence each other [12].

Silver cord: it is a silver-coloured, elastic cord which joins a person's physical body to its astral body (a manifestation of the physical body that is less distinct). During sleeping and immediately after death, a cloudlike faint mist forming above the body. It streams from the body, usually from the navel, although various people have various outlets for the silver cord.

The silver cord in metaphysical studies and literature, also known as the sutratma or life thread of the antahkarana, refers to a life-giving linkage from the higher self (atma) down to the physical body. It also refers to an extended synthesis of this thread and a second (the consciousness thread, passing from the soul to the physical body) that connects the physical body to the etheric body, onwards to the astral body and finally to the mental body [13].

The umbilical cord is a very intricate device, a very complex affair indeed, but it is as a piece of string compared to the complexity of the silver cord. This cord is a mass of molecules rotating over an extremely wide range of frequencies, but it is an intangible thing—so far as the human body is concerned. The molecules are too widely dispersed for the average human sight to see it. Many animals can see it, because animals see on a different range of frequencies—and hear on a different range of frequencies than humans. Dogs, as you know, can be called by a 'silent' dog whistle, silent because a human cannot hear it—but a dog easily can. In the same way, animals can see the silver cord and the aura, because both these vibrate on a frequency which is just within the receptivity of an animal's sight. With practice, it is quite easily possible for a human to extend the band of receptivity (mottakelighet) of their sight, in much the same way as a weak man, by practice and by exercise, can lift a weight which normally would be far, far beyond his physical capabilities.

Scientists trying to measure the distance of the moon broadcast on a very narrow beam—a waveform to the surface of the moon. That is much the same as the silver cord between the human body and the human Overself; it is the method whereby the Overself communicates with the body on Earth [14] (Fig. 9.13).

The astral body and the physical body are connected together by the silver cord. This latter is a mass of molecules vibrating at a tremendous speed. It is in some ways similar to the umbilical cord, which connects a mother to her baby; in the mother, impulses, impressions, and nourishment flow from her to the unborn baby. When the baby is born and the umbilical cord is severed, then the baby dies to the life it knew before, that is, it becomes a separate entity, a separate life, it is no longer a part of the mother, so it 'dies' as part of the mother and takes on its own existence (Fig. 9.14) [15].

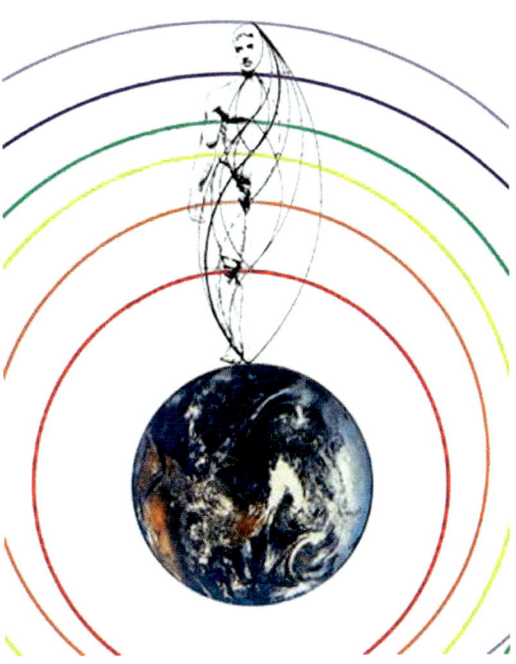

Fig. 9.13 Silver cord

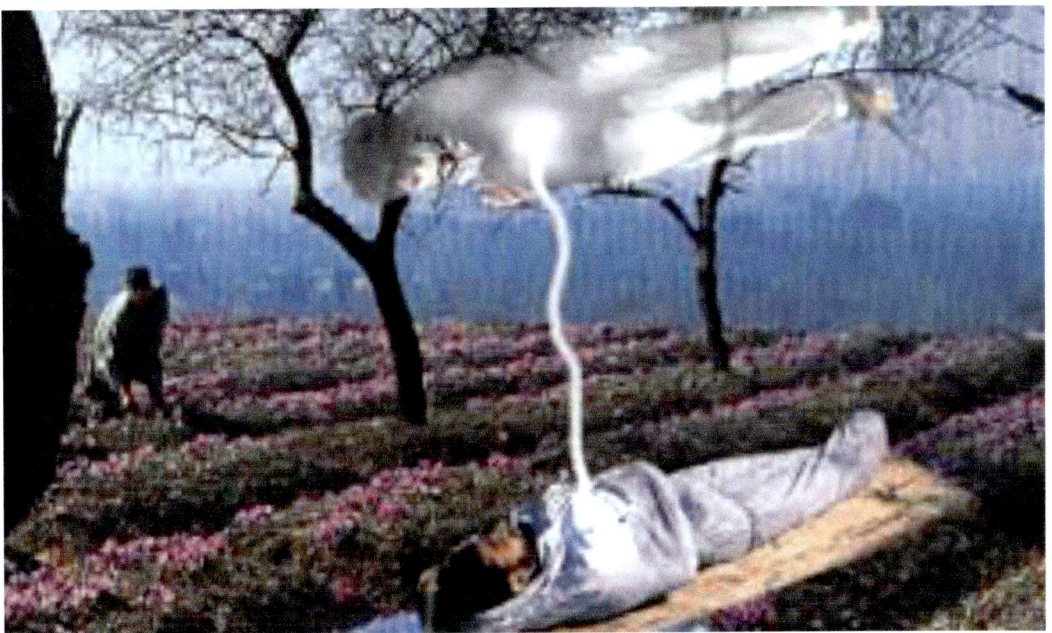

Fig. 9.14 Umbilical mystery

References

1. Al Maxey (Creation Magazine, June, 1996).
2. Browne T. Pseudodoxia epidemica, vol. 2. Chicago: University of Chicago Press; 1964.
3. Gosse PH. Evolution (biology). In: Omphalos: an attempt to untie the geological knot. London: J. Van Voorst; 1857. p. 376.
4. Jason H. Collins. Silent risk issues about the human umbilical cord, 2nd Edition, 2014.
5. Longrigg J. Greek rational medicine: philosophy and medicine from Alcmaeon to the Alexandrians. London: Psychology Press; 1993.
6. Geza Roheim A. Revised and expanded version of one of the author's first psychoanalytic studies, this was originally published in Hungarian: *Az filet fonala* (The Thread of Life).
7. Ethnographia; 1916. Novack AH, Mueller B, Ochs H. Umbilical cord separation in the normal newborn. Am J Dis Child. 1988;142(2): 220–3
8. Kruyt: Het Wezen van het Heidendom te Posso. (The Essence of Posso Paganism). Medizinische Nederlander Zend. Gen., 1903, XLVIII, pp. 21–35.
9. de Groot JJM. Les Fêtes-annuellement celébrées à Emoui. Annales Musée Gamete. 1886;II:476.
10. Grube W. Religion und Kultus der Chinesen. Leipzig: Verlag von Rudolf Haupt; 1910. p. 168.
11. Opler ME. Childhood and youth in Jicarilla apache society. Los Angeles: Publications of the Frederick Webb Hodge Anniversary Publication Fund; 1945. p. 5.
12. Iona Miller: Schumann resonance, psychophysical regulation & psi (part I). J Conscious Explor Res. 4(6): 2013.
13. Burger B. Esoteric anatomy: the body as consciousness. Chapter 8, North Atlantic Books IIO. Box 12327 Berkeley, California; 2012. http://www.weare1.us/Golden_Ratio.html.
14. Smed JA. Out-of-body experience studies. The Monroe Institute; 2013. www.monroeinstitute.org.
15. Blackmore S. Out-of-body experience. In: Gregory RL, editor. The oxford companion to the mind. 2nd ed. Oxford: Oxford University Press; 2004.

Part II

Umbilical Cord

Embryology

10

The umbilical cord begins to form between 4 and 6 weeks, as the embryonic disc takes a cylindrical shape. Located at the lower third of the embryo, the proximal portion of the umbilical cord begins to form and develops as a sac. The proximal portion of this sac houses the guts until the 10th week of gestation. At this time the umbilical cord is short, usually shorter than the head-to-tail (crown-rump) length of the embryo, and of proportionately large diameter. It is not able to tolerate rotation about itself or the formed embryo (Fig. 10.1).

This initial stalk develops in the centre of the implantation site, which is the reason the cord presents at the centre of the placenta. By 10 weeks, the intestines leave the proximal cord and return to the abdominal cavity, the elongation of the cord begins and the location of the umbilicus (belly button) positions in the middle third of the embryo. The elongation of the umbilical vein and arteries coincides with the development of Wharton's jelly, an umbilical cord connective tissue. The development of the umbilical cord is closely related to that of the amnion. Throughout the last days of the 2nd week postcoitus, the blastocystic cavity is filled by a loose meshwork of mesoderm cells, the extraembryonic mesoblast, which surrounds the embryoblast (day 13) [1], the embryoblast at that time is composed of two vesicles: the amniotic vesicle and the primary yolk sac (Fig. 10.2).

When these two vesicles are in contact with each other, they form the double-layered embryonic disc. During the following days the extra-embryonic mesoderm cells are rearranged in such a way that they line the inner surface of the trophoblastic shell as chorionic mesoderm. They also cover the surface of the two embryonic vesicles. Between the two mesoderm layers, the exocoelom cavity forms. It largely separates the embryo, and its mesodermal cover from the chorionic mesoderm. The exocoelom is bridged by the mesoderm in only one place, which lies basal to the amniotic vesicle. This mesenchymal connection is referred to as the connecting stalk. It fixes the early embryo to the membranes and is the forerunner of the umbilical cord [1]. During the same period (around day 18 p.c.), a duct-like extension of the yolk sac, originating from

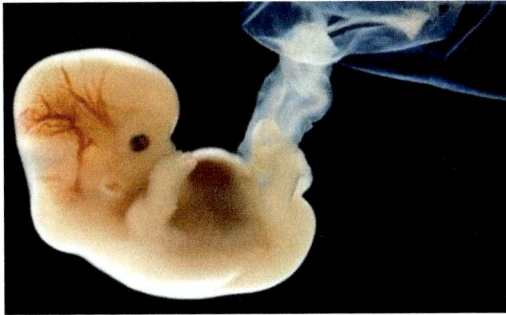

Fig. 10.1 Umbilical cord at 54 days embryo, it is short and wide

M. Fahmy, *Umbilicus and Umbilical Cord*, https://doi.org/10.1007/978-3-319-62383-2_10

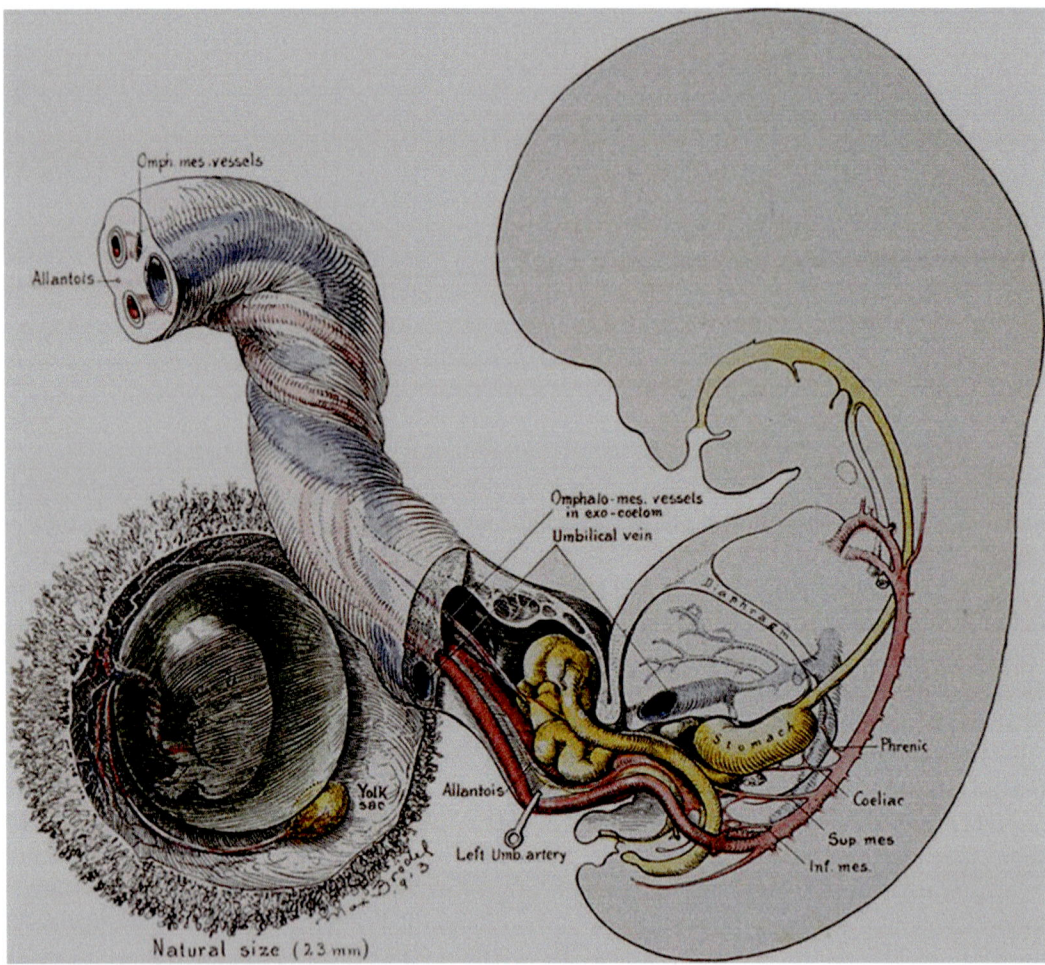

Fig. 10.2 Diagram of the early structures of the umbilical cord, the cord is thick and short with a herniated midgut

the future caudal region of the embryo, develops into the connecting stalk. This structure is the transitory allantois, the primitive extraembryonic urinary bladder (Fig. 10.2).

The three subsequent weeks are characterized by three developmental processes:

1. The embryo rotates in such a way that the yolk sac vesicle, originally facing the region opposite the implantation site, is turned toward the implantation pole.
2. The amniotic vesicle enlarges considerably, extending around the embryo.
3. The originally flat embryonic disc is bent in the anteroposterior direction and rolled up in the lateral direction. It thus 'herniates' into the

amniotic vesicle. As the embryo bends, it subdivides the yolk sac into an intraembryonic duct (the intestines) and an extraembryonic part (the omphalomesenteric duct), which is dilated peripherally to form the extraembryonic yolk sac vesicle.

Both the allantois and the extraembryonic yolk sac extend into the mesenchyme of the connecting stalk. Between days 28 and 40 post conception, the expanding amniotic cavity has surrounded the embryo so far that the connecting stalk, the urachus, and the yolk sac are compressed to a slender cord, which is then covered by amniotic epithelium (day 28). They thus form the umbilical cord. The cord lengthens as the embryo 'prolapses' backward into the amniotic sac [2]. During the same process of expansion, the amniotic mesenchyme locally touches and finally fuses with the chorionic mesoderm, thus occluding the exocoelomic cavity. This process persists until the end of the first trimester when, at approximately 12 weeks, the amniotic cavity completely occupies the exocoelom so that amniotic and chorionic mesenchyme have fused everywhere.

During the third week p.c., the extraembryonic yolk sac, the omphalomesenteric duct that connects with the embryonic intestines and the allantois become supplied with fetal vessels. All mammals use either allantoic or yolk sac vessels for the vascularization of the placenta. In human allantoic vessels, two allantoic arteries originating from the internal iliac arteries and one allantoic vein that enters the hepatic vein invade the placenta and become connected to the villous vessels.

The allantoic participation in placental vascularization is the reason for the term chorioallantoic placenta. In contrast, in the choriovitelline or vitelline placentation (e.g. that of rodents and bats), the yolk sac vessels establish fetoplacental vascular connections.

References

1. Heifetz S. Pathology of the umbilical cord. In: Lewis SH, Perrin E, editors. Pathology of the placenta. 2nd ed. New York: Churchill Livingstone; 1999. p. 107–35.
2. Hertig AT. The placenta: some new knowledge about an old organ. Obstet Gynecol. 1962;20:859–66.

Anatomy of the Umbilical Cord

11.1 Cord Length

The cord is believed to elongate until as late as 36 weeks although rapid change occurs until 28 weeks and then slows. The final length of the umbilical cord averages about 61 cm, or 24 in., with wide variations detected. As it was suggested by Leonardo da Vinci, the umbilical cord has usually the same length as the baby.

So why human UC is 61 cm?, the umbilical cords of whales, porpoises, goats and other mammals are relatively shorter than the human cord.

Walker and Rye of Cambridge surmised in the British Medical Journal in 1960 that prehistoric humans evolved length for protection. Nature's purpose was to allow the mother to pick up the newborn without disturbing the placenta. The event of breast feeding would then separate the placenta—an event which could attract predators. Having the fetus in tow would allow escape for mother and child [1].

Today, cord length correlates to several 'outcomes'. Cords too short and cords too long predispose the fetus to intrauterine dangers. It is considered that cord less than 32 cm is 'absolutely' short and more than 32 cm is 'relatively' short.

The length of the cord was determined by the amount of amniotic fluid, and increased length between bursts was observed with advancing age. The most of the cord's length is achieved by the 28th week of pregnancy. By the fourth month, it has grown to between 16 and 18 cm and, by the sixth month, to between 33 and 35 cm. It was also suggested that there may be a relation between cord length and umbilical arterial pressures.

Absent umbilical cord: There are rare cases of 'achordia', which have mostly been associated with abdominal wall defects or with acardiac fetuses. Most of these infants actually have a diminutive cord rather than no cord at all. Rupture of short cords and of cords with entanglement has been reported.

11.2 Long Umbilical Cord
(Fig. 11.1)

An excessively long cord poses problems because the fetus may become entangled in it, or the cord may prolapse, especially after the membranes rupture. In general, long cords have more pronounced spiralling, and it may be inferred from this fact also that the excessive length results from increased fetal movements. Umbilical cords measuring up to 300 cm have been reported [2]. One would think that such excessively long and spiralled cords would also require greater perfusion pressure, but this has not been confirmed, and some studies suggest that it is not true.

Looping about the neck and extremities was found in 23% of overall obstetrical cases, and it was more common with excessively long cords.

© Springer International Publishing AG 2018
M. Fahmy, *Umbilicus and Umbilical Cord*, https://doi.org/10.1007/978-3-319-62383-2_11

Fig. 11.1 Abnormally long UC

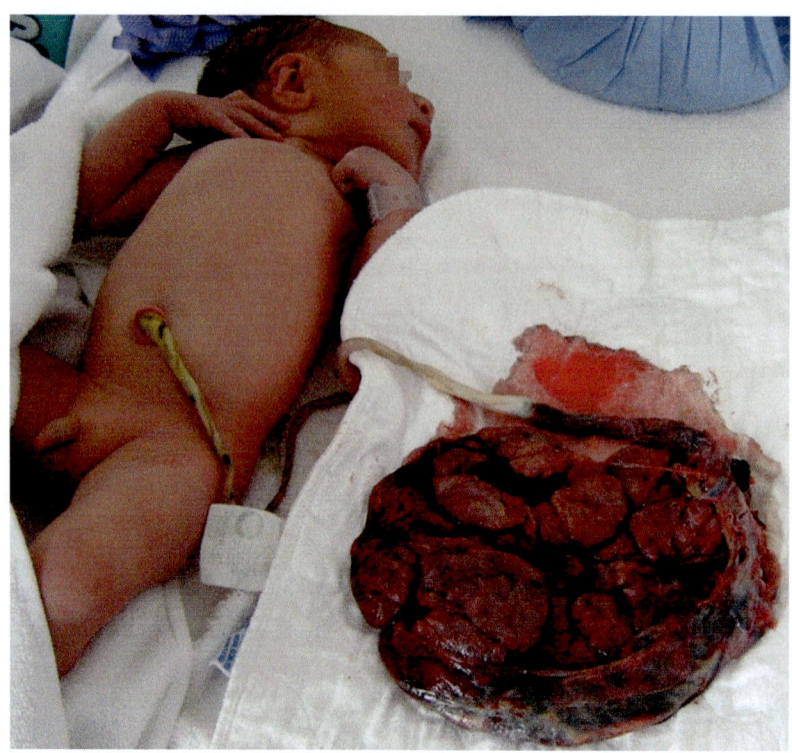

11.3   Abnormal Length and Nuchal Cord

When UC circled once about the neck, the cord was 76.5 cm long, and when circled twice about the neck it was 93.5 cm.

The possible relation between long cords and excessive fetal movements is more difficult to assess because of the deficiency of quantitative data on prenatal movements. It would also be of great interest to obtain more information as to whether children associated with long umbilical cords remain to be 'hyperactive' in later life; Naeye suggested that this may be so [3].

Excessively long cords were significantly more common with right spirals, with excessive spiralling, true knots, thromboses in fetal vessels, congestion and meconium staining.

Nuchal cords: (cord encirclement) It is an abnormal condition commonly associating long cord, where the cord loops around the fetal neck; it may be associated with or cause fetal growth restriction, in a survey of 11,201

deliveries; 19% of deliveries had one encirclement of the cord around the neck, 5.3% had two loops, 1.2% had three and 0.2% had four cord encirclements [4].

Nuchal cord was not correlated with the 1-year neurologic status, or stillbirths, but nuchal cords were increased with true knots, the frequency of knots and encirclement is 0.5% and an encirclement of 14.2% was found with cords ranging from 27 to 122 cm in length.

Infants born with nuchal cords are more often deprived of placental blood transfusion because their cords are severed by the obstetrician before extraction, and they are significantly more anaemic than controls, presumably because of reduced venous return from the placenta secondary to compression of the umbilical vein [5].

Tight nuchal cords may be the cause of hypovolemic shock of the newborn. Nuchal cord entanglement may have serious sequelae for the fetus. Cerebral palsy is a probable consequence of this prenatal problem [4].

Fetomaternal hemorrhage and pulmonary hemorrhages may have resulted from increased pulmonary perfusion because of tight nuchal cords.

It is now possible to make the diagnosis antenatally with ultrasonography, particularly when malposition and hydramnios suggest this possibility.

Causes of or associations with cord prolapse that were undertaken indicated a high caesarean section rate, a 10% mortality and high prematurity and breech rates. The haemodynamic response with fetal heart rate monitoring is of particular importance for the cases with occult prolapse.

The compressed umbilical cord may show profound pathologic changes, such as hemorrhage, and even rupture at the site of compression (Chap. 13).

It leads occasionally to thrombosis, found when multiple sections are taken, but thrombi ensue more commonly in the surface chorionic vessels. That cord compression may have serious fetal neurologic consequences.

Clapp et al. [6] determined the occurrence of nuchal cords prospectively from 24 weeks on and found it to increase from 12 to 37%.

Hydramnios and male fetuses had a greater propensity. Finally, a statistical study of 926 cases with excessively long cords (+70 cm) was performed by Baergen et al. [7]; they found a significantly increased risk of brain imaging abnormalities and/or abnormal neurological follow-up; in addition, mothers with a history of an excessively long umbilical cord are at increased risk of a second long cord.

11.4   Conditions Associated with Short Cord

The first pregnancy tends to generate a shorter cord than subsequent pregnancies.

The concept changes, however, when cord insertion site and cord entanglement are considered. This idea is called a relatively short cord. Very short cords less than 20 cm are associated with genetic malformations.

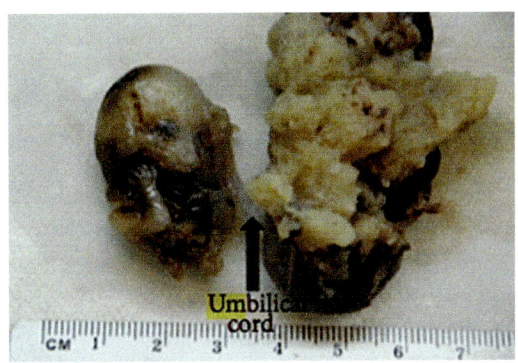

Fig. 11.2   Extremely short UC

Males have slightly longer cords than females (58.46 versus 56.90 cm in vertex; 53.78 versus 52.51 cm in breech) (Fig. 11.2).

Infants with Down syndrome (trisomy 21) have significantly shorter cords (45.1 versus 57.3 cm for controls); this may be due to the reduced fetal activity in utero [8].

Likewise, with breech presentations, the cord is shorter by some 4.5 cm than with births from a vertex presentation and 7.9 cm shorter in twins [9].

Lethal bony malformations such as osteogenesis imperfecta had significantly reduced cord lengths.

Prenatal alcohol administration to rats shortens the cords, as does atenolol (a beta-blocker) given to rabbits. Shorter cords have since been found in offspring who suffer the fetal alcohol syndrome [10].

There was slight correlation between cord length and fetal and placental weights.

When cord lengths were evaluated for IQ, short cords showed a higher incidence of neurologic abnormalities. Cord length may also influence fetal position; breech-positioned fetuses have shorter cords due to less activity [11].

When the fetus is constrained, as occurs, for instance, with amnionic adhesions and in ectopic pregnancies, the cord is short.

Cords less than 15 cm were often associated with abdominal wall defects and evisceration, spinal and limb deformities and other lesions [12].

Umbilical cord circumference and diameter are also important measurements. On average, normal umbilical cords are 3.7 cm in circumference with a range of 3–5 cm.

The diameter range of 1.0–3.0 cm can suggest an abnormal cord with edema, tumor or hernia. Dimensions greater than 6-cm circumference should prompt an examination of the cord and fetus. Are shorter cords thicker than longer cords? Although rarely published, it appears that this may be the case.

Before cutting any thick cord, it should be checked to ensure that the fetal intestine is not present within the cord.

Epithelium of the cord: The cord is covered by amnionic epithelium, which is contiguous with the surface of the placenta and the fetal skin, near the umbilicus, the cord epithelium is largely unkeratinized, and stratified squamous epithelium provides the transition from the abdominal wall to the cord's surface. Farther away from the umbilicus, the epithelium transforms into a stratified columnar epithelium (two to eight layers) and finally into a simple columnar epithelium. The latter continues developing into the simple columnar to cuboidal epithelium of the placental amnionic surface. The basal cells of the stratified parts of the amnion resemble the amnionic epithelium of the membranes, whereas the superficial cells sometimes are squamous, poor in organelles and pyknotic.

The amnion of the cord is structurally similar to that described for the membranes, the one difference being that the amnion of the membranes is easily detached whereas the amnion of the cord grows firmly into the central connective tissue core and cannot be dislodged. The connective tissue of the cord is derived from the extraembryonic mesoblast [13].

Parry and Abramovich [14] found two principal cells types, with intermediates. In contrast to earlier theories, they suggested that these cells do not have any water regulatory function. Thus, if there is larger water content in the proximal portion of the cord, it must have other underlying causes. In this context it is interesting to note that Gebrane-Younes and coworkers [15], based on the ultrastructure of the umbilical endothelium and other wall components, have suggested a considerable fluid transudation out of the umbilical vessels into the amnionic fluid.

In general, the amnion of the cord is structurally similar to that described in the membranes; and there are no indications that this is different for its basic functions.

Wharton's jelly: Wharton's jelly is a specialized tissue serving many purposes for the developing fetus. Its specialized cells contain gelatin-like mucus that encases fibres. These properties give it an elastic and cushion effect, which can tolerate the vibration, bending, stretching and twisting of an active fetus.

In addition, it holds the vessels together, may regulate blood flow, plays a role in providing nutrition to the fetus, stores chemistry for the onset of labour and protects the supply line.

Umbilical cords without much Wharton's jelly are more prone to compression, and its complete absence is usually associated with fetal death.

If an umbilical cord is twisted or knotted, it is more likely to tighten where there is less resistance, such as an area low in Wharton's jelly. It is believed that males have more Wharton's jelly content than do females and that good nutrition increases the amount.

Wharton's jelly tends to reduce with gestational age and can disappear when pregnancies go beyond 40 weeks. Because these cases tend to have fetal heart rate changes, the level of Wharton's jelly is a consideration when obstetricians plan the deliveries of pregnancies low on amniotic fluid.

Wharton's jelly is derived from the extraembryonic mesoblast. McKay et al. [16] referred to this jelly-like material of the exocoelom as a 'thixotropic gel' (gels or fluids that are thick or viscous and under static conditions will flow) because it liquefies when touched. The incorporation of this mesenchyme into the cord substance and the sub-amnionic layers probably accounts for their mucoid and compressible structures. The Wharton's jelly also seems to be an erectile tissue, as the filled umbilical cord is a relatively firm, rigid structure and that with expansion and contraction of the vasculature, its thickness and turgidity vary, and this characters enable Wharton's jelly to perform its protective function for the umbilical vessels.

This jelly is composed of a ground substance of open-chain polysaccharides (hyaluronic acid;

carbohydrates with glycosyl and mannosyl groups) distributed in a fine network of microfibrils. Immunohistochemically, the interstitial collagen types I, III, and VI, as well as the basal lamina molecules collagen type IV, laminin, and heparan sulfate, were found in this connective tissue. Immunoreactivities for these extracellular matrix molecules were accumulated around cleft-like territories 'stromal clefts' in Wharton's jelly; the stromal clefts themselves were occupied by homogeneous ground substance, which was devoid of collagens and basal lamina molecules but probably contained ample proteoglycans. These fibre-free stromal clefts must not be misunderstood as lymphatic vessels that exist neither in the cord nor in the placenta [17].

Wharton's jelly contains evenly distributed spindle-shaped fibroblasts with long extensions and numerous mast cells. These cells can be stained selectively, surround the vessels densely and are also found underneath the cord surface.

Electron microscopic and immunohistochemical studies revealed that the stromal cells embedded into the collagen meshwork were myofibroblasts rather than typical fibroblasts. Myofibroblasts are fibre-producing cells that have contractile properties similar to those of smooth muscle cells; the stromal cells of Wharton's jelly depending on their location within the cord show different degrees of differentiation from mesenchymal cells to myofibroblasts [18] (Fig. 11.3).

There are surprisingly few macrophages in the umbilical cord. Even when the cord is deep green due to meconium staining and when meconium-filled macrophages are readily seen in the membranes, only relatively few activated and pigmented macrophages are seen in the cord substance. Similarly, after intrafunicular bleeding, hemosiderin is not formed in situ.

The tensile properties of the cord have been reported; there are no significant differences in these tensile parameters with respect to the sex of the baby, but there was a significant positive correlation between the tensile breaking load and the birth weight of the baby. The average tensile breaking load is 2.49 times the weight of the baby at birth [19].

Recent studies by sonographers have concerned the variable thickness (diameter) of the umbilical cord, attributed to Wharton's belly contents, as it varies considerably and, at times, can be shown to have prognostic value; the diameter increases with gestational age to about 32 weeks; fetuses with chromosomal anomalies and those with other placental abnormalities had larger volumes of cords [20].

Cysts, for instance, may cause much enlargement (vide infra) and make the cord heavier, and

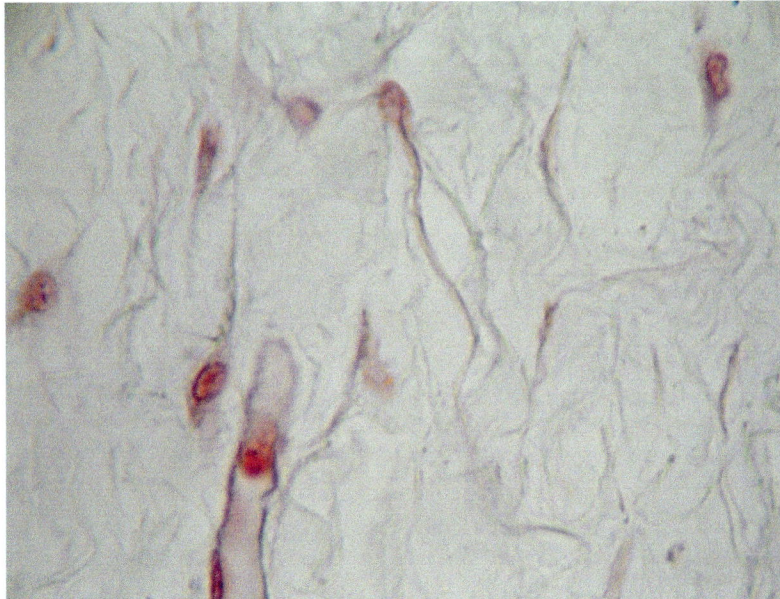

Fig. 11.3 Histology of Wharton's jelly

in many placentas of pregnancies in diabetics, the cord appears thicker and more waterlogged (Chap. 14).

Umbilical vessels: There are normally two arteries and one vein in the human umbilical cord (Fig. 11.4). An originally developed second umbilical vein atrophies during the second month of pregnancy. In rare cases (1%), there is only one umbilical artery, an anomaly that may be associated with multiple fetal malformations; local fusion of the two arteries has also been reported [21].

The arrangement of umbilical vessels is different in many other species, for example, two arteries and two veins are found in the nine-banded armadillo, with many subtle variations; other animals may have an admixture of yolk sac (vitelline) vessels. Cats may have four vessels of each type. The notion of a 'double umbilicus' is based on a single observation of a somewhat displaced, doubled umbilical vein found in an adult, with puckering of the skin. In rare cases, there were two umbilical veins, and a portion of the cord was separated, giving it a partially split appearance. The persistence of a second (right) umbilical vein within frequently (18%) malformed fetuses had

been described. Thus, the findings are limited to sonographic intra-fetal findings [22].

The mean intravital diameter of the arteries is around 3 mm, with a slight tendency to increase towards the placenta. The venous diameter is around twice this size (Fig. 11.5).

Human Umbilical Vessels Differ in Many Ways from the Major Vessels of the Body: The endothelial cells of both the arteries and the veins

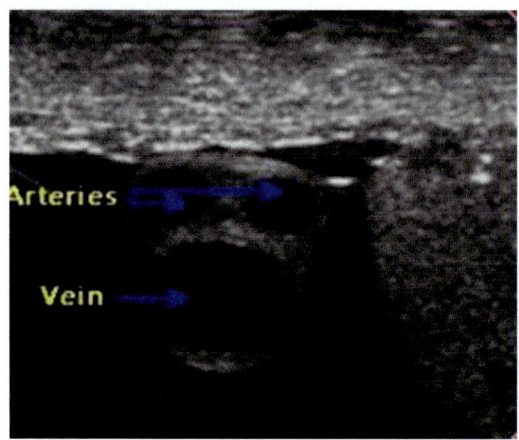

Fig. 11.5 Doppler ultrasound of umbilical cord presentation at 32 weeks

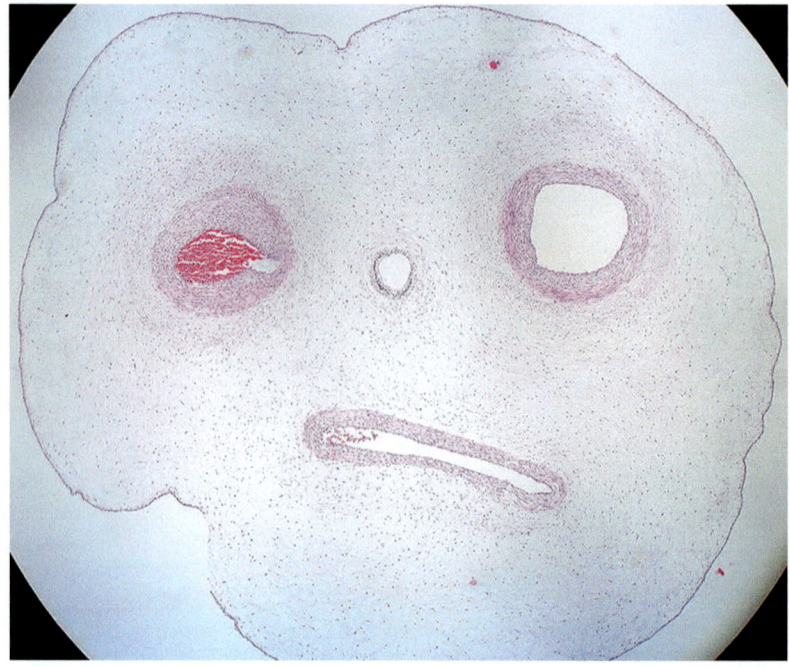

Fig. 11.4 Cross section of mature umbilical cord, near its placental insertion showing a sparsely cellular Wharton's jelly, an umbilical vein and two arteries H&E

are unusually rich in organelle and thus structurally different from the endothelium of the villous vessels. Gebrane-Younes et al. [23] have given a careful account of the ultrastructure of the endothelium; they described ultrastructural evidence that transudation of fluid through the umbilical vessel walls contributes to the formation of amnionic fluid.

The arteries possess no internal elastic membrane and have much less elastica in general than other arteries. The vein, on the other hand, has an elastic subintimal layer. The muscular coat of the arteries consists of a system of crossing spiralled fibres (Fig. 11.6).

Desmin-positive smooth muscle cells are largely concentrated on the outer layer of the media. In contrast, the inner media smooth muscle cells are poorly differentiated with few myofilaments. They hardly can contribute actively to postpartal closure of the cord arteries. The venous muscular coats are thinner than those of the arteries and composed of more separate layers of longitudinal or circular fibres. Media smooth muscle cells of the cord and adjacent chorionic vessels are major placental storage sites for glycogen.

Each umbilical vessel is surrounded by crossing bundles of spiralled collagen fibres that form a kind of adventitia. The umbilical vessels of human umbilical cords lack vasa vasorum. Fetuses beyond 20 weeks of gestation, however, have vasa vasorum in the intraabdominal portions of their umbilical arteries [24].

After delivery, umbilical cords show irregular constrictions of the arteries, but the mechanism is not completely clear. It is known that increased transmural pressures exerted on the umbilical arteries led to vasoconstriction. In addition, many substances induce vasodilatation or vasoconstriction of the umbilical vessels. Vasodilators include serotonin, angiotensin, oxytocin, prostaglandins, nitrous oxide and atrial natriuretic peptide. Vasoconstrictors include angiotensin II, 5-hydroxytryptamine (5-HT), thromboxane, neuropeptide Y and endothelin-1. The functions of these vasoconstrictors are still under discussion, and they may function as mediators of closure of the placental circulation at birth.

Abnormal umbilical vessels anastomosis: An important macroscopic feature of umbilical arteries is the presence of an anastomosis between the two arteries near the surface of the placenta. The older literature and more recent studies have shown that 96% of cords have some sort of arterial anastomosis [25]. Most were seen 1.5 cm from the placental insertion and were either truly

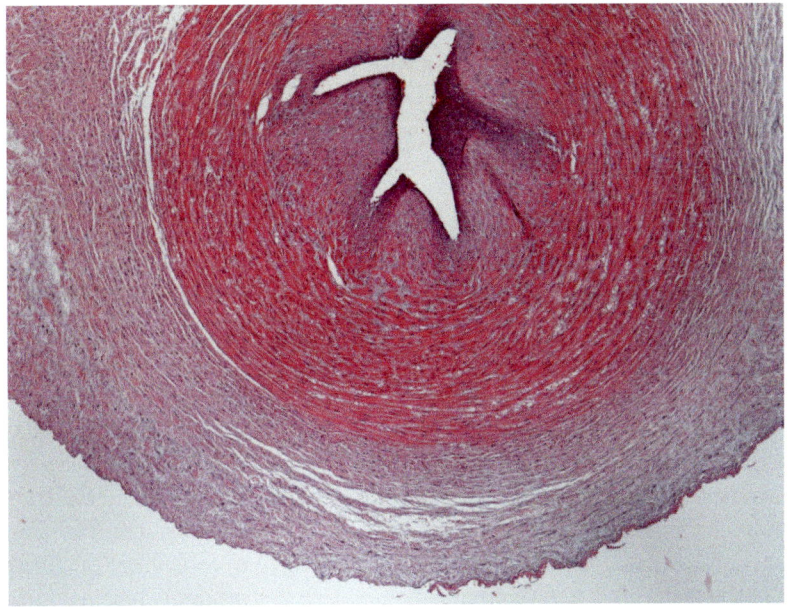

Fig. 11.6 Histological appearance of the umbilical artery, with two layers of smooth muscle cells without a prominent internal elastica or adventitia

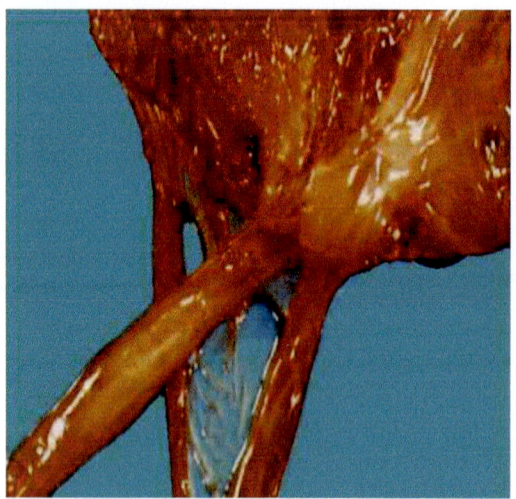

Fig. 11.7 Aberrant anastomosis between umbilical arteries near the placenta

anastomotic vessels or the two arteries fused. On rare occasions, two such communicating vessels exist (Fig. 11.7).

Fujikura [26] measured the distance of the anastomosis from the placental surface; it ranges from 0.5 to 6 cm. Like Hyrtl [27], who attached much importance to this communication, which is believed to be meaningful for an equalization of flow and pressures between the two arteries and for the uniform distribution of blood to the different lobes of the placenta. A better understanding of the functional importance of Hyrtl's anastomosis has come from numerous sonographic studies that employed Doppler flow evaluation.

These have taken on a significant importance in prenatal evaluations now and have, for instance, detected a difference in the size of the two arteries and are commonly used to anticipate fetal growth and its impairment.

Often the looping of umbilical vessels is the cause for 'false knots' of the cord. In most cases, local loops of the arteries, or sometimes even the vein, cause knot-like dilation of the cord.

Sometimes focal varicosities of the veins or perivascular accumulations of connective tissue result in a similar external appearance. Finally, there are the 'valves (nodes) of Hoboken' [28], named after a seventeenth-century Dutch

anatomist. These crescentic folds in the inner wall of umbilical arteries are present after delivery, but that they do not exist in vivo.

11.5 Innervation of Umbilical Cord

There is general agreement about UC innervation that no nerves traverse the umbilical cord from fetus to placenta and that the placenta has no neural supply [29].

A number of investigators, however, have since investigated this apparent lack of nerves, and some have come to different conclusions. Thus, Kernbach [30] studied the amnion with Cajal stains and considered the powdery Nissl substance of extravillous trophoblast cells to represent sympathicoblasts with nerve fibres. He also believed that he had identified nerves in the amnion.

Fox and Jacobson [31] stained various segments of umbilical cords from abortuses and term placentas with methylene blue and observed fibres in all segments of all cords. The fibres were most easily seen in Wharton's jelly but surrounded and entered the vascular walls. Fox and Jacobson interpreted the fibres to be neural elements. It is possible that these structures relate to the vagal fibres described in embryos by Pearson and Sauter [32], which are thought to be instrumental in closing the ductus venosus after birth. The same authors subsequently investigated the sacral portions of embryos and found convincing evidence of neural supply of umbilical arteries. Some neural elements terminate before entering the cord, whereas others penetrate it. This report was contrary to the older literature, which was reviewed.

Ellison [33] then took up the topic and studied the cords with a thiocholine technique. He demonstrated acetylcholinesterase-positive nerve endings in the proximal 20 cm of umbilical cord, but the placental side invariably gave negative results. The illustrations of tiny nerves present around the umbilical vessels appear convincing. Because they frequently showed degenerative changes, they were interpreted as having a primarily prenatal function.

Electron microscopic investigation for innervation of the human umbilical cord has generally been negative, with no evidence of nerve fibres in the cord vessels, but they were present within the fetus and the immediate vicinity of the umbilicus, so the umbilical cord is considered to be a model of a nerve-free effector organ.

Immunohistochemical examination of cords obtained from the first, second and third trimester and using a panel of antibodies directed against neural and glial structures also failed to identify any nerve tissues in the middle and placental segment of the human umbilical cord [34].

Presence of nerve fibres within the umbilical cord, specially near to its fetal end, could be interpreted as not representing misplaced embryonic rests but as the result of in situ differentiation of local stem cells [35].

References

1. Stefos T, Sotiriadis A, Vasilios D, et al. Umbilical cord length and parity–the Greek experience. Eur J Obstet Gynecol Reprod Biol. 2003;26:41–4.
2. Arvy L, Pilleri G. Le Cordon Ombilical. Funis Umbilicalis. Bern: Verlag Hirnanatomisches Institut, Ostermundigen; 1976.
3. Naeye RL. Umbilical cord length: clinical significance. J Pediatr. 1985;107:278–81.
4. Soernes T. Umbilical cord encirclements and fetal growth restriction. Obstet Gynecol. 1995;86:725–8.
5. Shepherd AJ, Richardson CJ, Brown JP. Nuchal cords as a cause of neonatal anemia. Am J Dis Child. 1985;139:71–3.
6. Clapp JF, Stepanchak W, Hashimoto K, Ehrenberg H, Lopez B. The natural history of antenatal nuchal cords. Am J Obstet Gynecol. 2003;189:488–93.
7. Baergen RN, Malicki D, Behling C, Benirschke K. Morbidity, mortality, and placental pathology in excessively long umbilical cords: retrospective study. Pediatr Dev Pathol. 2001;4:144–53.
8. Moessinger AC, Blanc WA, Marone PA, Polsen DC. Umbilical cord length as an index of fetal activity: experimental study and clinical implications. Pediatr Res. 1982;16:109–12.
9. Soernes T, Bakke T. The length of the human umbilical cord in vertex and breech presentations. Am. J. Obstet. Gynecol. 1986;154:1086–7.
10. Calvano CJ, Hoar RM, Mankes RF, Lefevre R, Reddy PP, Moran ME, Mandell J. Experimental study of umbilical cord length as a marker of fetal alcohol syndrome. Teratology. 2000;61:184–8.
11. Gilbert-Barness E, Drut MR, Grange DK, Opitz JM. Developmental abnormalities resulting in short umbilical cord. Birth Defects Orig Artic Ser. 1993;29(1):113–40.
12. Gilbert E. The short cord syndrome. Pediatr Pathol. 1986;5:96.
13. Hempel E. Die ultrastrukturelle Differenzierung des menschlichen Amnionepithels unter besonderer Berücksichtigung des Nabelstrangs. Anat Anz. 1972;132:356–70.
14. Parry EW, Abramovich DR. Some observations on the surface layer of full-term human umbilical cord epithelium. J Obstet Gynaecol. 1970;77:878–84.
15. Gebrane-Younes J, Minh HN, Orcel L. Ultrastructure of human umbilical vessels: a possible role in amniotic fluid formation? Placenta. 1986;7:173–85.
16. Hertig AT, Richardson MV. Studies of the function of early human trophoblast. II. Preliminary observations on certain chemical constituents of chorionic and early amniotic fluid. Am J Obstet Gynecol. 1955;69:735–41.
17. Nanaev AK, Shirinsky VP, Birukov KG. Immunofluorescent study of heterogeneity in smooth muscle cells of human fetal vessels using antibodies to myosin, desmin and vimentin. Cell Tissue Res. 1991;266:535–40.
18. Mitchell KE, Weiss ML, Mitchell BM, Martin P, Davis D, Morales L, Helwig B, Beerenstrauch M, Abou-Easa K, Hildreth T, Troyer D, Medicetty S. Matrix cells from Wharton's jelly form neurons and glia. Stem Cells. 2003;21:50–60.
19. Pennati G. Biomechanical properties of the human umbilical cord. Biorheology. 2001;38:355–66.
20. Ghezzi F, Raio L, Di Naro E, Franchi M, Buttarelli M, Schneider H. First-trimester umbilical diameter: a novel marker of fetal aneuploidy. Ultrasound Obstet Gynecol. 2002;19:235–9.
21. Kelber R. Gespaltene "solitäre" Nabelschnurarterie. Arch Gynakol. 1976;220:319–23.
22. Bell AD, Gerlis LM, Variend S. Persistent right umbilical vein—case report and review of literature. Int J Cardiol. 1986;10:167–76.
23. Gebrane-Younes J, Minh HN, Orcel L. Ultrastructure of human umbilical vessels: a possible role in amniotic fluid formation? Placenta. 1986;7:173–85.
24. Sexton AJ, Turmaine M, Cai WQ, Burnstock G. A study of the ultrastructure of developing human umbilical vessels. J Anat. 1996;188:75–85.
25. Arts NFT. Investigations on the vascular system of the placenta. General introduction and the fetal vascular system. Am J Obstet Gynecol. 1961;82:147–58.
26. Fujikura T. Fused umbilical arteries near placental cord insertion. Am J Obstet Gynecol. 2003;188:765–7.
27. Hyrtl J. Die Blutgefäße der menschlichen Nachgeburt in normalen und abnormen Verhältnissen. Wien: Braumüller; 1870.
28. Hoboken W. Anatomia secundinae. Ultrajecti: Ribbium; 1669.
29. Spivack M. On the presence or absence of nerves in the umbilical blood vessels of man and guinea pig. Anat Rec. 1943;85:85–109.

30. Kernbach M. Existe-t-il du tissu nerveux dans le placenta? Rev Fr Gynécol. 1969;64:357–61.
31. Fox H, Jacobson HN. Innervation of the human umbilical cord and umbilical vessels. Am J Obstet Gynecol. 1969;103:384–9.
32. Pearson AA, Sauter RW. The innervation of the umbilical vein in human embryos and fetuses. Am. J. Anat. 1969;125:345–52.
33. Ellison JP. The nerves of the umbilical cord in man and the rat. Am J Anat. 1971;132:53–60.
34. Fox H, Khong TY. Lack of innervation of human umbilical cord. An immunohistochemical and histochemical study. Placenta. 1990;11:59–62.
35. Drut R, Quijano G. Heterotopic neurons in the umbilical cord. Pediatr Dev Pathol. 2005;8:124–7.

Physiology, Ultrastructure, Ultrasonography and Pharmacology of the Umbilical Cord

12

12.1 How the Human Umbilical Cord Works?

Umbilical cord blood vessels are without branches; this is unique compared to the large blood vessels of the adult body, the aorta and vena cava. Its properties, therefore, are different in some respects and alike in others. The umbilical cord has two-way traffic: the arteries carry blood pumped by the heart away from the fetus, and this circulation surrounds the vein normally; the umbilical vein returns blood to the fetus from the placenta rejuvenated with oxygen and nutrients and devoid of waste products.

How this happens is still surrounded by mystery. The fetal heart cannot expand or work harder because it is surrounded by a fluid-filled lung, like pushing against a water bed. Therefore, as the fetus steadily grows exponentially and three-dimensionally, how does it accommodate the increased blood volume it needs over time? As the fetus grows, the cord elongates and grows in diameter. The fetus has to work against a larger column of fluid and tissue resistance at the placental end. It has been estimated that by 31 weeks, the umbilical cord must carry 70 quarts of blood per day, moving at 4 miles an hour.

This remarkable organ also must participate in fetal growth milestones; additionally, it may act as an assist pump to the fetal heart. This assist pump may be designed to help the fetus over difficult growth proportions which may exist at 20, 24, 28 and 32 weeks—times that are known for premature labour to appear. The extra stress on the fetus may require that the cord be designed correctly so that it can have properties of an assist mechanism or pump. This theory, proposed in the 1950s, requires that the arteries surround the vein in the proper architecture. If this is so, then future research into this issue may explain fetal effects secondary to cord design. To date, no assist pump property has been detected in the umbilical cord.

How blood flow is regulated in addition to being carried by the umbilical cord is unclear. Cord length does not significantly affect blood flow dynamics; however, blood flow must meet some resistance for the circulation to work. As a result, the umbilical arteries are surrounded with four layers of smooth muscle to maintain a certain amount of muscular tone. The umbilical vein is not as musculated. The system operates fully dilated, but stimuli from chemistry or hormones can affect the system and cause constriction. This must happen at birth to reduce blood loss.

In larger mammals, the cord must constrict from the placenta to the fetus to avoid anaemia. In the human, similar mechanisms may be available chemically. Regulation of blood flow, vessel constriction at birth and blood loss prevention may be the roles of these vessel-active substances; some of these substances originate in the placenta.

Researchers using ultrasonography recently have been able to measure umbilical blood flow

© Springer International Publishing AG 2018
M. Fahmy, *Umbilicus and Umbilical Cord*, https://doi.org/10.1007/978-3-319-62383-2_12

with colour Doppler imaging. This technique allows visualization of the blood vessels based on the movement of the blood itself. These studies also suggest that the umbilical vein, arteries and placenta act as an assist pump of sorts to the fetal heart [1]. Measurement of blood flow allows the obstetrician to determine whether enough blood volume is circulating in the placenta to provide nutrition and oxygen to the fetus. Under certain conditions this blood flow can be reduced, and circulation in the placenta altered to create a growth-affected fetus, intrauterine growth retardation (IUGR). In essence, it is a way of determining the fetus' blood pressure.

These findings become important because, in addition to the potential for fetal harm or stillbirth, important lifetime tendencies are emerging. The fetus seems to have the ability to set its vital signs for its adult life. If stressed, the IUGR fetus sets blood pressure and heart function, which can predispose the fetus to adult heart attack. These mechanisms are just beginning to be understood, and the umbilical cord may be an important part of the mystery [2].

12.2   Ultrastructure of Umbilical Cord

12.2.1 Umbilical Cord Design

The complexity of umbilical cord built has long been of interest to anatomists. A look at all mammals shows a variety of design adaptations. In humans, it has been determined that there are several designs. What these differences mean to the fetus is unknown.

Attempts by several scientists to understand how the umbilical cord works have taught us that the cord is more like an organ rather than a rigid conduit (pipeline).

Not all cords are alike. Just as there are different kinds of hair (curly/straight, thick/thin), there are different kinds of cords.

Most cords (99%) have three vessels, although some (1%) have only two, and even less have four.

The relationship between the normal vein and two arteries is usually parallel, and this parallel configuration can vary, however, and may imply effects which can alter blood supply to the fetus. Variances include arteries that are together or separated with each artery lateral to the vein (Fig. 12.1). Another variance is arteries that wind around the vein while the vein remains central in the cord. This is sometimes referred to as spiralled arteries, but helical is the preferred term. The vein can also parallel the arteries in a helical configuration, and the vein can wind around the arteries.

Several researchers have concentrated on these differences and suggest that umbilical cords of absolutely straight designs may be more prone to disruptions of blood flow.

The location of umbilical cord attachment to the fetus and placenta is also important. Placental attachments can be in the centre, off centre, on the edge or in the membranes. Membranous insertions of the umbilical cord are called velamentous insertions; these placental cord designs have flaws which can lead to cord tears (Chap. 13).

Umbilical attachment of the cord can vary and predispose the infant to hernias at the umbilicus and "constriction" of the cord (Fig. 12.2).

Amniotic bands can interfere with both ends of the umbilical cord; the amniotic membrane can leave remnants in the form of fibrous bands which can stiffen and occlude the blood circulation through the cord. These events are reproductive mishaps that have no current remedy. In order to begin the process of creating solutions to umbili-

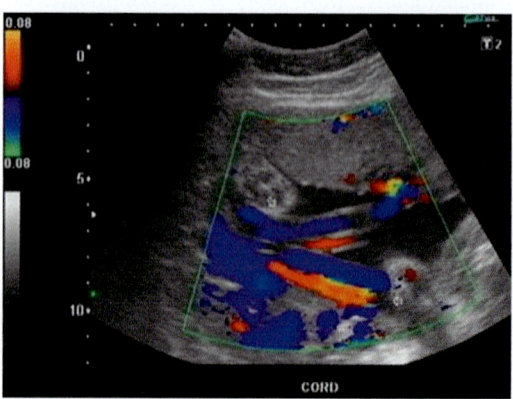

Fig. 12.1 Doppler ultrasound of umbilical cord with hypocoiled umbilical cord

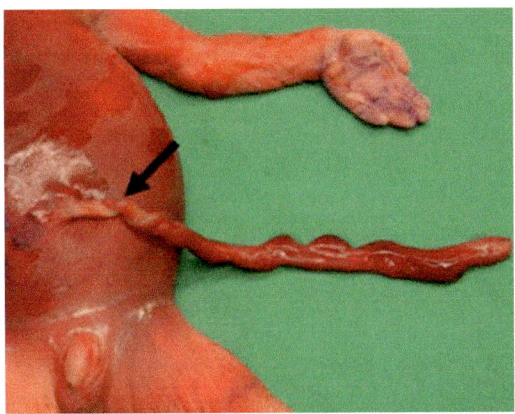

Fig. 12.2 Preterm stillborn infant with UC constriction near the fetal end

cal cord-related complications, understanding cord function and design must be thorough.

12.2.2 Spiral Turns of the Cord

The umbilical cord is usually spiralled, a quality referred to as 'chirality'. A counterclockwise spiral (left) exceeds that of the opposite direction by a ratio of 7:1. The helices may be seen by ultrasonographic examination as early as during the first trimester of pregnancy [3].

Some believe that these helices are of no practical value whatsoever. Helices are readily seen by the ninth week of gestation. They usually number up to 40, but as many as 380 turns have been described [4]. The number is already well established early in pregnancy, and it increases only insignificantly during the third trimester.

It therefore follows that the cord length grows not by increased spiralling but by increasing the pitch between each turn of the spiral. It is uncommon to find an absence of spirals in the cord, but when this occurs, it has an ominous prognosis, 4.3% of newborns lacked cord twists had a significantly higher increase in perinatal mortality and other problems. The umbilical coiling index (number of coils divided by length of cord; average 0.21/cm) may identify the fetus at risk [4]. When the index fell below the tenth percentile, more chromosomal errors, fetal distress and meconium staining were identified.

The excessive coiling was associated with cocaine usage and increased frequency of premature labour (Fig. 12.3). Reduced coiling was a predictor of problems with labour and delivery. Uncoiled cords were present in 4.9%; their mean coiling index was 0.19/cm, and the cords of the uncoiled specimens were not unusually short.

Black patients had significantly less coiling than white patients. Infants with fixation of their bodies to the placental surface (due to amnionic bands) have not only relatively short cords but also few or no umbilical helices [5].

A complex fetal anomaly with undercoiled, short umbilical cord and suggested decreased fetal motion have occurred. The same is true for species with elongated embryos in elongated uterine horns (e.g. whales), a situation that hinders embryonic rotation. Only infants with single umbilical arteries had a significant reduction of spirals. No other anomalous development correlated, and one or the other twist was not more commonly associated with perinatal morbidity or mortality.

It is interesting that an occasional cord may have helices in opposite directions.

The spirals of the cord have been studied in 5000 cords by morphometry and histology [6]. A left twist was found in 79% with a left/right ratio of 3.7:1.0; in twins, the left direction was found in 61%, and mixed spiralling occurred in 26% (Fig. 12.4).

Fetuses with single umbilical arteries had a 1.5:1.0 left/right ratio. These authors also gave figures for cord dry mass and weight/length ratios. Fletcher [7] found a 76.5% left-handed spiral and a right-handed twist in 15.5%, but mixed in 6.5% of normal pregnancies.

12.3   Contractility of Umbilical Vessels

There has been much interest in the mechanisms of closure of umbilical vessels after birth. There are an irregular constrictions of arteries occurred at irregular intervals, with increased transmural pressures exerted on the umbilical arteries, which led to vasoconstriction. Throughout the last 2 weeks of pregnancy, the cord vessels show increasing responsiveness to mechanical irrita-

Fig. 12.3 Preterm with over coiled long UC

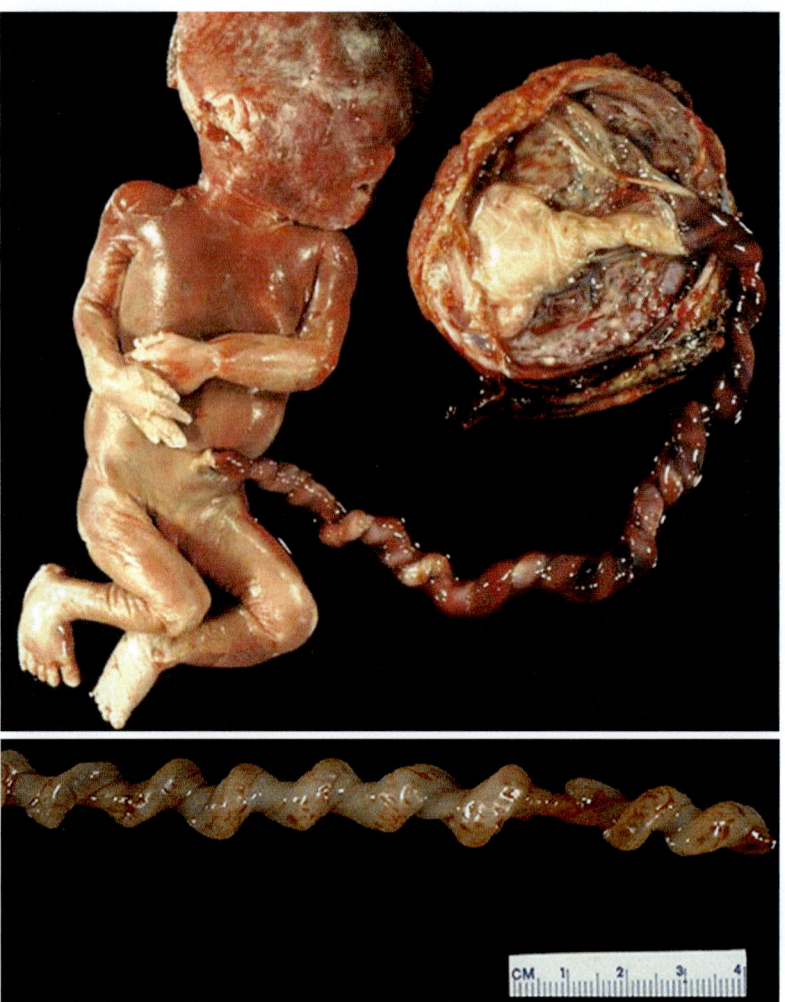

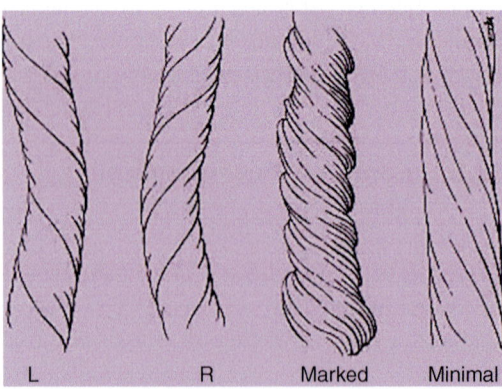

Fig. 12.4 Different types of cord twists including left (L), right (R), minimal and marked twisting

tion, which is not present during the preceding periods of pregnancy. This response and other mechanisms indirectly confirm the absence of a neural mechanism operating in cord vessels [8].

Electron microscopic observations led Röckelein and Scharl [9] to the assumption that an endotheliomuscular interaction, mediated by the endotheliomuscular interdigitations, may play an important role in postnatal arterial closure mechanism. As a consequence of muscular contraction, a cytoplasmic prolapse of smooth muscle cells into the endothelial cells, may causing a kind of 'hydrops' of the latter. Seemingly hydropic endothelial cells of umbilical arteries deeply protruding into the arterial lumens and partly occluding those have been seen by many authors.

The umbilical vessels are exquisitely sensitive to various endocrine mediators, such as serotonin, angiotensin and oxytocin [10].

Moreover, smooth muscle contractility of the vessel walls is influenced in paracrine loops by substances produced within the neighbouring endothelial cells. Among these mediators, prostaglandins have been shown to be produced within the umbilical vascular endothelium. Despite earlier observations to the contrary, it is now known that the endothelium of the umbilical vein produces far more prostaglandins than does that of the arteries. There is, however, little production of prostaglandins in placental surface vessels.

The synthetic rate of prostaglandins PGI2 and PGE2 was significantly reduced in smoker and diabetic pregnant as compared to those from normal control mothers. Because both prostaglandins are potent vasodilators and platelet aggregation inhibitors, so the impaired placental perfusion in smoking and diabetic mothers may be mediated by the altered umbilical endothelium [11]. The cord (presumably its amnionic surface) is the major source of PGE2 in the gestational sac during labour. Another vasodilator that has attracted much attention is nitric oxide, which is produced from the conversion of L-arginine to citrulline by nitric oxide synthase (NOS). This enzyme has been detected immunohistochemically not only in villous syncytiotrophoblast but also in fetal villous and umbilical endothelium. A reduction in this enzyme's activity has been correlated with abnormal umbilical artery waveforms.

Atrial natriuretic peptide (ANP) is another potent vasodilator that additionally seems to be involved in fetal fluid haemostasis. Its binding sites have been detected in umbilical smooth muscle cells [12]. Immunoreactivity for the peptide itself and its messenger RNA have been found in the umbilical endothelium.

Vasoconstrictor substances found in umbilical endothelium and comprise angiotensin II, 5-hydroxytryptamine (5-HT) and thromboxane, neuropeptide Y (NPY) as well as endothelin-1 and endothelin-2 detected only in fibroblasts and amnionic epithelium of human cords rather than in endothelium. Binding sites for endothelin-1 have been described in the media of umbilical vessels, the activity of the arteries exceeding that of the vein [13].

The functions of these vasoconstrictors are still under discussion. NPY and angiotensin II, which are found most abundantly in the endothelial cells, cause relatively weak or no responses on the term umbilical artery in vitro. When immature vessels were more sensitive to angiotensin II, arachidonic acid and oxytocin, term vessels reacted more to vasopressin, norepinephrine, PGD2 and PGE2. In vitro, 5-HT and endothelin-1 were found to be powerful vasoconstrictors on all levels of fetoplacental circulation. The latter substances are also under discussion as mediators of closure of placental circulation at birth.

These findings shed new light on the highly complex mechanisms of autoregulation, not only of the umbilical circulation but also of the villous circulation, as most of these mediators have been described also in the walls of the larger chorionic and villous vessels [14]. Further studies will have to elucidate the complicated interactions of these substances, as they are very likely to be involved in abnormal conditions, such as intrauterine growth restriction (IUGR) and a high Doppler resistance index.

The vessels of patients with preeclampsia, growth-retarded fetuses and diabetes, as well as those of smoking mothers, show reduced prostacyclin production. Similar effects have been found in vitro. Degeneration of endothelium from umbilical vessels had earlier been shown to occur in smoking mothers. Other effects of smoking on the placenta have been discovered as well. One example is that the steroid production is altered; others are trophoblastic degeneration and microvascular changes, and several other effects have been observed. Although it is attractive to consider that prostaglandins are the principal mediators of umbilical vascular responses, some evidence has been adduced that there may be considerable differences among species. Alcohol leads to a dose-dependent contractile response in umbilical arteries in vitro, but oestrogens dilate the vessels [15].

References

1. Di Naro E, Raio L, Ghezzi F, Franchi M, Romano F, D'Addario V. Longitudinal umbilical vein blood flow changes in normal and growth-retarded fetuses. Acta Obstet Gynecol Scand. 2002;81(6):527–33.
2. Benoit R, Copel J, Williams K. Does single umbilical artery (SUA) predict IUGR? Am J Obstet Gynecol. 2002;187:208. (abstract 546)
3. Dudiak CM, Salomon CG, Posniak HV, Olson MC, Flisak ME. Sonography of the umbilical cord. Radiographics. 1995;15:1035–50.
4. Strong TH, Jarles DL, Vega JS, Feldman DB. The umbilical coiling index. Am J Obstet Gynecol. 1994;170:29–32.
5. Spatz WB. Nabelschnur-Längen bei Insektivoren und Primaten. Z Säugetierkd. 1968;33:226–39.
6. Blackburn W, Cooley NR, Manci EA. Correlations between umbilical cord structure-composition and normal and abnormal fetal development. In: Saul RA, editor. Proceedings of the greenwood genetics conference, vol. 7. Clinton: Jacobs Press; 1988. p. 180–1.
7. Fletcher S. Chirality in the umbilical cord. Br J Obstet Gynaecol. 1993;100:234–6.
8. Shepherd JT. Bayliss response in the umbilical artery. Fed Proc. 1968;27:1408–9.
9. Röckelein G, Scharl A. Scanning electron microscopic investigations of the human umbilical artery intima: a new conception on postnatal arterial closure mechanism. Virchows Arch A. 1988;413:555–61.
10. LeDonne AT, McGowan L. Effect of an oxytocic on umbilical cord venous pressure. Obstet Gynecol. 1967;30:103–7.
11. McCoshen JA, Tulloch HV, Johnson KA. Umbilical cord is the major source of prostaglandin E2 in the gestational sac during term labor. Am. J. Obstet. Gynecol. 1989;160:973–8.
12. Salas SP, Power RF, Singleton A, Wharton J, Polak JM, Brown J. Heterogeneous binding sites for a-atrial natriuretic peptide in human umbilical cord and placenta. Am J Physiol. 1991;261:R633–8.
13. Cai WQ, Bodin P, Sexton A, Loesch A, Burnstock G. Localization of neuropeptide Y and atrial natriuretic peptide in the endothelial cells of human umbilical blood vessels. Cell Tissue Res. 1993;272:175–81.
14. Okatani Y, Taniguchi K, Sagara Y. Amplifying effect of endothelin-1 on serotonin-induced vasoconstriction of human umbilical artery. Am J Obstet Gynecol. 1995;172:1240–5.
15. De Sa MF, Meirelles RS. Vasodilating effect of estrogen on the human umbilical artery. Gynecol Investig. 1977;8:307–13.

Congenital Anomalies of the Umbilical Cord

13

13.1 Placental Attachment (Site of Cord Insertion)

The umbilical cord normally inserted on the placental tissue itself, more often near or at the centre than elsewhere, as shown in Fig. 13.1. In nearly 7% of term placentas, it has a marginal insertion, which, in the English-language literature, is often referred to as a 'battledore' placenta (Fig. 13.2).

In about 1% of placentas, the umbilical cord inserts on the membranes, referred to as velamentous or membranous insertion (Fig. 13.3). Here, the umbilical vessels course over the free membranes and, having lost their protection by Wharton's jelly, and are more vulnerable to trauma and disruption.

Not only are the sites of insertion variable, the insertion itself may take an abnormal shape. Thus, the branching of vessels can occur before the cord comes to the surface of the placenta in the 'furcate cord' insertion (Fig. 13.4). At times, the cord runs parallel to the placental surface or in the membranes before its vessels branch, the "interposition" is usually covered by a membrane (Fig. 13.5).

The fetal end of the umbilical cord may also be anomalous, as is found primarily in infants with gastroschisis (short cords) or with omphalocele. Some of these anomalies are associated with significant disturbances in fetal growth.

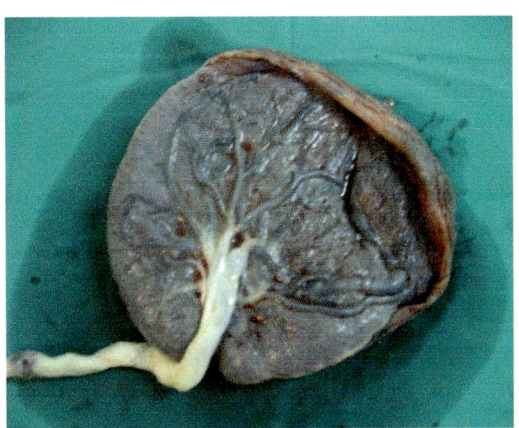

Fig. 13.1 Central cord insertion

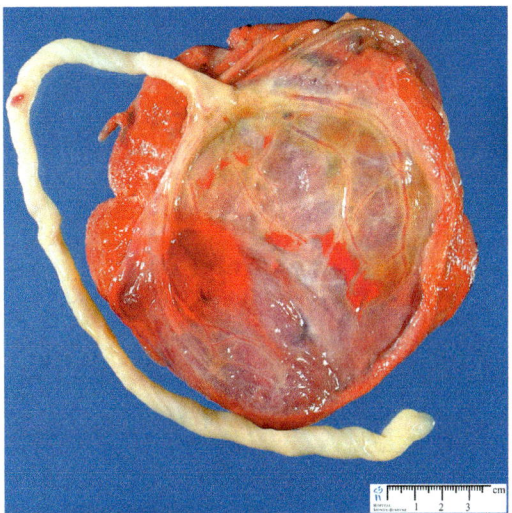

Fig. 13.2 Marginal cord insertion

© Springer International Publishing AG 2018
M. Fahmy, *Umbilicus and Umbilical Cord*, https://doi.org/10.1007/978-3-319-62383-2_13

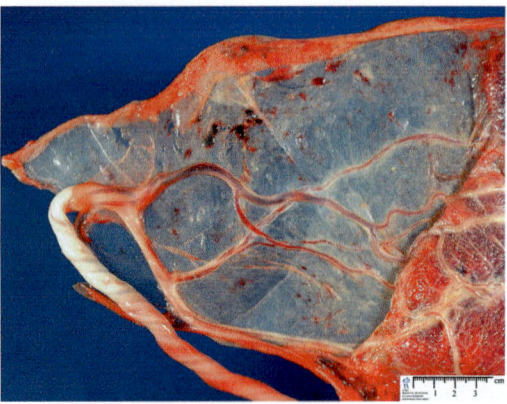

Fig. 13.3 Velamentous cord insertion

13.2 Velamentous Cord Insertion
(Fig. 13.3)

It is also called a membranous insertion of the umbilical cord. It has been of great interest to understand the pathogenesis of velamentous and marginal insertions of the umbilical cord. There are two mutually contradictory theories: abnormal primary implantation (polarity theory) and trophotropism.

Velamentously inserted cords are associated with twinning and single umbilical artery (SUA).

Velamentous and marginal cords are almost invariably present in higher multiple births. They are common when intrauterine devices (IUDs) are found in the placental membranes.

The incidence of different types of cord insertion varies throughout numerous reported series because in the interpretation of what is truly a marginal or already a velamentous insertion, or merely an excessively eccentric one, but the frequency is around 1% of singleton term deliveries [1].

The cord may insert reasonably close to the edge of the placenta or far away from it (Fig. 13.4).

The close insertion is much more common than the extreme situation, where the cord inserts at the apex of the membranous sac. In the latter configuration, the long membranous course of the vessels makes them even more vulnerable to injury. It should be pointed out though that a

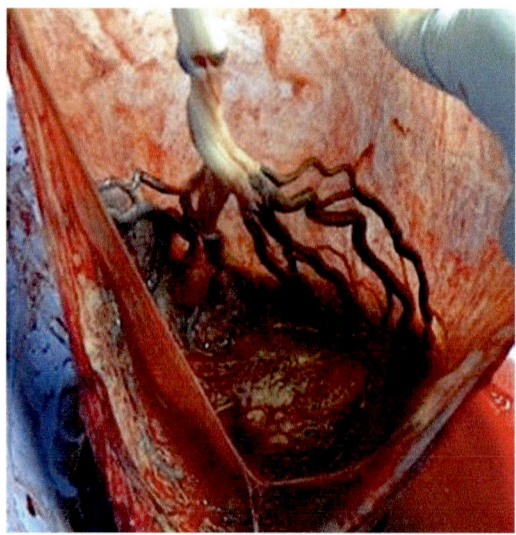

Fig. 13.4 Extensive umbilical vessels branching at the site of placental insertion

membranous course of fetal blood vessels is not reserved to a velamentous insertion of the cord.

Quite often there are such membranous vessels issuing from marginally inserted cords, and they have the same serious prognosis. Also, membranous fetal vessels are not synonymous with vasa praevia. The latter condition exists only when the membranous vessels course over the internal os uteri, previous to (ahead of) the fetal head during delivery. In multiple gestations, the velamentous cord insertion often arises on the dividing membranes, and the membranous vessels are then similarly prone to disruption.

It is founded that velamentous cord insertion is more common in placentas of the twin-to-twin transfusion syndrome and suggested that this may impact the severity of the growth restriction to the donor twin. Thrombosis of arteries and veins has both been seen in this insertional anomaly, and thrombi may be associated with neonatal purpura and fetal death [2].

Some of these pregnancies have led to prenatal haemorrhages and abortion [3]. Moreover, one can sonographically observe eccentric expansion of the placenta during the course of advancing pregnancy, which would leave the cord insertion site behind.

13.3 Furcate Cord Insertion
(Fig. 13.5)

Furcate cord insertion is a rare abnormality in which the umbilical vessels separate from the cord substance prior to reaching the surface of the placenta. They lose the protection afforded by Wharton's jelly and are prone to thrombosis and injury. The condition was first described by Hyrtl [6], and much discussion was devoted to its differentiation from velamentous insertion. Fatal haemorrhage is commonly associated with this condition. The furcate and velamentous cord had varices and numerous mural thrombi; many of the placental vessels had degenerations and calcifications in their walls [4].

There also exists a rare description of a double cord with separate vessel duplication or a bifurcated cord with placental duplication in a single tone pregnancy (Fig. 13.6).

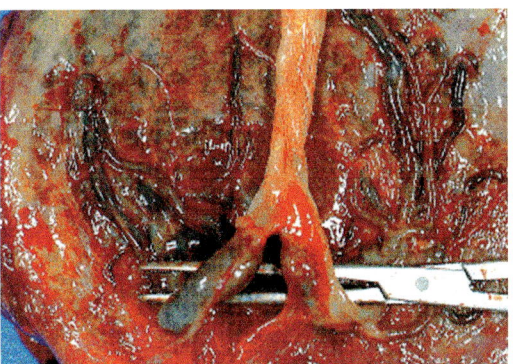

Fig. 13.5 Furcate insertion of umbilical cord

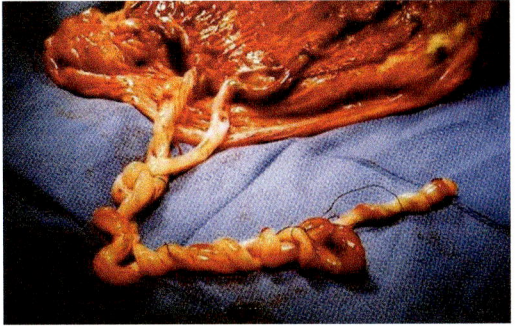

Fig. 13.6 Duplicated umbilical cord in a singleton pregnancy

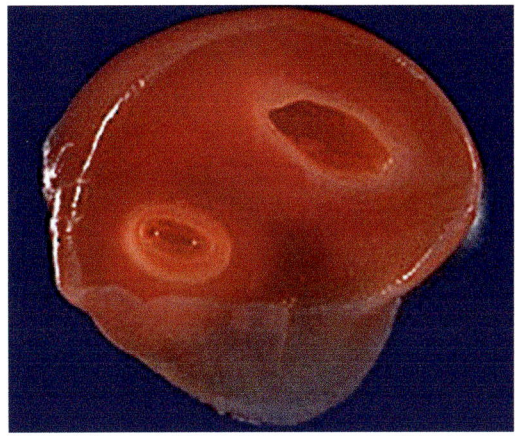

Fig. 13.7 Single umbilical artery

13.4 Single Umbilical Artery
(Fig. 13.7)

Single umbilical artery (SUA) is the commonest true congenital anomaly of humans. An enormous literature has been created in efforts to explain its nature and significance. Single umbilical artery was apparently first described by Vesalius at 1943. It did not attract further notice until the 40 cases listed by Otto [5] and the later attention by Hyrtl [6], who summarized 70 cases in his interesting monograph. Since then, there has been a veritable flood of information on SUA, which can now be easily detected prenatally by ultrasonography. Considering its incidence of about 1% in newborns, Heifetz compiled all data and reported there being a 0.63% frequency [7].

References

1. Ebbing C, et al. Velamentous or marginal cord insertion and the risk of spontaneous preterm birth, prelabor rupture of the membranes, and anomalous cord length, a population-based study. Acta Obstet Gynecol Scand. 2017;96(1):78–85.
2. Collins JH. Umbilical cord accidents: human studies. Semin Perinatol. 2002;26:79–82.
3. Golden AS. Umbilical cord-placental separation: a complication of IUD failure. J Reprod Med. 1973;11:79–80.

4. Walkup DWM. A rare case of duplicated placenta and bifurcated umbilical cord in a singleton pregnancy. J Diagn Med Sonography. 2001;17(5):280–5. doi:10.1177/875647930101700507.

5. Otto AW. Lehrbuch der pathologischen Anatomie des Menschen und der Thiere. Berlin: Ruecker; 1830.

6. Hyrtl J. Die Blutgefäße der menschlichen Nachgeburt in normalen und abnormen Verhältnissen. Wien: Braumüller; 1870.

7. Heifetz SA. Single umbilical artery: a statistical analysis of 237 autopsy cases and review of the literature. Perspect Pediatr Pathol. 1984;8:345–78.

Umbilical Cord Cysts

14

Cystic lesions originate from embryonic vestiges remaining as a consequence of the incomplete obliteration of the urachus and omphalomesenteric duct, are more often single than multiple and are usually isolated, even though with association with other congenital anomalies, usually of the gastrointestinal tract, and other syndromes. The presence of multiple umbilical cord cysts is associated with an increased risk of miscarriage, aneuploidy and congenital anomalies. Additionally, pseudocysts have also been described, originating as a result of myxoid degeneration of the Wharton's jelly secondary to persistent patent urachus, urachus cysts or abdominal wall defects. They can be single (commoner) or multiple.

Incidence: They may be seen in 1–3% of pregnancies. Many cases are seen in the first trimester and often resolve at or before term [1].

Clinically: Cysts can occur at any location along the umbilical cord, but they are usually located towards its fetal insertion, cysts are irregular in shape, containing a clear fluid and located between the vessels and umbilical veins can be identified from the cyst wall specially in large pseudocyst and giant umbilical cord [2] (Fig. 14.1). The cyst sizes can be variable ranging from a few millimetres up to 8 cm. Giant umbilical cord considered as a large pseudocyst may be fusiform with a smooth regular surface (Fig. 14.2) or irregular and gives the picture of multiple cysts of different sizes and shapes (Fig. 14.3).

True cysts are less common and are located towards the anterior abdominal, usually eccentric, near to the fatal abdominal wall, but pseudocyst is usually seen in continuity of the cord (Fig. 14.4).

True cysts are formed of embryonic remnants or communicated with vestige structures, urachal or vitellointestinal remnants (Fig. 14.6).

It could be almost impossible to differentiate a true cyst from a pseudocyst on sonographic grounds.

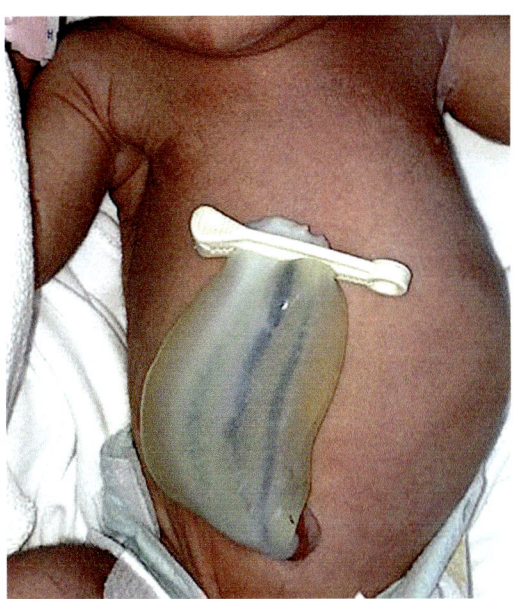

Fig. 14.1 A large pseudocyst of the umbilical cord with prominent vessels seen clearly from the thin cyst wall

© Springer International Publishing AG 2018
M. Fahmy, *Umbilicus and Umbilical Cord*, https://doi.org/10.1007/978-3-319-62383-2_14

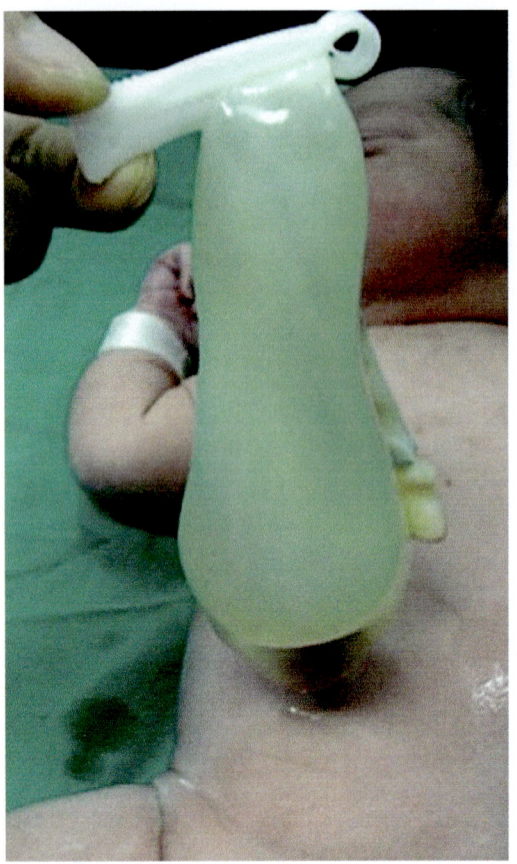

Fig. 14.2 Giant umbilical cord (pseudocyst) with smooth thick wall

14.1   Differential Diagnosis

Umbilical arterial aneurysm (UAA), which shows flow on colour Doppler US, may be wrongly diagnosed as a cord cyst.

After delivery the differential diagnosis is between an umbilical pseudocyst and an allantoic cyst with a patent urachus, which can be distinguished by ultrasound; as it shows the channel communicating from the umbilicus to the bladder. Bladder outlet obstruction can be excluded by a micturating cystourethrogram preoperatively or by an intraoperative cystoscopy [3].

Umbilical cord cyst has to be differentiated from congenital hernia of umbilical cord (Chap. 32), small omphalocele (Chap. 34) and cord haemangioma (Sect. 17.1), but cyst may be associated with such anomalies (Figs. 14.5 and 14.7).

14.2   Pathology

Umbilical cord cysts can represent either a true or false cysts:

- True cysts: have an epithelial lining, actually a flat or cuboidal uroepithelium, and it could be:

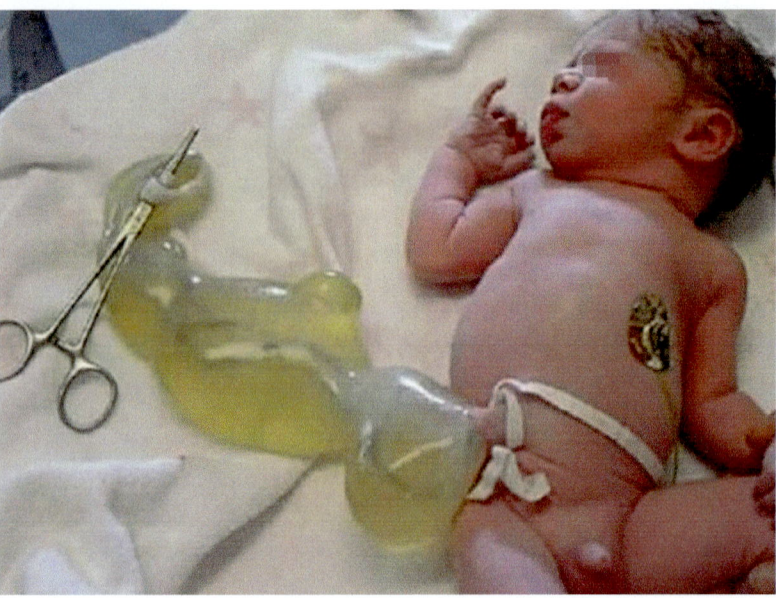

Fig. 14.3 Multiple pseudocysts with different sizes, giving the picture of giant cord

Allantoic cyst (urachal)

Omphalomesenteric duct cyst

- False cysts (pseudocysts): are more common than the true cysts, have no epithelial lining and represent localized edema, liquefaction or degeneration of Wharton's jelly.

Pseudocysts are also associated with chromosomal anomalies and other congenital anomalies.

The exact mechanism of formation of the umbilical cord pseudocyst remains unknown. One hypothesis suggests that prolonged reflux of hypoosmolar fetal urine into the Wharton's jelly via a patent urachus might cause localized edema and formation of pseudocysts. Laboratory evidence has been provided by Tsuchida and Ishida, as they infused the human umbilical cords with distilled water, 0.9% saline, 3% saline or 10% saline. Enlargement of the cords occurred when

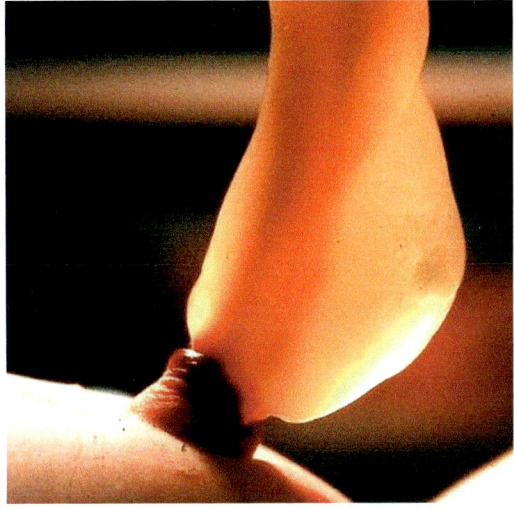

Fig. 14.4 True small umbilical cyst associated at the fetal end of the cord

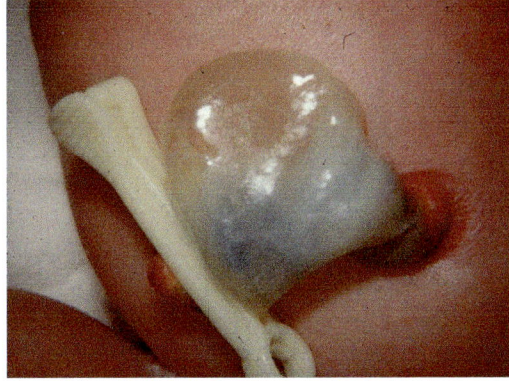

Fig. 14.6 Umbilical cyst associated with a patent urachus

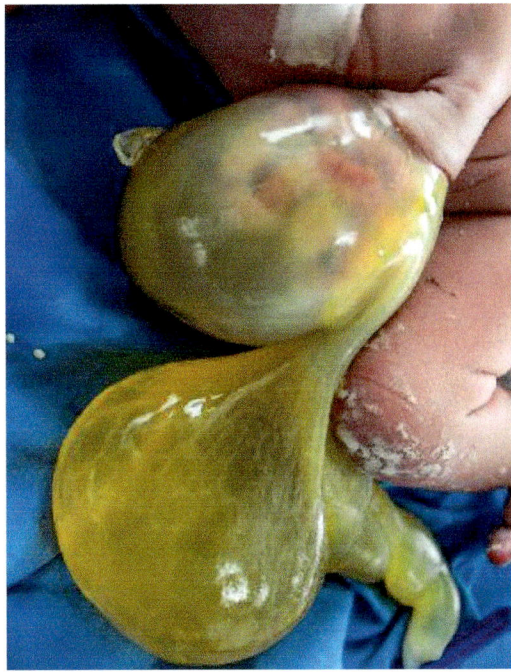

Fig. 14.5 Umbilical cyst on the top of an omphalocele

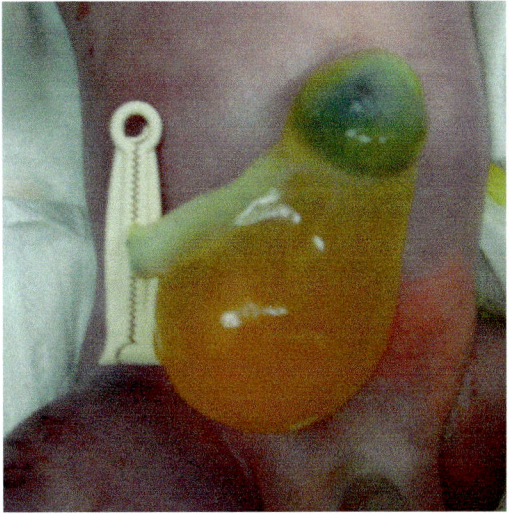

Fig. 14.7 Congenital hernia of the cord with a true umbilical cyst

infused with distilled water or 0.9% saline. They concluded that prolonged reflux of hypoosmolar fetal urine into the umbilical cord via a patent urachus produces the swollen cord noted at delivery [4].

14.3   Associated Anomalies

There are increased associations (especially when there are additional sonographic abnormalities and if the cyst persist to the third trimester) with certain chromosomal/structural anomalies. Nearly 20% of cord cysts of any type are associated with structural or chromosomal anomalies: [5]

Aneuploidic conditions such as:

Trisomy 18

Trisomy 13

Association with other cord anomalies like omphalocele, patent urachus and congenital hernia of umbilical cord (Figs. 14.4, 14.5, 14.6, and 14.7)

Prune belly syndrome (Fig. 14.8)

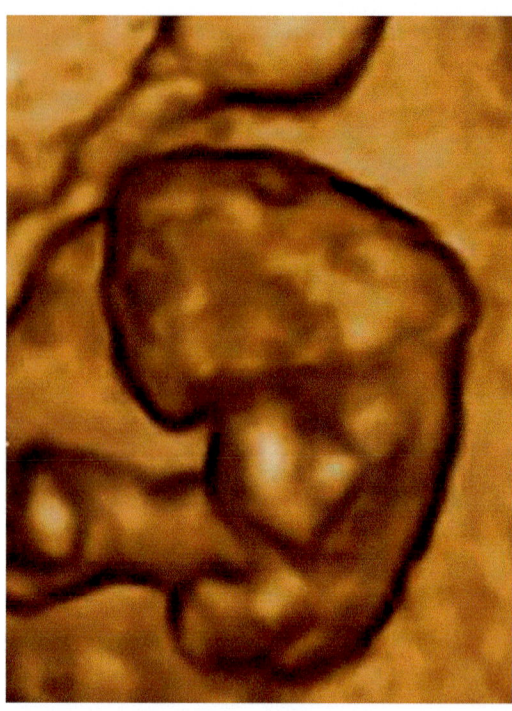

Fig. 14.9 3-D US revealing a small umbilical cyst at the fetal end of the cord

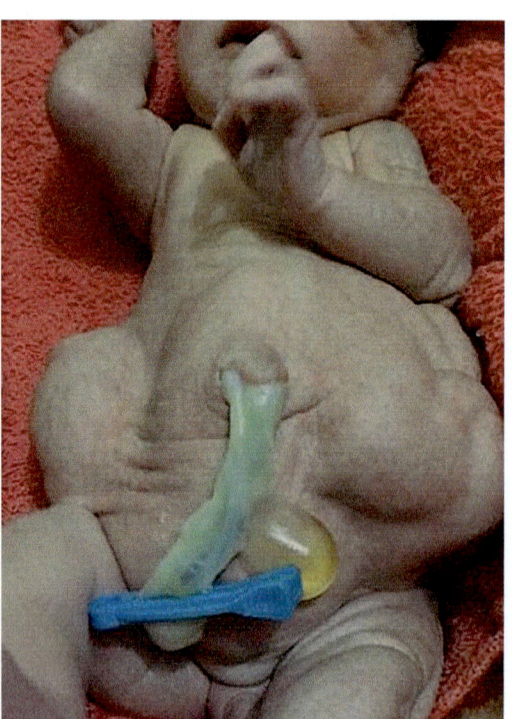

Fig. 14.8 A small umbilical cyst near the placental end in a case of prune belly syndrome

14.4   Radiographic Features

Antenatal ultrasound diagnoses almost all cysts, and detection of a giant U cord prenatally should lead to close monitoring of the mother and fetus because of possible vascular compression by the cystic mass particularly at the term and during labour, resulting in fetal compromise. Workup including amniocentesis with fetal karyotype to diagnose or to exclude chromosomal and other associated anomalies is indicated, once U cyst (s) is diagnosed (Fig. 14.9).

Giant umbilical cord can easily be diagnosed on prenatal scans and is unmistakable postnatally [6].

14.5   Treatment and Prognosis

Ghezzi et al. [7] proposed that while single cysts in the first trimester are associated with a favourable pregnancy outcome, the presence of multiple umbilical cord cysts is associated with an increased risk of miscarriage and aneuploidy.

A simple umbilical pseudocyst requires no treatment but needs to be differentiated from an allantoic cyst with persistent patent urachus.

Intrauterine fetal death is the reported complication due to cord cysts because of compression of umbilical vessels causing intrauterine compromise of blood flow. If a large cyst is present, delivery can be undertaken as soon as fetal lung maturity is achieved.

The natural history of these cysts is to resolve by the end of the first trimester. The longer the cyst persists, the more likely it is to be associated with a congenital anomaly. However, if no other anomaly is found, the prognosis is excellent, most advocate a detailed sonographic assessment to be performed if an umbilical cord cyst is seen [8].

A transient cyst which resolves on subsequent imaging is considered to carry an excellent prognosis.

Concerning factors include:

Multiple cysts

Presence of other sonographic abnormalities

Persistence during serial sonographic assessment or persistence into the second or third trimester

Surgery is usually required, not for the condition itself but for the cause of the condition. Although it is an uncommon anomaly, operative exploration must be carried out to repair the commonly associated urachal remnant [9].

Cases detected antenatally should be referred early to a specialized centres to diagnose possible associated anomalies. All cases of true cyst without an obvious omphalocele or cord hernia should be considered as a case of patent urachus until proven otherwise. Gynaecologists, paediatricians and midwives, especially in developing countries, should be aware about cases of U cord cysts, which were not diagnosed antenatally and discovered only at the time of delivery, to apply cord clamp sufficiently distal to the cyst and to refer the case to a specialist who had a reasonable experience to deal with congenital anomalies.

References

1. Heredia F, Jeanty P. Umbilical cord anomalies. http://www.TheFetus.net/.
2. Wildhaber BE, Antonelli E, Pfister RE. The giant umbilical cord, case report. Arch Dis Child Fetal Neonatal Ed. 2005;90:F535–6. doi:10.1136/adc.2005.076380.
3. Managoli S, Chaturvedi P, Vilhekar KY. Umbilical cord allantoic cysts in a newborn with vacterl association. Indian J Pediatr. 2004;71(5):419–21.
4. Tsuchida Y, Ishida M. Osmolar relationship between enlarged umbilical cord and patent urachus. J Pediatr Surg. 1969;4:465–7.
5. Ross JA, Jurkovic D, Zosmer N, Jauniaux E, Hacket E, Nicolaides KH. Umbilical cord cysts in early pregnancy. Obstet Gynecol. 1997;89(3):442–5.
6. Nobuhara KK, Lukish JR, Hartman GE, Gilbert JC. The giant umbilical cord: an unusual presentation of a patent urachus. J Pediatr Surg. 2004;39:128–9.
7. Ghezzi F, Raio L, Di Naro E, et al. Single and multiple umbilical cord cysts in early gestation: two different entities. Ultrasound Obstet Gynecol. 2003;21(3):215–9. doi:10.1002/uog.68.
8. Svigos J, Khurana S, Munt C, et al. Presentation of an umbilical cord cyst with a surprising jet: a case report of a patent urachus v1; ref status: indexed; 2013. http://f1000r.es/xx.
9. Wildhaber BE, Antonelli E, Pfister RE. Giant umbilical cord. Arch Dis Child Fetal Neonatal Ed. 2005;90(6):535–6.

Umbilical Cord Knots

15

Umbilical cord knots are clinically significant, with an associated fetal mortality, which may reach up to 10% [1] (Fig. 15.1).

Incidence: Browne (1925) reported that true knots occur with a frequency of 0.4–0.5%. A 0.35% incidence of true knots was detected among 2000 consecutive deliveries [2].

Cases Commonly Associated with True Cord Knot: Excessively long umbilical cords are apt to become knotted.

True knots are not rare in twins.

Cord torsion.

Cord knot encountered in vessels of the twin-to-twin transfusion syndrome.

Pathology and Sequels.

Much venous distention was evident behind the first knot.

Knot may be single or multiple; Collins [3] also described triple knots associated with fetal demise and other cord abnormalities (Fig. 15.2).

Knots in the umbilical cord may not only cause fetal death, but also they may lead to significant prepartum hypoxia with lasting damage.

Knots cause compression of Wharton's jelly at the site of knotting.

When an umbilical knots examined microscopically, it is a common finding to have a mural thrombosis in the vein. Venous distention distal to the knot is a characteristic finding in knots with clinical significance, as the tendency of the unknotted cord to curl if the knot had been present for some time. Not every knot causes the same damage.

The normal pressure in the umbilical vein (10 mmHg) was raised to 20 mm by one slack knot; two knots raised it to 60 mm [4].

The venous stasis that occurs with true knots of the umbilical cord often results in thrombosis of placental surface veins.

Mural thrombosis or complete occlusion may be found, some even being calcified. In addition, the veins are frequently thickened and may exhibit 'cushions'.

Etiology: The precise etiology was not demonstrated.

It frequently related to the unusual construction of the placental vessels, especially their deficiency of an elastic membrane.

Elevated umbilical venous pressure definitely results in knots formation.

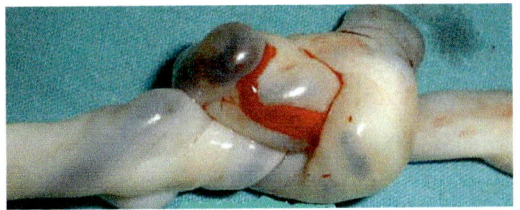

Fig. 15.1 True cord knot

M. Fahmy, *Umbilicus and Umbilical Cord*, https://doi.org/10.1007/978-3-319-62383-2_15

Fig. 15.2 Umbilical cord with two knots

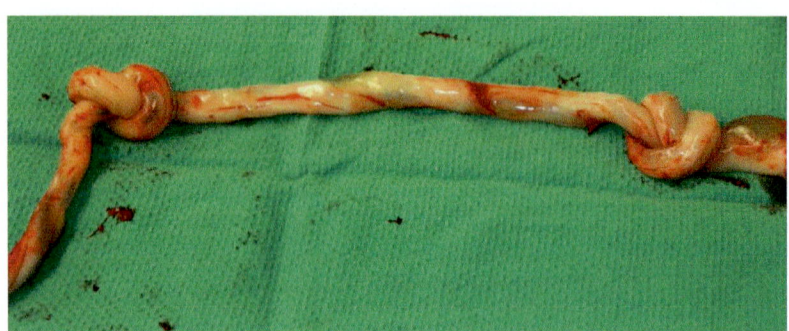

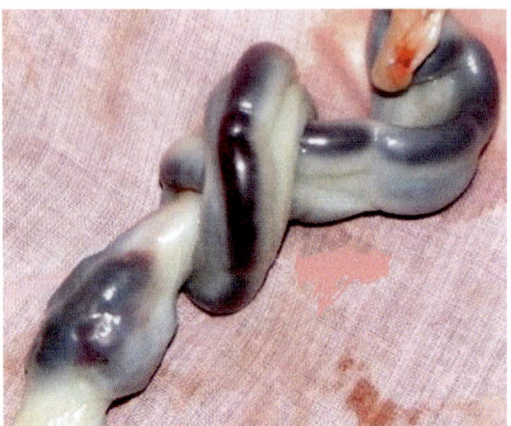

Fig. 15.3 True knot near the fetal end of the cord

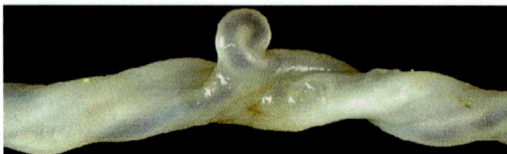

Fig. 15.4 False cord knot

exaggerated looping of umbilical cord vessels that causes focal dilatation of the cord. On US scans, these exaggerated loops appear as a bulge in the umbilical cord or a knoblike protuberance on it. The loops are apparent only in certain scanning planes [6].

Knotting is commonly observed in monoamnionic/monochorionic (MoMo) twins and a cause for their excessive mortality.

UC knots may be detected near to the placental end of the cord, but cases of knots at the fetal end are also reported (Fig. 15.3).

15.1   False Knots (Fig. 15.4)

False UC knots should not be listed as knots at all. This term has become so customary.

Definition: Local redundancies of umbilical vessels (mostly the vein), rather than knots, and they are often large [5].

False knots are relatively common variants of cord anatomy and are not clinically significant. It is important to differentiate them from true knots, cord cyst and other vascular cord anomalies. The term false knot usually indicates

References

1. Scheffel T, Langanke D. Die Nabelschnur-komplikationen an der Universitäts Frauenklinik von 1955 bis 1967. Zentralbl Gynäkol. 1970;92:429–34.
2. Chasnoff IJ, Fletcher MA. True knot of the umbilical cord. Am J Obstet Gynecol. 1977;127:425–7.
3. Collins JC, Muller RJ, Collins CL. Prenatal observation of umbilical cord abnormalities: a triple knot and torsion of the umbilical cord. Am J Obstet Gynecol. 1993;169:102–4.
4. Maher JT, Conti JA. A comparison of umbilical cord blood gas values between newborns with and without true knots. Obstet Gynecol. 1996;88:863–6.
5. Arvy L, Pilleri G. The cetacean umbilical cord; studies of the umbilical cord of two Platanistoidea: Platanista gangetica and Pontoporia blainvillei. In: Pilleri G, editor. Investigations on Cetacea, vol. VII. Berne: Brain Anatomy Institute; 1976. p. 91–103.
6. Hertzberg BS, et al. False knot of the umbilical cord: Sonographic appearance and differential diagnosis. J Clin Ultrasound. 1988;16(8):599–602.

Umbilical Cord Prolapse

16

Umbilical cord prolapse continues to be a catastrophic and stressful event not only for the patient but also for the physician; early diagnosis and prompt delivery usually result in a satisfactory outcome.

Definition: Umbilical cord prolapse is a rare life-threating emergency that has a perinatal mortality rate of 50% [1]; it occurs when the umbilical cord descends in advance of the presenting fetal part during or just before labour. This may be overt where the cord protrudes into the cervix, occult where the cord becomes compressed between the fetus and the uterine wall, or it may be a frank breech presentation with prolapsed cord (Fig. 16.1).

Incidence: The incidence of umbilical cord prolapse varies between 0.14 and 0.62% [1].

Predisposing factors to umbilical cord prolapse:

- Fetal malpresentation and breech presentation accounted for 36.5% of the umbilical cord prolapse cases.
- Preterm delivery, low birth weight, contracted pelvis and multiparity
- Babies with birth weight less than 1250 g had a 19-fold increase and multiparous mothers a twofold increase in risk [2].
- Polyhydramnios
- Amnioinfusion is associated with a higher incidence of umbilical cord prolapse [3].
- Previous studies have found an association of excessively long umbilical cords (ELUCs)

with true knots, cord entanglements, prolapse and torsion [4].

Perinatal complications have been reported with both excessively long and excessively short cord. The average UC length at term has been reported to be 61 cm, ELUCs are reported to be from 70 to 80 cm in length, while cords longer than 80 cm were more common, with a reported incidence of 3.7% [5]. Long umbilical cord may lead to cord prolapse, cord entanglement or nuchal cord.

In twin pregnancies, cord prolapses occur more frequently in the second twin to be delivered, with 9% in the first twin and 14% in the second twin.

Types of cord prolapse (Fig. 16.1):

A—Complete occult prolapse.
B—Cord presenting in front of the fetal head may be seen in the vagina (overt).
C—Frank breech presentation with prolapsed cord.

The first signs of umbilical cord prolapse usually:

A severe, prolonged, fetal bradycardia
A change from a normal fetal monitor tracing to severe variable decelerations

Overt prolapse occurs when the umbilical cord is protruding from the vagina or is palpated during a vaginal exam. Occult prolapse occurs

M. Fahmy, *Umbilicus and Umbilical Cord*, https://doi.org/10.1007/978-3-319-62383-2_16

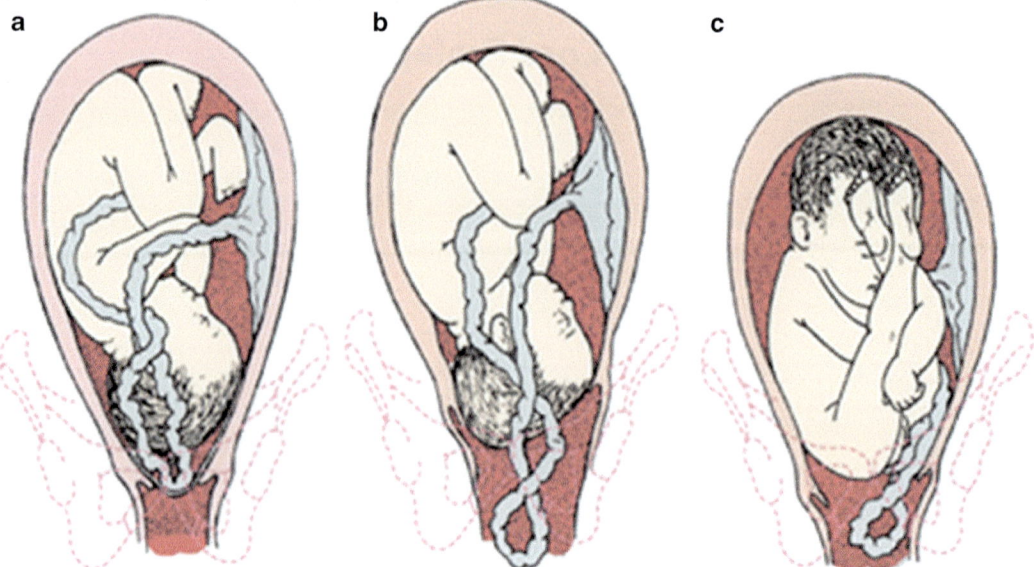

Fig. 16.1 Different types and grades of cord prolapse, (**a**) occult in head presentation, (**b**) overt in head presentation and (**c**) overt in breech presentation

when the cord is not visible or palpable, but it is located between the presenting part and the pelvis or cervix.

Sequels: Umbilical cord prolapse can result in increased morbidity for the fetus and the mother. Prompt diagnosis and intervention is essential if the fetus is to survive.

Cord prolapse is one of the important umbilical cord accidents (UCA), which is responsible for at least 1% of IUGR fetuses born at 38 weeks [5]. Doppler ultrasound can diagnose precisely the degree of cord prolapse and any associated congenital anomalies or a threatening risks (Fig. 16.2).

Management: The gold standard for treatment of umbilical cord prolapse in the setting of a viable pregnancy typically involves immediate delivery by the quickest and safest route possible. This usually requires caesarean section, especially if the woman is in early labour. Occasionally, vaginal delivery will be attempted if clinical judgement determines, that is, a safer or quicker method.

Maternal positions, which may be helpful in cases with minimal fetal risk, include:

- Knee–chest position—patient on her knees with her head and arms resting on the bed (Fig. 16.3)
- Trendelenburg position

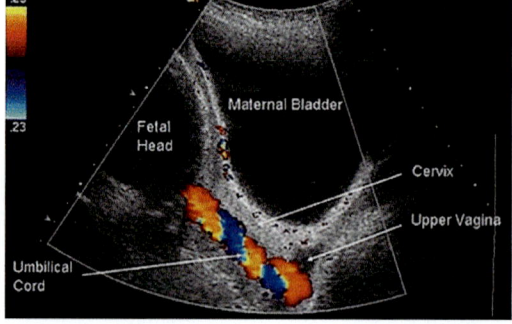

Fig. 16.2 Doppler US demonstrating cord prolapsing down to the middle third of vagina

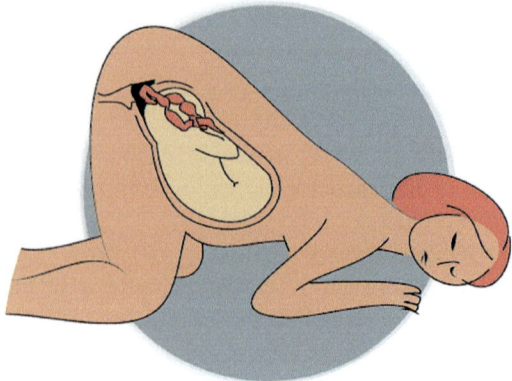

Fig. 16.3 Mother's position which may be helpful to decrease the risk on the fetus in cord prolapse

• Modified Sims position—patient in side-lying position with hips elevated on pillows

One of the leading treatments of umbilical cord compression is amnioinfusion.

When umbilical cord compression is minor, the method of treatment is to increase the mother's oxygen, in order to increase the blood flow through the umbilical cord. In more severe cases of umbilical cord compression, there should be constant monitoring of the baby to assess if there are signs of distress, in which case emergency caesarean section should be taken.

References

1. Baergen RN, et al. Morbidity, mortality, and placental pathology in excessively long umbilical cords: retrospective study. Pediatr Dev Pathol. 2001;4:144–53.
2. Koonings PP, Paul RH, Campbell K. Umbilical cord prolapse, a contemporary look. J Reprod Med. 1990;35:690–2.
3. Dilbaz B, et al. Risk factors and perinatal outcomes associated with umbilical cord prolapse. Arch Gynecol Obstet. 2006;274(2):104–7.
4. Roberts WE, Martin RW, Roach HH, Perry KG, Martin JN, Morrison JC. Are obstetric interventions such as cervical ripening, induction of labor, amnioinfusion, or amniotomy associated with umbilical cord prolapse. Am J Obstet Gynecol. 1997;176:1181–5.
5. McLennan H, Price E, Urbanska M, Craig N, Fraser M. Umbilical cord knots and encirclements. Aust N Z J Obstet Gynaecol. 1988;28:116–9.

Umbilical Cord Tumors

17.1 Umbilical Cord Teratoma

Teratoma often occurring in the gonads, their occurrence in extragonadal sites is rare with umbilical cord being one such rare site.

Incidence: Few cases and limited case series had been published with cord teratoma; the credit of the first case report goes to Budin, at 1878 [1]. I assume that some cases may escape proper early diagnosis, as the teratoma may compromise normal fatal progression and end with fatal death.

Clinically: On average, normal umbilical cords are 3.7 cm in circumference with a range of 3–5 cm. A larger cord diameter can suggest an abnormal cord with oedema, tumor or hernia. Dimensions greater than 6 cm circumference should prompt an examination of the cord and fetus [2]. Teratomas may grow to large sizes and can disrupt umbilical vessels and fetal blood flow.

Antenatal ultrasound showing an umbilical cord swelling with a homogeneous character and absence of an intratumoral flow, intercessional calcification may be seen. Umbilical cord teratomas are identified at varying ages of gestation, ranging from 17 weeks to term, it have a very polymorphic presentation and can reach a considerable size, the smallest with a diameter of 1.8 cm and the largest with the size of an infant's head had been reported. They were observed along the whole length of the cord, fixed by a short pedicle when they were small or more widely attached when they were large. The largest teratomas were seen in the central part of the umbilical cord. They are frequently covered with skin and can be solid, cystic, cartilaginous or bony structures characterized by distinct calcification. Many cases had been presented with variable sizes of abdominal wall defect in the form of omphalocele; as the presence of the progressively growing neoplastic swelling at the base of the cord may interfere with proper return of bowel to the abdominal cavity, and leads to exampholas and bowel herniation (Fig. 17.1). Most of the reported cases were in females, and most were recognized after term delivery.

Histopathology: Teratomas are most probably derived from ectopically located germ cells; at the histological level, it is a developmental benign neo-

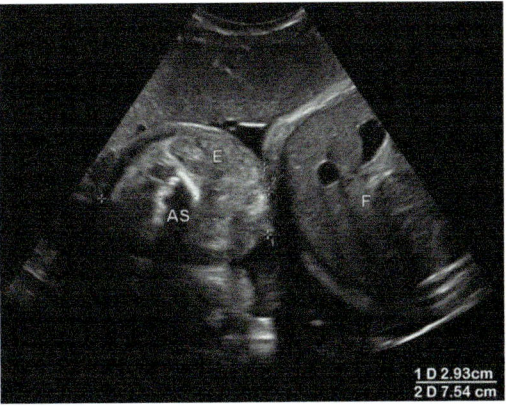

Fig. 17.1 Ultrasound image at 28 weeks' gestation showing exomphalos (E) and acoustic shadowing (AS), which was recognized retrospectively to be due to bone component of teratoma. *F* fetus

© Springer International Publishing AG 2018
M. Fahmy, *Umbilicus and Umbilical Cord*, https://doi.org/10.1007/978-3-319-62383-2_17

Fig. 17.2 A typical case of large umbilical cord teratoma (T), with a small omphalocele (E) and a normal umbilical cord (UC). 'This photo reproduced after kind permission from Dr. David Keene, Royal Manchester Children's Hospital, Manchester, UK [6]'

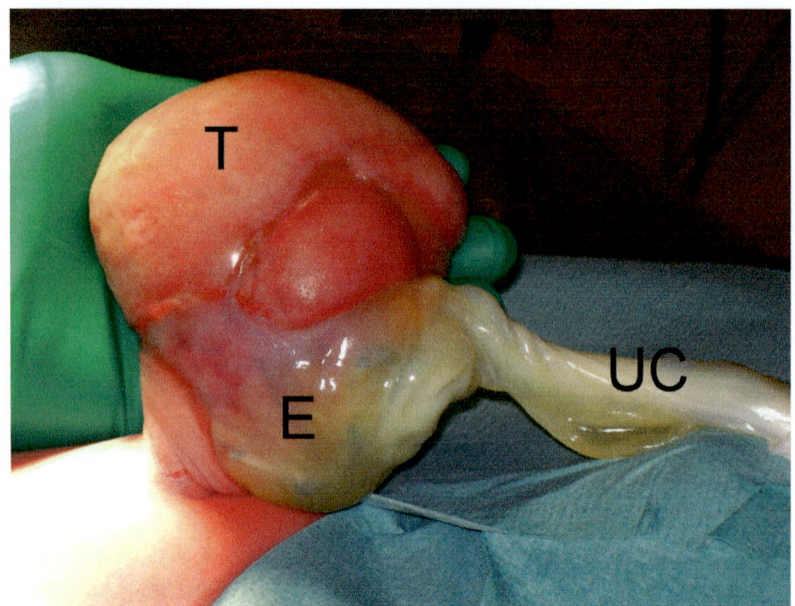

plasm with tissues from the three germinal layers, having different cellular and organoid components derived from more than one germ layer. Adipose tissue, connective tissue, smooth muscle, nervous tissue, glial tissue, glandlike structures and cysts covered by squamous or columnar lining were the most frequent histological structures observed [3].

Tissues were mature in most of the reported cases, but in some instances immature areas were observed with a slightly premature infant. Rarely, they contain malignant tissue; therefore, serial tumor markers and imaging are required during the first few years of life [4].

Associated Anomalies: Concurrent malformations are described in about half of published cases, with large as well as small teratomas; commonly encountered anomalies include:

- Known midline defects associated with umbilical teratomas include exomphalos, exstrophy of the urinary bladder and myelomeningocele [4–6].
- Single umbilical artery.
- Trisomy 13 [5].
- Review of 11 reported cases reveals that four of them were local regional involving the abdominal wall and/or abdominal organs. This preferential, but not exclusive, locoregional distribution

seems particular to congenital teratomas and has already been described for the sacrococcygeal region as well as for the heart and pericardium, the stomach and the retroperitoneal region [2].

Complications:

- Rupture of cord vessels is a particular danger associated with UC teratomas, which may have a fatal outcome.
- Cord tumors are a significant cause of cardiac failure in the fetus ('high-output heart failure').
- Cord teratoma is always benign; but in some cases locoregional involving the abdominal wall and/or abdominal organs may be detected.
- Despite the large volume of some tumors, few obstetrical complications have been reported.

Diagnosis: Antenatal diagnosis of an umbilical cord tumor can be challenging in the presence of an exomphalos. The initial ultrasound features may have suggested the presence of only a large exomphalos; however, acoustic shadowing that indicated bone and narrowing of the umbilical cord between the mass and the abdominal wall were suggestive of a tumor (Fig. 17.2).

Management: Outcome in cord teratomas is determined by the extent of resection of the tumor and the presence of foci of yolk sac tumor in the neoplasm. The presence of associated anomalies and surgical complications after correction of the congenital malformations also affects the outcome in these cases. Teratoma itself could be shelled out easily, which usually attached only at the umbilical ring, and abdominal wall could be closed primary [7]. Strict follow-up is indicated for detection of any recurrence or sequel.

17.2   Haemangioma of Umbilical Cord

Nomenclature: The word "haemangioma" is derived from the ancient Greek αἷμα (blood), ἀγγεῖον (vessel) and ογκος (mass or tumor). Other terms used for cord haemangioma: angiomyxoma, myxangioma, haemangiofibromyxoma or myxsarcoma.

Incidence: Umbilical cord tumors are rare, with haemangiomas and teratomas accounting for the most common tumors. Haemangiomas of the umbilical cord are extremely rare benign vascular tumors, not always detected prenatally. There is no association between fetal gender, maternal age, race or gravidity and cord haemangioma development. From 1951 to date, only 44 cases have been reported [8].

Pathology: Theoretically cord haemangioma may arise from umbilical, omphalomesenteric or allantoic vessels [9].

A possible hereditary predisposition to this vascular anomaly is still under discussion. Review of 37 reports in the literature from 1951 through 2005 revealed that most of these lesions were referred to as haemangioma and rarely as angiomyxoma, myxangioma or haemangiofibromyxoma because of the myxoid appearance of the commonly associated oedematous degeneration of the Wharton's jelly [10].

The typical microscopic appearance is that of capillaries embedded in myxoid stroma, which is probably a degeneration of Wharton's jelly [11].

Relation between cord and placental haemangiomas: The frequency of umbilical cord haemangioma disorder is much lower than that of placental haemangiomas. Although cord hae-

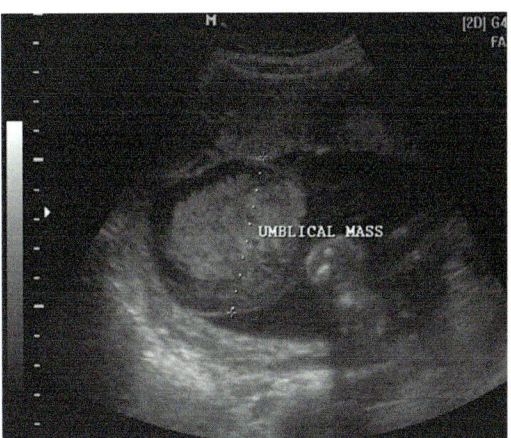

Fig. 17.3 Antenatally detected UC haemangioma

mangiomas are very similar to placental haemangioma with regard to origin and nature, the clinical significance of cord haemangioma is better defined than placental haemangioma. Also unlike the placental haemangiomas, cord haemangiomas have been associated with maternal hydramnios [12].

Clinically: U cord haemangioma may be presented in one of these occasions:

- Most cases (80%) are diagnosed precisely antenatally, which was suspected when an echogenic, heterogeneous (composed of solid and cystic areas) fusiform mass is visualized within the umbilical cord. The placental end of the cord was the preferred site of location, and the umbilical artery the commonest vessel of origin [8] (Fig. 17.3).
- During delivery and before cord cut, the tumor presents as a fusiform or spindle-shaped swelling in the cord with the presence of an angiomatous nodule, surrounded by oedema of the Wharton's jelly ranging in size from 0.2 to 18 cm in diameter, and if the case is not diagnosed antenatally by the gynaecologist, it is challenging for the clinician to suspect haemangioma of the cord and to differentiate it from other umbilical cord swellings (Fig. 17.4).
- Small haemangioma may be detected in the cord without obvious cord oedema and with a normal cord calibre.

- After fall down of umbilical stump, haemangioma may be presented as a reddish cystic swelling covered by amnion, and it may gave a false impression of umbilical polyp. In such case, Doppler US and angio-MRI may be indicated to diagnose haemangioma precisely, before any attempt for excision, and also to detect any other associated visceral haemangiomas (Fig. 17.5).
- Haemangioma of the umbilicus in older child or adult is discussed in (Sect. 30.2)

Associated anomalies: UC haemangioma has been associated with increased alpha-fetoprotein (AFP), hydramnios, congenital anomalies and

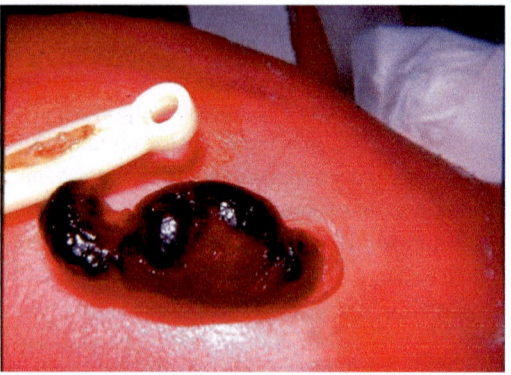

Fig. 17.4 A fusiform UC haemangioma at the fetal end of the cord

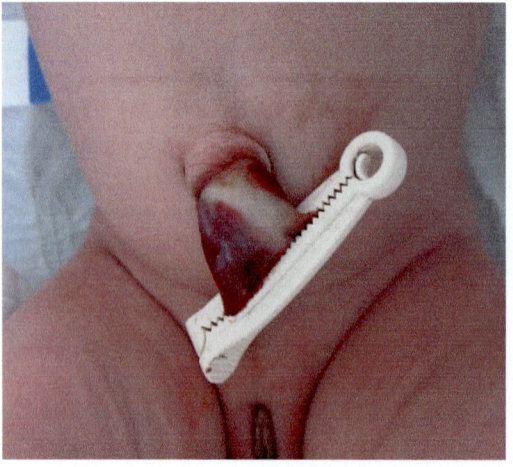

Fig. 17.5 UC haemangioma, not detected neither ante- or postnatally and presented as a round rubbery irreducible umbilical mass with the umbilical vessels displaced towards the bottom; cord stump had not yet fallen off

increased perinatal mortality. Impaired umbilical circulation has been proposed as the predisposing factor for fetal compromise [13].

The cause of elevated maternal serum alpha-fetoprotein level in association with umbilical cord haemangioma is unclear, gastrointestinal malformations, hypospadias and vascular birthmarks had been reported [14].

UC haemangioma has been described also in association with cutaneous vascular malformations, single umbilical artery and other malformations, such as heart malformations, anencephaly, skin malformations, various syndromes and, cutaneous/systemic haemangiomas [14].

Differential diagnosis: Antenatally, the differential diagnosis of umbilical cord haemangioma should include umbilical vessels abnormalities like varicosity, aneurysms and thrombosis [15]. Varicose umbilical vein and umbilical artery venous malformations (AVM) have been reported in few cases, and the condition may be discovered incidentally by routine physical examination or can present as haemorrhagic shock after clamping of the umbilical cord. It is usually associated with cardiomegaly and heart failure or liver failure which may complicates undetected cases with reluctant management [16].

Umbilical artery aneurysm is an extremely rare vascular anomaly associated with poor fetal outcome, comprehending chromosomal aberration, progressive oligohydramnios and fetal death due to acute umbilical venous compression.

Haematoma of the umbilical cord (bleeding into the substance of the cord) is usually an accidental event secondary to cordocentesis done for diagnostic purposes, while spontaneous haematoma remains very rare and it may imitates haemangioma.

Differential diagnosis after delivery should comprise umbilical cord teratoma, other rare cord tumors and cysts. Umbilical cord polyp, hernia into the cord, vitellointestinal and urachal remnants as well as small omphalocele should be considered during diagnosis of cord haemangioma (Fig. 17.6).

Angiomyxoma is a rare tumor of the umbilical cord and considered by some authors as a variant of haemangioma; it is associated with increased perinatal morbidity and mortality and differentiated from haemangioma by the presence of massive degeneration of Wharton's jelly [15].

Sequel and complications: A majority of antenatally diagnosed haemangiomas are small and are usually asymptomatic. However, if they are large, then the following signs and symptoms may be present:

- Excessive bleeding/haemorrhage within the gastrointestinal tract resulting in fetal distress.

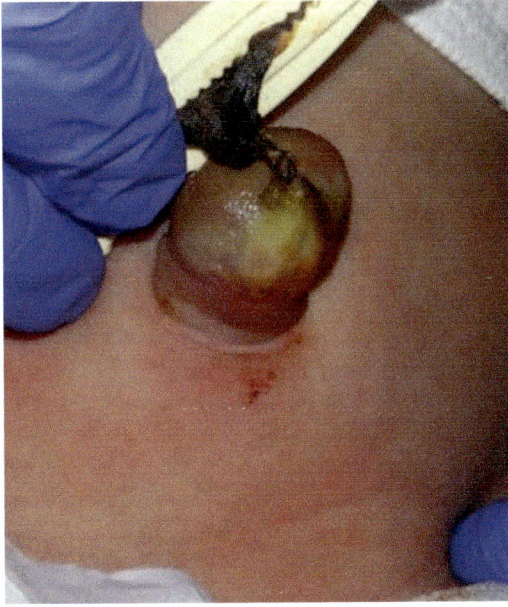

Fig. 17.6 A case of hernia of umbilical cord looks like cord haemangioma

- Decreased blood flow to the fetus.
- Umbilical vessels thrombosis with cord twist secondary to cord haemangioma (Fig. 17.7).
- A high perinatal mortality and morbidity rate has been reported with haemangiomas of umbilical cord. Impaired umbilical circulation is considered as the predisposing factor for fetal demise. It is associated with premature delivery, cardiac failure, severe fetal haemorrhage, IUGR and intrauterine death [10].
- Episodes of proximal obstruction of umbilical artery blood flow, and transient fetal pleural and pericardial effusions had been reported.

Only 46% of the cases resulted in the delivery of a normal healthy infant, and fetal morbidity was recognized in 54% of the cases [17].

Bleeding from the haemangioma may be detected within the cord immediately after delivery, and if the case was not previously diagnosed antenatally, it will be extremely difficult to differentiate it from cord haematoma (Fig. 17.8).

Management: Close antenatal follow-up is mandatory, with serial US examinations and Doppler studies, which should involve AFI (amniotic fluid index) and tumor size. The examination should be at 4 weeks intervals up to 32–34 weeks and every 1–2 weeks thereafter depending on the findings [10].

Early induction of delivery has to be considered for fetal growth restriction with abnormal fetal surveillance and if pulmonary maturity is

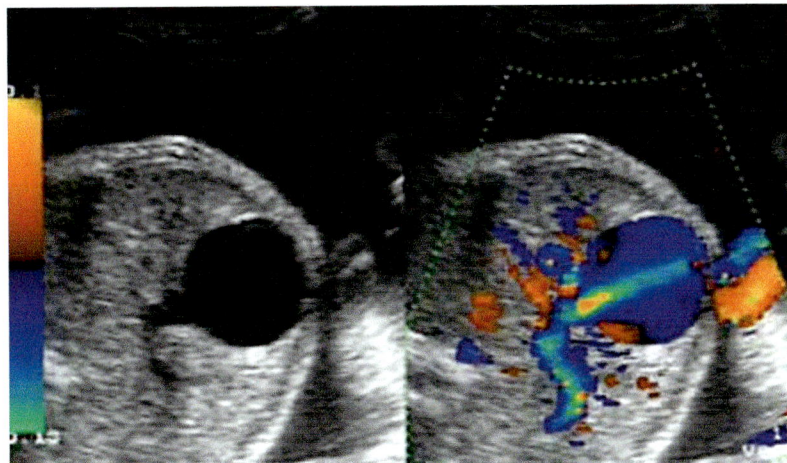

Fig. 17.7 Umbilical vessels thrombosis with cord twist secondary to cord haemangioma

Fig. 17.8 Bleeding inside a cord haemangioma, making it looking like hamartoma

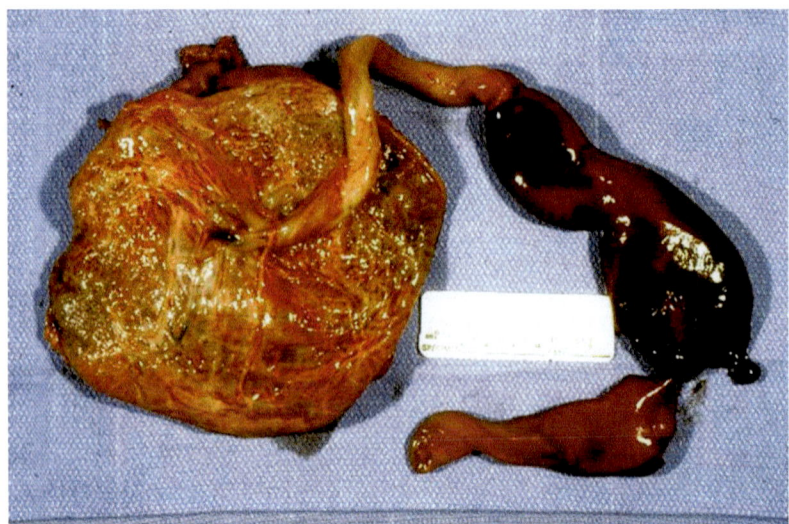

assumed. These cases highlight possible mechanisms for fetal decompensation as well as the importance of a multifaceted approach to the management of an umbilical cord mass using multiple tools for fetal assessment.

No specific treatment may be necessary for haemangiomas of umbilical cord that are small in size, since the condition is not associated with any signs and symptoms, just a careful cord cut and clamping with workup to rule any other associated anomalies.

Larger haemangiomas may require treatment, and the healthcare provider may decide on the course of action on a case-by-case basis. Histopathological examination of the severed cord is mandatory to confirm the diagnosis, and if haemangioma is suspected or confirmed, the newborn should be monitored for any cardiac or other anomalies.

17.3 Umbilical Cord Haematoma

Cord haematomas can arise during pregnancy which may lead to fetal death or may occur during labour and giving rise to fetal distress as evidenced by cardiotocographic (CTG) abnormalities.

Incidence: Umbilical cord haematoma is a rare cause for stillbirths with a reported rate of around 1:5500 [18]. With the advance in application of fetal intervention for diagnosis and treatment of congenital anomalies, it is expected to see more cases of cord haematomas.

Historical background: Hyrtl first described this finding in 1871; little is known about its etiology and pathogenesis [19].

Etiology: Reviewing the published cases of U cord haematoma reveals three main etiological conditions, in which the cord haematoma may take place, but still many cases remain unexplained:

- Spontaneous haematoma
- Haematoma secondary to other cord or placental anomalies and diseases
- Iatrogenic haematoma

Spontaneous haematoma: Spontaneous formation of a haematoma without any associated cord anomalies and without previous fetal intervention is possible, and the following risk factors have been reported: short UC, cord prolapse, velamentous cord insertion and fetal clotting disorders [20].

Secondary haematoma: Umbilical cord haematoma may occur secondary to congenital infections by different pathogens, twisting and traction of cord, true cord knots, vessel wall abnormalities, umbilical cord cysts, trauma and post-term babies [21].

Either congenital weakness of a cord vessel wall or varix may be associated with cord haematoma.

The decrease of Wharton's jelly which occurs in postmaturity is postulated to predispose the cord to vessel torsion [22].

Iatrogenic haematoma: Iatrogenic causes secondary to amniocentesis, in utero transfusions, diagnostic cordocentesis and fetal blood sampling for the investigation of fetal anaemia. Specialized genetic investigations are possible through UC puncture; even ultrasound-guided puncture of the UV may end with haematoma [23].

Since the majority of the reported haematomas occurred near the umbilicus, it is postulated that traction on either a short or relatively short cord, due to looping around the fetal parts, may be responsible for this location of the haematoma during descent of labour and delivery.

Mechanical trauma of cord between fetal and maternal tissues may weaken the vessel wall when placental blood is forced into the umbilical vein during uterine contractions. Increasing pressure may then cause rupture of the weakened vessel wall [24].

Clinically: The need for detailed examination of placenta, membranes and cord has to be emphasized, as majority of the stillbirths classified as unexplained could actually be due to a cord pathology. This clear identification also helps in better counselling of the patients and relieves their stress. It is also necessary to try to identify a cause as many of these can be recurrent and appropriate identification will help in prevention of the same [25].

Haematomas of the cord are usually single and arise from the umbilical vein. They vary in size from 1.3 cm to the size of a child's arm, and, although usually situated near the umbilicus, they may be located anywhere along the cord (Fig. 17.9).

Rupture of umbilical vein accounts for the majority of the haematomas and in around 10% umbilical artery ruptures [26].

Complications: The perinatal loss associated with this condition is greater than 50% [27].

Case reports of cord haematomas giving rise to fetal heart rate abnormalities in labour have been reported. Even after emergency caesarean section, many neonates developed hypoxic

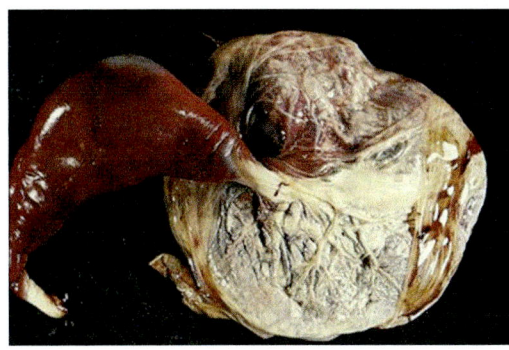

Fig. 17.9 Umbilical cord haematoma involving the entire cord

ischaemic encephalopathy and died in the neonatal period [26].

Haematoma if large enough, can compress UC vessels and impair fetal circulation, and fetal death is caused as a result of anoxia due to compression of fetal vessels by the haematoma or by exsanguination of fetal blood.

The procedural risk of abortion is 1% (fetus without malformations) [27].

References

1. Budin P. Note sur une tumeur du cordon ombilical. Prog Med. 1878;2:550–1.
2. Satgé DCL, Laumond M-A, Desfarges F, Chenard M-P. An umbilical cord teratoma in a 17-week-old fetus. Prenat Diagn. 2001;21:284–8.
3. Kreyberg L. A teratoma-like swelling in the umbilical cord possibly of acardius nature. J Pathol Bacteriol. 1958;75:109–12.
4. Smith D, Majmudar B. Teratoma of the umbilical cord. Hum Pathol. 1985;16:190–3.
5. Hargitai B, Csabai L, Bán Z, Hetényi I, Szucs I, Varga S, Papp Z. Rare case of exomphalos complicated with umbilical cord teratoma in a fetus with trisomy 13. Fetal Diagn Ther. 2005;20(6):528–33.
6. Keene DJB, Shawkat E, Gillham J, Craigie RJ. Rare combination of exomphalos with umbilical cord teratoma. Ultrasound Obstet Gynecol. 2012; 40:481.
7. Chavali LV, Vijaya Bhaskar R, Bhaskar Reddy J. Immature teratoma at umbilicus region presenting as exomphalos: a case report with review of literature. Indian J Med Paediatr Oncol. 2014;35(3): 231–3.
8. Iglesias-Deus A, et al. Umbilical cord and visceral hemangiomas diagnosed in the neonatal period. Medicine (Baltimore). 2016;95(42):e5196.

9. Shalev E. Placenta and umbilical cord. In: Chervenak FA, Isaacson GC, Camp-bell S, editors. Ultrasound in obstetrics and gynaecology, vol. 2. Boston: Little, Brown and Company; 1993. p. 1083–97.

10. Sathiyathasan S, Jeyanthan K, Hamid R. Umbilical hemangioma: a case report. Arch Gynecol Obstet. 2011;283(Suppl 1):15–7.

11. DeCosta EJ, Gerbie AB, Andresen RH, Gallanis TC. Placental tumors: hemangioma; with special reference to an associated clinical syndrome. Obstet Gynecol. 1956;7:249–59.

12. Heifetz SA, Rueda-Pedraza ME. Hemangiomas of the umbilical cord. Pediatr Pathol. 1983;1(4):385–98.

13. Daniel-Spiegel E, Weiner E, Gimburg G, Shalev E. The association of umbilical cord hemangioma with fetal vascular birthmarks. Prenat Diagn. 2005;25:300–3.

14. Papadopoulos VG, Kourea HP, Adonakis GL, Decavalas GO. A case of umbilical cord hemangioma: Doppler studies and review of the literature. Eur J Obstet Gynecol Reprod Biol. 2009;144(1):8–14.

15. Smulian JC, Sarno AP, Rochon ML, Loven VA. The natural history of an umbilical cord hemangioma. J Clin Ultrasound. 2016;44(7):455–8.

16. Meyer M, Barsness KA. Umbilical arteriovenous malformation: a case report and literature review. Pediatr Surg Int. 2013;29(8):851–3.

17. Cardarella A, Buccoliero AM, TaddeiA SL, Taddei GL. Hemangioma of umbilical cord: report of a case. Pathol Res Pract. 2003;199:51–5.

18. Gualandri G, Rivasi F, Santunione AL, Silingardi E. Spontaneous umbilical cord hematoma: an unusual cause of fetal mortality: a report of 3 cases and review of the literature. Am J Forensic Med Pathol. 2008;29(2):185–90.

19. Hyrtl J. The hazards of umbilical cord haematoma. Med J Aust. 1871;1:648. Cited by Roberts-Thomson, M.E. (1973).

20. Arora PK, Mohandas S, McAndrew S. spontaneous umbilical cord hematoma. J Pediatr. 2017;184:233–233.e1.

21. Sepulveda W, Wong AE, Gonzalez R, Vasquez P, Gutierrez J. Fetal death due to umbilical cord hematoma: a rare complication of umbilical cord cyst. J Matern Fetal Neonatal Med. 2005;18(6):387–90.

22. Toland OJ, Mann HJ, Helsel CM. Hematoma of the Umbilical Cord: A case report. Obstet Gynecol. 1959;14:799.

23. Tongsong T, Wanapirak C, Kunavikatikul C, et al. Cordocentesis at 16–24 weeks of gestation: experience of 1,320 cases. Prenat Diagn. 2000;20:224–8.

24. Berry SM, Stone J, Norton ME, et al. Fetal blood sampling. Am J Obstet Gynecol. 2013;209:170–80.

25. Abraham A, Rathore S, Gupta M, Benjamin SJ. Umbilical cord haematoma causing still birth a case report. J Clin Diagn Res. 2015;9(12):QD01–2.

26. Sizun J, Soupre D, Broussine L, Giroux JD, Piriou P, Ventrillon E, et al. Spontaneous umbilical cord hematoma, a rare cause of acute fetal distress. Arch Pédiatr Organe Off Soc Fr Pédiatr. 1995;2(12):1182–3.

27. Irani PK. Haematoma of the umbilical cord. Br Med J. 1964;2(5422):1436–7.

Rare Anomalies of the Umbilical Cord

18

Generally the anomalies of the umbilical cord are rare; recently with the wide use of accurate ultrasound techniques and routine scanning for each pregnant women, it becomes possible to diagnose many rare cord anomalies; very rarely MRI is indicated to diagnose precisely some suspected cases; most of this cord anomalies are reported with twins and chromosomal anomalies. Some specific anomalies like cord cyst, haemangioma, knots and tumors were discussed before.

False knots, which are actually a vascular redundancies, often appear as varicosities in the umbilical cord. However, real varix formations are rare. When present, they show marked, focal thinning of the wall of the umbilical vein that may be associated with muscle necrosis. Fetal death may occur from fetal haemorrhage or compression of the aneurysmally dilated veins. When elastic stains are done on such cords, it has been repeatedly found that the elastic fibres of the vein are focally deficient.

The umbilical cord may rupture, either completely or partially. This will inevitably lead to bleeding and often results in cord haematomas. Excessively short cords may rupture during descent, but velamentous cord insertion is the most frequent antecedent of this complication. Rupture has also been reported in association with varices, cord entanglement, trauma from amniocentesis or therapeutic intrauterine transfusion

and severe acute funisitis. If rupture occurs, it is most often at the site of its placental attachment, but can occur anywhere. Spontaneous cord complete rupture is an uncommon event; most ruptures are partial and cause local haematomas or haemorrhage.

Necrosis of umbilical vessel walls may result from chronic and severe meconium exposure. The cord will usually be discoloured green or greenish brown. On occasion, they are the sequelae of thrombosis, but they may occur without it. Necrosis of umbilical arteries and a linear ulceration of Wharton's jelly have been described associated with intestinal atresia. Obviously, this leads to haemorrhage into the umbilical cord and amniotic fluid, with resultant fetal anaemia and the potential for fetal exsanguination. Segmental thinning of umbilical vessels has also been described as a focal thinning of the vessel wall with virtual absence of the vascular media. It is seen predominantly in the umbilical vein and has been associated with congenital malformations and fetal distress.

The cord may show various discolourations similar to those seen in the fetal membranes. Green discolouration may be present in meconium exposure; brown discolouration is usually due to hemosiderin from old haemorrhage and yellow discolouration from maternal bilirubinemia, and red-brown discolouration is usually secondary to haemolysis after fetal death.

M. Fahmy, *Umbilicus and Umbilical Cord*, https://doi.org/10.1007/978-3-319-62383-2_18

18.1   Thrombosis of Umbilical Vessels

Pathologic Features: The incidence of umbilical vessel thrombosis is 1 in 1300 deliveries, 1 in 1000 perinatal autopsies and 1 in 250 high-risk gestations. Venous thromboses are more common than arterial thromboses, but the latter are more often lethal. Old thrombi in umbilical vessels, primarily the vein, may calcify, and occasionally massive calcification has made it difficult to ligate the cord at delivery [1].

Pathogenesis: Thrombosis of umbilical vessels most frequently occurs near term. It may develop due to velamentous insertion, inflammation, varices, entanglement, knotting, torsion, abnormal coiling, amnionic bands, maternal diabetes and funipuncture. Coagulation problems caused by thrombophilias of mother or infant are sometimes the cause. The formation of thrombi with velamentous insertion of the cord is readily understandable. It is also easy to understand that thrombosis of cord vessels may occur in varices and from knotting as well as the entangling of cords in monoamnionic twins [2].

Clinical Features and Implications: Thrombosis can compromise the circulation and lead to growth restriction, fetal death or neurologic injury. Thrombi may also break off and potentially embolize to the fetus or to the placenta, where they may cause infarction. More remarkable are the thrombi that occur in the absence of all these more readily understood complications, and they are perhaps the most common. Very frequently thromboses of vessels in the cord are associated with similar events in the villous ramifications. Thrombosis due to coagulation defects has been associated with extensive CNS lesions in the infants as well as stroke and neonatal thrombosis [3].

18.2   Strictures or Coarctation of the Umbilical Cord

Synonyms: Constriction of the umbilical cord, umbilical cord occlusions and fibrosis circumscripta of the umbilical cord.

Definition: Coarctation is characterized by a localized narrowing of the cord with disappearance of the Wharton's jelly, thickening of the vascular walls and narrowing of their lumens. Generally, torsion of the umbilical cord is present [4] (Fig. 18.1).

Incidence: Approximately 30 cases have been described in the literature. However, this may not represent the real incidence of this entity [5].

Etiology and Pathology: The mechanisms responsible for coarctation of the umbilical cord are not understood. Edmonds suggested that coarctation and subsequent torsion are a postmortem event caused by necrobiosis of the Wharton's jelly [4].

Weber [6] pointed out the following objections to this hypothesis: (1) live-born fetuses have been reported to have constrictions, and (2) coarctations are extremely rare in stillbirths. Perhaps this complication should be viewed as a local failure of Wharton's jelly development that creates a weak point in the umbilical cord. Fetal motion could lead to torsion around this point. The site of the torsion is generally close to the fetus. A localized edematous area is frequently reported distal to the torsion point. Multiple strictures along the length of the umbilical cord can be found [6].

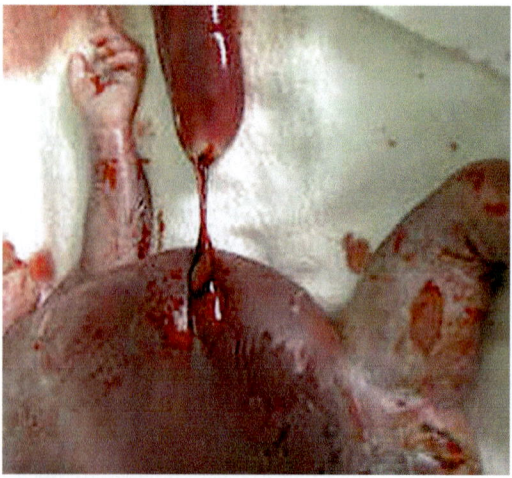

Fig. 18.1 Coarctation of the umbilical cord, with a proximal cord oedema

Diagnosis: To date, this condition is difficult to diagnose with ultrasound, although recognition should be possible.

Associated Anomalies: The following anomalies have been reported with coarctation of the umbilical cord: oesophageal atresia and tracheoesophageal fistula, cleft lip, anencephaly, anophthalmia and exophthalmos, polyhydramnios, ventricular septal defect and trisomy 18 and generalized subcutaneous edema; usually detected in such cases, they may be a sequel of venous congestion.

Prognosis: Most reported cases of coarctation result in stillbirths. However, this may represent reporting biases. Recurrences in subsequent pregnancies have not been noted in the literature [7].

18.3 Umbilical Vein Varix

Fetal intra-abdominal umbilical vein varix is a focal variceal dilatation of the umbilical vein. Its clinical importance has not yet been clearly established, but it has been reported to be associated with increased fetal malformations, chromosomal abnormalities and increased death rates [8] (Fig. 18.2). The umbilical vein was considered dilated when the measurement was above two standard deviation of the mean for gestational age (Fig. 18.2). Association of the presence of umbilical vein varix and fetal anomalies and/or obstetrical complications has been reported in literature [9].

Additional sonographic abnormalities were detected prenatally in 31.9%, most commonly anomalies of the cardiovascular system (including structural and functional abnormalities), hydropic features and anaemia. Chromosomal abnormalities were detected in 12%, and recently it has been suggested that this prenatal finding should be considered as a soft marker for aneuploidy. Mortality associated with the umbilical vein varix has been reported between 24 and 44% [10].

In the presence of umbilical vein varix, fetal echocardiography and detailed ultrasound study of fetal anatomy are needed to exclude associated anomalies. Isoimmunization should be ruled out, and consideration of karyotyping should be discussed. Serial follow-up scans are needed to exclude the onset of hydrops or thrombosis of the varix. A close fetal monitoring by serial colour Doppler and ultrasonographic examinations should be performed [11].

Sepulveda [12] concludes that fetuses with varix of the intra-fetal umbilical vein should be considered at risk for poor outcome. However, if no other anomalies are present, the prognosis is generally good.

Differential diagnosis: Differential diagnosis includes other abdominal cysts such as choledochal, mesenteric or urachal cysts. The presence of intra-abdominal umbilical vein varix can be confirmed by colour Doppler finding of turbulent flow in the cystic mass.

Prognosis: A varix of intra-fetal umbilical vein is considered a poor prognostic sign; but if no associated anomalies are present, the prognosis is generally good.

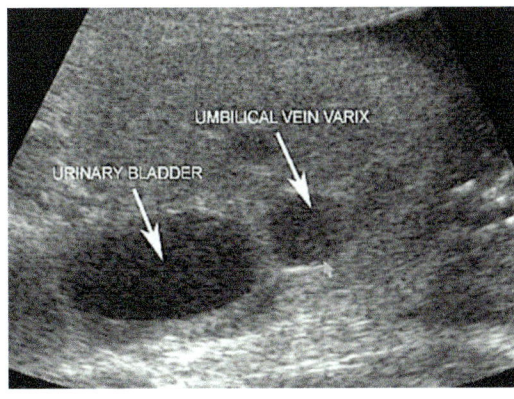

Fig. 18.2 US of umbilical vein varix

18.4 Umbilical Artery Aneurysm
(Fig. 18.3)

Aneurysm of the umbilical cord is an extremely rare vascular anomaly. The mechanisms leading to the formation of aneurysm of the umbilical vessels are poorly understood, although congenital thinning of the vascular wall could be the most probable etiologic factor. It seems likely that Wharton's jelly plays a critical role in preventing aneurysmal dilatation of the umbilical vessels even if a significant weakness of the arterial or venous wall develops [13].

Aneurysms are a relatively frequent finding in placental surface vessels, with a prevalence of up to 2% being reported at detailed examination of the chorionic vessels; all aneurysms were located near the placental cord insertion, where the umbilical vessels branch into the chorionic plate and therefore loose the protection of Wharton's jelly.

Nevertheless, in spite of the rarity of this condition, the prenatal diagnosis of an umbilical artery aneurysm is a significant finding because of its high association with fetal life-threatening complications such as thrombosis and compression of neighbouring vessels. These complications are not only restricted to umbilical artery aneurysms as they can also occur in cases of umbilical vein aneurysm or varix, where fetal distress and unexpected intrauterine death have also been reported [14].

Recently umbilical artery aneurysm can be picked up early by ultrasound and Doppler (Fig. 18.4).

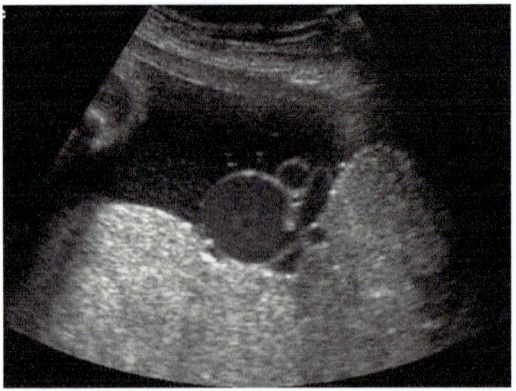

Fig. 18.4 US showing an umbilical artery aneurysm

References

1. Fritz MA, Christopher CR. Umbilical vein thrombosis and maternal diabetes mellitus. J Reprod Med. 1981;26:320.
2. Colgan TJ, Luk SC. Umbilical cord torsion, thrombosis and intrauterine death of a twin fetus. Arch Pathol Lab Med. 1982;106:101.
3. Woifman WL, Purohit DM, Self SE. Umbilical vein thrombosis at 32 weeks' gestation with delivery of a living infant. Am J Obstet Gynecol. 1983;146:468.
4. Edmonds HW. The spiral twist of the normal umbilical cord in twins and in singletons. Am J Obstet Gynecol. 1954;67:102.
5. Tavares-Fortuna JF, Lourdes-Pratas M. Coarctation of the umbilical cord: a cause of intrauterine fetal death. Int J Gynaecol Obstet. 1978;15:469.
6. Weber J. Constriction of the umbilical cord as a cause of fetal death. Acta Obstet Gynecol Scand. 1963;42:259.
7. Speck G, Palmer RE. Torsion of the umbilical cord: a cause of fetal death. South Med J. 1961;54:48.
8. Ipek A, Kurt A, Tosun O, Gumus M, Yazicioglu KR, Asik E, Tas I. Prenatal diagnosis of fetal intra-abdominal umbilical vein varix: report of 2 cases. J Clin Ultrasound. 2007;36(1):48–50.
9. Fung TY, Leung TN, Leung TY, Lau TK. Fetal intra-abdominal umbilical vein varix: what is the clinical significance? Ultrasound Obstet Gynecol. 2005;25(2):149–54.
10. Mulch AD, Stallings SP, Salafia CM. Elevated maternal serum alpha-fetoprotein, umbilical vein varix, and mesenchymal dysplasia: are they related? Prenat Diagn. 2006;26(8):659–61.
11. Volpe G, Resta L, Volpe P, Stefanelli R, Minervini M, Volpe N, Buonadonna L, Gentile M. Varix of the extra-hepatic portion of the fetal intra-abdominal umbilical vein: pathogenesis, prenatal sonographic diagnosis, and perinatal outcome. Minerva Ginecol. 2006;58(1):17–23.

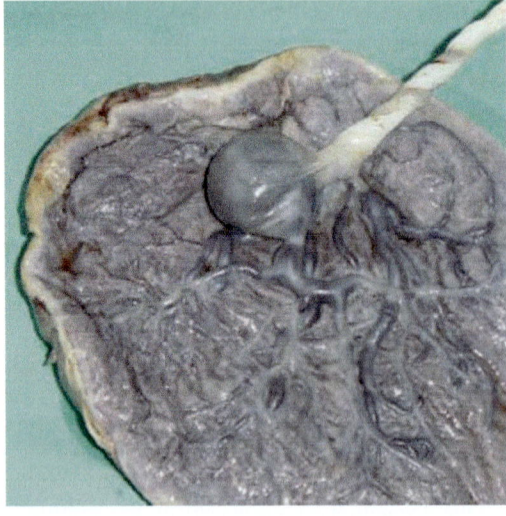

Fig. 18.3 A well-circumscribed aneurysm near the placental end of the cord

12. Sepulveda W, Mackenna A, Sanchez J, Corral E, Carstens E. Fetal prognosis in varix of the intrafetal umbilical vein. J Ultrasound Med. 1998;17(3):171–5.

13. Benirschke K, Kaufmann P. Pathology of the human placenta. 4th ed. New York: Springer; 2000. p. 373–5.

14. Sepulveda W, Corral E, Kottmann C, Illanes S, Vasquez P, Monckeberg MJ. Umbilical artery aneurysm: prenatal identification in three fetuses with trisomy 18. Ultrasound Obstet Gynecol. 2003;21(3): 292–6.

Part III

Normal Umbilicus

Embryology

The umbilical cord begins to form between 4 and 6 weeks, as the embryonic disc takes a cylindrical shape; located at the lower third of the embryo, the proximal portion of the umbilical cord begins to form and develops as a sac herniation, which houses the guts until the tenth week of gestation. At this time the umbilical cord is short, usually shorter than the head-to-tail (crown-rump) length of the embryo and of proportionately large diameter. It is not able to tolerate rotation about itself or the formed embryo. This initial stalk develops in the centre of the implantation site, which is the reason the cord presents at the centre of the placenta.

By 10 weeks, the intestines leave the proximal cord and return to the abdominal cavity, the elongation of the cord begins and the location of the umbilicus (belly button) positions in the middle third of the embryo. The elongation of the umbilical vein and arteries coincides with the development of Wharton's jelly, an umbilical cord connective tissue.

Embryologically, the fascial margins of the umbilical defect are formed by the third week of fetal life when the fourfolds of the somatopleure tend to fold inward. An umbilical cord is produced in the fifth week. By the tenth week of embryonic life, abdominal contents return from their location outside in the coelom into the developing abdominal cavity. The vitelline duct and the allantois regress by the fifteenth to sixteenth week. If any of these processes are defective, umbilical malformations will be manifested.

19.1 Separation of the Umbilical Cord

Normal Separation: The umbilical cord of the newborn usually separates and sloughs by the end of the second postnatal week (Fig. 19.1).

However, a wide variation exists in the age at which cord separation occurs in healthy infants with regard to ethnicity, geographical location and methods of cord care (Chap. 14).

The time at which the umbilical cord separates is often a cause of concern to parents; several studies in both developing and developed countries have followed healthy newborns to determine the effect of perinatal factors such as birth weight, gestational age, type of delivery and neonatal complications on umbilical cord separation. A study of 911 neonates by Oudesluys-Murphy et al. [1] determined the mean time of cord separation as 7.4 days (SD, 3.3; range, 1–29 days).

In 1993, a follow-up of 293 consecutive healthy term newborns by Rais-Bahrami et al. [2] estimated the mean age at cord separation to be 10.9 days. Other studies have reported the mean age at cord separation to range between 5.8 and 10.9 days [3].

Although the precise mechanism of cord separation is not known; drying, infarction, collagenase activity, necrosis and granulocyte influx may all influence the time at which it occurs. Superimposed bacterial infection of the umbilicus may delay this process. Perinatal fac-

© Springer International Publishing AG 2018
M. Fahmy, *Umbilicus and Umbilical Cord*, https://doi.org/10.1007/978-3-319-62383-2_19

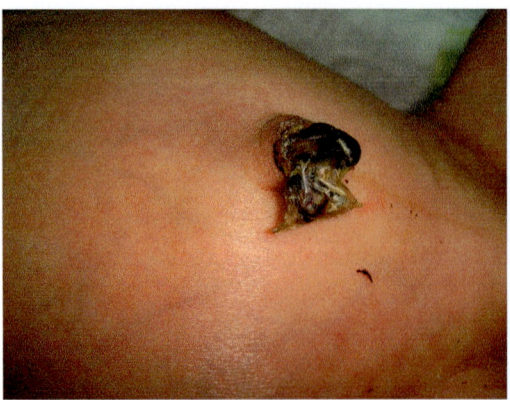

Fig. 19.1 Normal dried umbilical stump, before fallen down

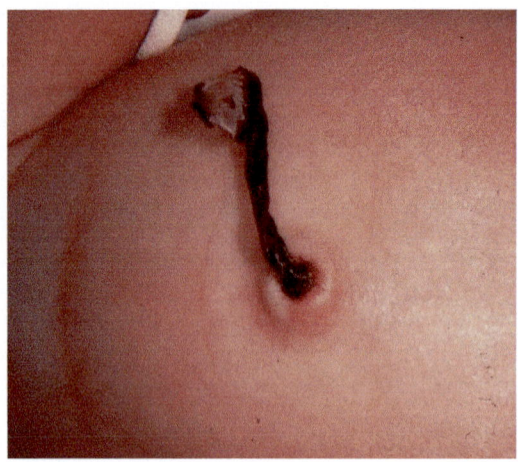

Fig. 19.2 Delayed cord separation

tors influencing the histology of the umbilical area have been studied in neonates who had died when cord separation was occurring or had just been completed. Histopathological results showed that the older the infant was at death, the greater was the degree of infiltration of polymorphonuclear cells into the area of separation of the umbilical cord. Granulocyte influx and phagocytosis play a role in the resorption of the umbilical cord base leading to involution, cord separation and healing [4].

The movement of neutrophils towards sites of inflammation and emigration from the bloodstream is mediated by various families of adhesion molecules including integrins and selectins.

19.2 Delayed Separation of the Umbilical Cord (Fig. 19.2)

A marked delay in cord separation raises the suspicion of leucocyte adhesion deficiency (LAD), a rare disorder leading to defective neutrophil function. Patients with LAD type I have been found to have a history of delayed umbilical cord separation and omphalitis in infancy. As this immunologic disorder has a high morbidity and mortality, screening and early detec-

tion are recommended. Also this has prompted increased referrals for screening for immune defects.

Overall, cord separation may be said to be delayed when it occurs after 2 weeks and is considered well beyond the normal limit when it occurs after 3 weeks of age [5].

When cord separation is delayed in healthy infants with no local or systemic infections, an important diagnostic consideration is a persistence of urachal or vitellointestinal duct anomalies (Chaps. 33 and 34).

References

1. Oudesluys-Murphy AM, Eilers GAM, de Groot CJ. The time of separation of the umbilical cord. Eur J Pediatr. 1987;146(4):387–9.
2. Rais-Bahrami K, Schulte EB, Naqvi M. Postnatal timing of spontaneous umbilical cord separation. Am J Perinatol. 1993;10(6):453–4.
3. Coffey PS, Brown SC. Umbilical cord-care practices in low- and middle-income countries: a systematic review. BMC Pregnancy Childbirth. 2017;17:68. doi:10.1186/s12884-017-1250-7.
4. Novack AH, Mueller B, Ochs H. Umbilical cord separation in the normal newborn. Am J Dis Child. 1988;142(2):220–3.
5. Wilson CB, Ochs HD, Almquist J, et al. When is umbilical cord separation delayed? J Pediatr. 1985;107(2):292–4.

Anatomy and Physiology of the Umbilicus

Size of the umbilicus: At 1975 Baroudi [1] described in his paper that a normal navel resembled a round, depressed scar and measured 1.5–2 cm in diameter. These characteristics were not based on any objective data taken from subjects. Three years later, in 1978, Dubou and Ousterhout [2] reported their measurements of umbilical size from 100 nonobese patients (no BMI reported). Of the 100 subjects, 36 were men and 64 were women, ranging in age from 18 to 69 years. The mean ± SD height and width of the umbilicus was 2.1 ± 0.6 cm and 2.3 ± 0.7 cm, respectively.

The umbilicus was located at a mean ± SD of −0.7 ± 1.3 cm in relation to the iliac crest (crest at zero). There were differences seen in the position between men and women. There were no statistical differences in measurements between the races.

The abdominal wall at the umbilical region is formed of:

1. The skin
2. The superficial fascia and more or less fat
3. The superficial sheath of the abdominal muscle
4. The rectus abdominis
5. The deep layer of the sheath
6. The subperitoneal connective tissue
7. The peritoneum

In the midline of the abdomen, the muscle layers are replaced by a thick cord of connective tissue, forming the linea alba, which, at the umbilicus, may reach 1 cm in breadth.

The umbilicus contains the obliterated orifices of three umbilical vessels, namely, one vein with a thin wall and wide lumen and two arteries with thick walls and narrow lumens. The vein lies at the 12 o'clock position, whereas the two arteries are located at the 4 and 8 o'clock positions when facing the umbilicus (Chap. 6).

Blood supply of the umbilicus: The middle of the anterior abdominal wall, including the umbilicus, is supplied by the branches of the superior and inferior epigastric arteries. The two epigastric arteries anastomose together on each side of the umbilicus and form an important alternative channel for blood flow in case of aortic coarctation. The superficial veins form a venous network radiating from the umbilicus. A few small veins called the paraumbilical veins connect this network with the portal vein through the umbilicus and along the ligamentum teres. This connection forms an important portosystemic venous anastomosis.

The two umbilical arteries form umbilical ligaments—one on each side of the median umbilical ligament. These arteries connect the superior vesical vessels with the umbilicus. These arteries function to support the urinary bladder anterolaterally [3].

Umbilical innervations: The ventral rami of the nerves T7–L1 supply the anterior abdominal wall through the lower five intercostal (T7–11) and subcostal (T12) nerves, as well as the iliohypogastric and ilioinguinal nerves carrying L1. The umbilicus is segmentally innervated by T10.

Lymphatic drainage: The lymph drainage of the skin of the abdominal wall above the umbilicus drains into the anterior (pectoral) axillary lymph nodes, whereas that below it drains into the superficial inguinal lymph nodes. The lymphatics of deep tissue, including the muscles and fascia above the umbilicus, drain into the parasternal lymph nodes, whereas that below the umbilicus pass through the external iliac lymph nodes to reach para-aortic nodes (Fig. 20.1).

Contents of the umbilicus: The umbilical scar contains four fetal structures: (1) the umbilical vein, which passes to the liver along the suspensory ligament; (2) and (3) the umbilical arteries, passing downward and outward to the bladder; and (4) the urachus, which passes to the bladder (Fig. 20.2).

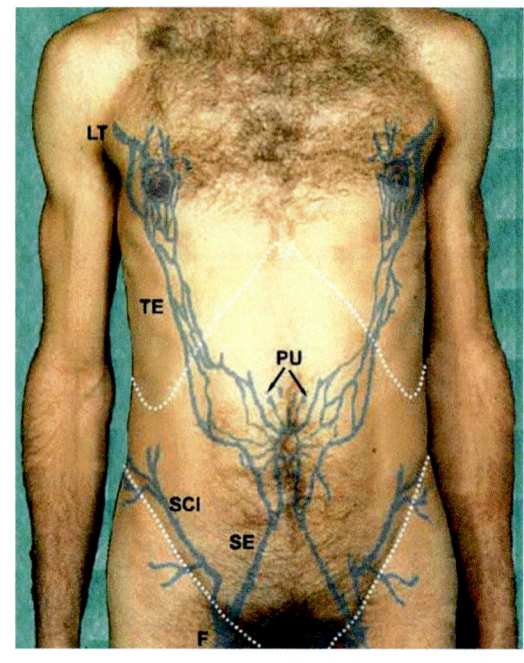

Fig. 20.1 Lymphatic drainage of umbilicus

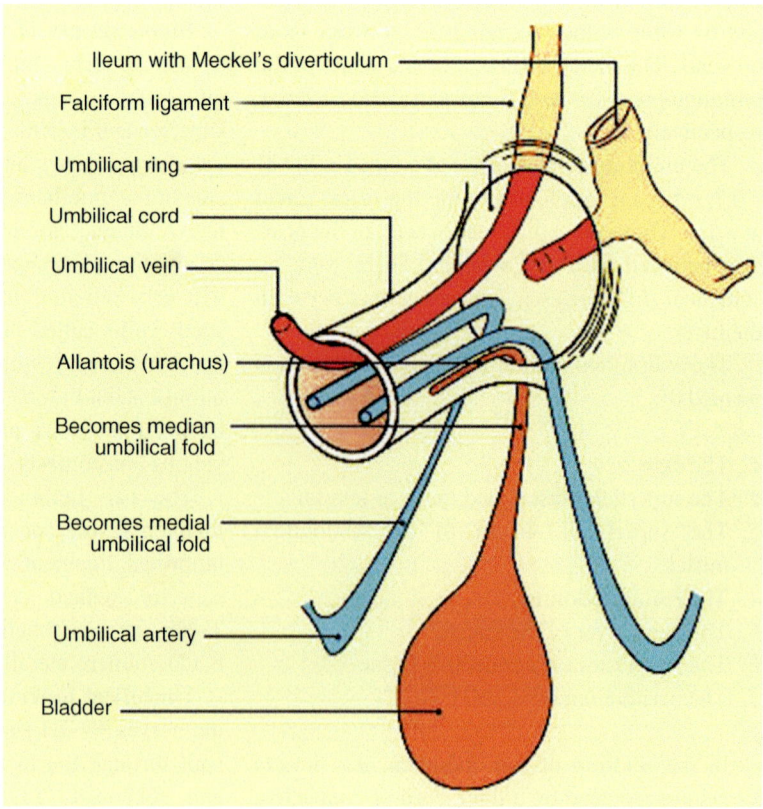

Fig. 20.2 Contents and potential embryonic remnants of the umbilicus

The umbilicus is usually infundibular in form and surrounded by an elevated outer margin, that is the cushion or base, at the bottom of which is a concealed scar left after the umbilical cord stump falls off; such scar (cicatrix) may be situated in or near a shallow skin depression, which is called the furrows. The mamelon can be more or less prominent and must be regarded as the remnants of the solid lower part of the umbilical cord, which contained the umbilical arteries and urachus. Finally, when the mamelon exists, its projection from the umbilical depression forms a natural surrounding furrow, which may more than one. Each mentioned component of the normal umbilicus may or may not be present, thus giving rise to a large variety of intermediary forms.

So the umbilicus is composed of four distinct anatomic structures (Fig. 20.3):

- Mamelon: Area of central hump.
- Cicatrix: Dense scar, which marks the intersection of fetal intra- and extraembryonic mesoderm.
- Cushion: Slightly raised skin margin around the mamelon and cicatrix; cushion may form a prominent skin folds or ridges.
- Furrows: The depression inside the cushion and surrounding the mamelon.

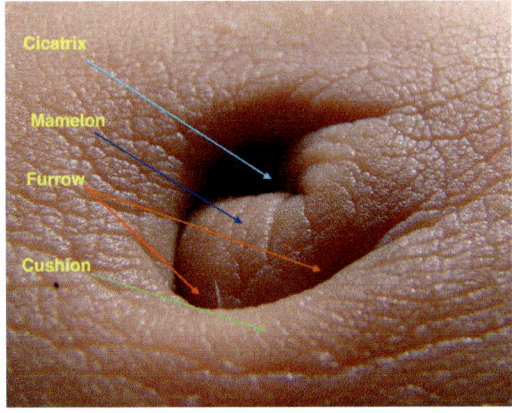

Fig. 20.3 Normal structural contents of the umbilicus, four distinct structures in normal umbilicus

Histologic appearance of the umbilicus: The umbilical pit is at first covered over with squamous epithelium but is devoid of papillae. Later the epithelium is identical with that of the outer skin; the scar, however, is usually lacking in sebaceous or sweat glands; this explains rarity of sebaceous cysts in the umbilicus.

Umbilical ring: The umbilicus lies over the umbilical ring, which is the last part of abdomen to close in fetus or after birth. In some conditions such as omphalocele, gastroschisis, bladder or cloacal exstrophy, prune belly syndrome and umbilical hernia, this defect is not closed and may be too large and may change the appearance and the position of the umbilicus.

The inner surface of the umbilicus is free and separated from the abdominal cavity by the parietal peritoneum which is covered by an umbilical fascia of variable thickness; this ring makes a reinforcement of the peritoneum. This opening with its borders measures about 1 cm or more in diameter, with its upper margin arched and its lower margin rectangular. The central orifice is about 2–4 mm in diameter, and it is closed solely by a ball of fat. The margins of the orifice are formed by the oblique fascia of the aponeurosis of the linea alba, to which they are added behind the fibres of the arch, so that there is formed a homogeneous mass. The upper border of the ring is free; the inferior border receives the insertion of the urachus in the umbilical arteries, which form in adult the median and two medial umbilical ligaments, respectively [4] (Fig. 20.4).

The vein is attached sometimes to the right or to the centre and may be divided into filaments. The fusion of these various cords with the base of the ring results in a fibrous nodule which is thick and very adherent to the skin. The parietal peritoneum covers the inner surface of the ring; it is only lightly adherent and in stout subjects is usually separated by adipose lobules. Sometimes it passes directly over the orifice and at other times is depressed [4]. At this point only the skin and peritoneum close the abdominal cavity (Chap. 28).

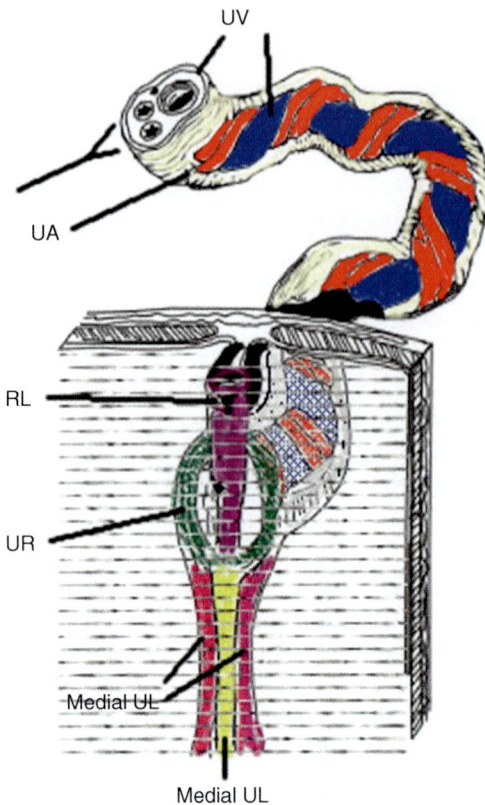

UV

UA

RL

UR

Medial UL

Medial UL

Fig. 20.4 *UR* umbilical ring, *UV* umbilical vein, *UA* umbilical arteries, *LR* ligamentum teres, *UL* umbilical ligaments

References

1. Baroudi R. Umbilicaplasty. Clin Plast Surg. 1975;2:431–48.
2. Dubou R, Ousterhout DK. Placement of the umbilicus in an abdominoplasty. Plast Reconstr Surg. 1978;61:291–3.
3. Snell R. Clinical anatomy by regions. 9th ed. New York: Lippincott; 2012.
4. Chang-Seok O, et al. Morphologic variations of the umbilical ring, umbilical ligaments and ligamentum teres hepatis. Yonsei Med J. 2008;49(6):1004–7.

Umbilical Position

The umbilicus is a prominent mark on the abdomen, with its position being relatively consistent among humans. The umbilicus itself typically lies at a vertical level corresponding to the junction between the L3 and L4 vertebrae, with a normal variation among people between the L3 and L5 vertebrae.

Umbilicus lies within a line from the lower border of the xiphisternum to the upper border of the pubis, the position of the umbilicus in newborns was 59.28 ± 5.2 (54.1–64.5) percent off this line, and it was independent of other anthropometric data, but this position shows a narrow window of variation in different races, it was measured on 50 neonates in England, and the normal position of the umbilicus was about 60% off the way from xiphisternum to the pubis and was independent of variables mentioned above [1].

The umbilicus is located more inferiorly in men compared with women and that on average the distance to the iliac crests is shorter in women, the latter of which is likely related to differing body types by sex, specifically the wider hips in women compared with men [2].

The umbilicus is displaced superiorly during pregnancy, and inferiorly by ascites and hepatosplenomegaly (Tanyol's sign). In such cases the positional shift of the umbilicus is revisable, and the umbilicus will resume its normal position once the primary diseases resolved (Fig. 21.1).

Many abdominal wall malformations and deformities are associated with abnormal umbilical position, usually a downward displacement, and the most common condition in which the umbilicus is usually ectopic inferiorly is the bladder, exstrophy cloacal exstrophy and OEIS syndrome (omphalocele, exstrophy of the cloaca, imperforate anus and spinal abnormalities) (Fig. 21.2).

Cases of prune belly syndrome may had an ectopic insertion of umbilical cord, and the resultant umbilicus may be higher up or lowdown in the linea alba (Fig. 21.3).

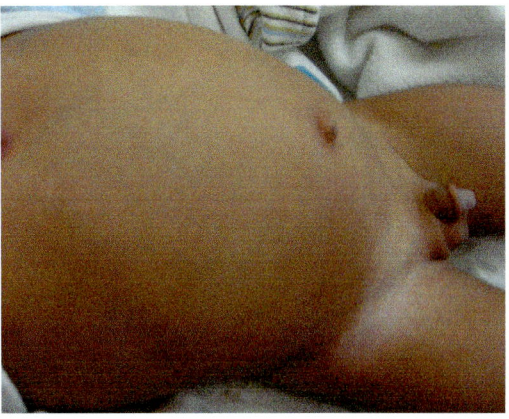

Fig. 21.1 Umbilicus shifted down secondary to abdominal distension with hepatosplenomegaly

© Springer International Publishing AG 2018
M. Fahmy, *Umbilicus and Umbilical Cord*, https://doi.org/10.1007/978-3-319-62383-2_21

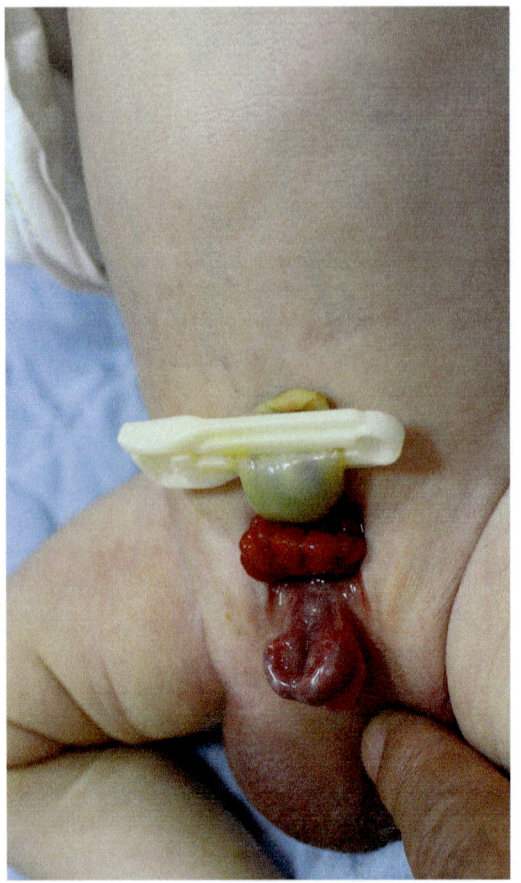

Fig. 21.2 Low seated umbilical cord with bladder exstrophy

Patients with achondroplasia had a low umbilicus, and few cases had been reported with low seated umbilicus without any detectable abdominal wall defects or other congenital anomalies (Fig. 21.4).

Abnormal umbilical appearance or location may be a finding in a genetic disorder such as:

- Robinow's syndrome, a rare inherited disorder of short stature and macrocephaly with frontal bossing, the umbilicus is high, flat and poorly epithelialized.
- Axenfeld–Rieger syndrome, a rare genetic disorder that includes malformations of the anterior chamber of the eye and teeth; the umbilicus is broad and prominent with a large stalk and redundant skin.
- In Aarskog–Scott syndrome, a disorder of multiple limb and genital abnormalities with short stature; the umbilicus can be either flat with radiating branches of the cicatrix or a deep longitudinally oriented ovoid depression [3].
- Syndromes associated with proboscoid umbilical hernia, which was described in Chap. 28, may be associated with abnormally lower umbilicus at the midline.

I never came across any reported case of ectopic umbilicus inserted away from midline.

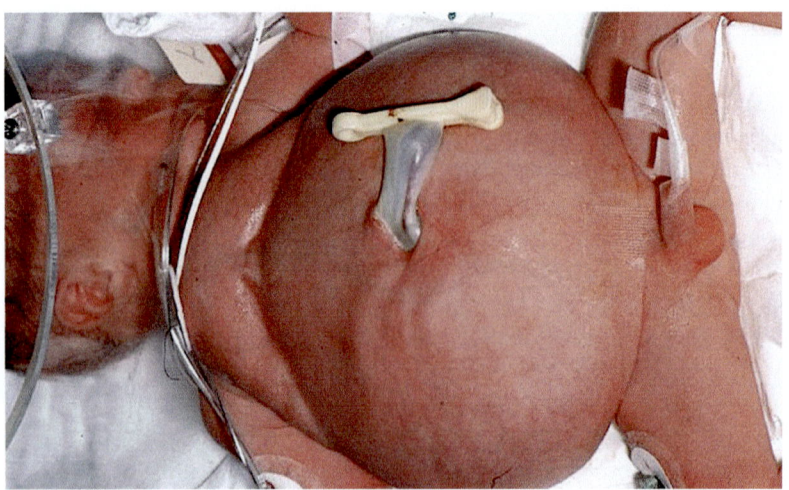

Fig. 21.3 A case of prune belly syndrome with abnormal and unusual higher position of the umbilicus

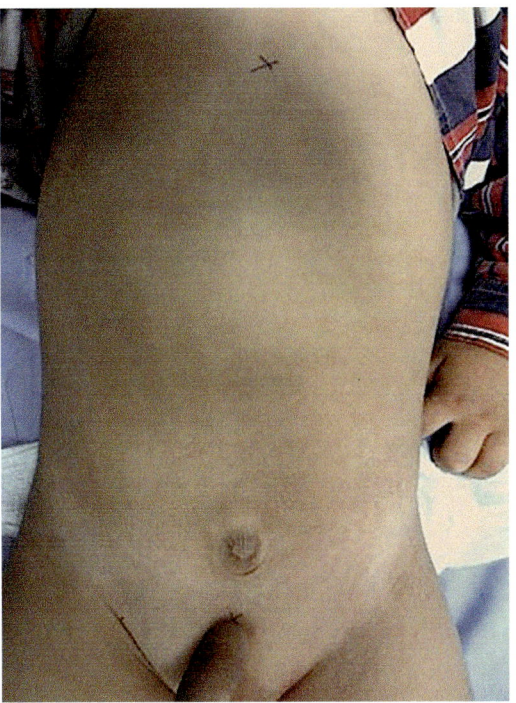

Fig. 21.4 Significant low positioned umbilicus without any other congenital anomalies

References

1. Williams AM, Brain JL. The normal position of the umbilicus in the newborn: an aid to improving the cosmetic result in exomphalos major. J Pediatr Surg. 2001;36:1045–6.
2. Yu D, Novicoff WM, Gampper TJ. The average size and position of the umbilicus in young men and women. Ann Plast Surg. 2016;76(3):346–8.
3. Tsukahara M, Fernandez GI. Umbilical findings in Aarskog syndrome. Clin Genet. 1994;45:260–5.

Umbilicus Types and Shapes

Early at 1904, Bert and Viannay [1] classified umbilicus to three main types:

- Transverse umbilicus
- Round umbilicus
- Vertical umbilicus

Thomas Stephen Cullen [2] described and illustrated in details, as many as 60 different forms of umbilicus which may be assumed under normal condition.

Cullen Mentioned an Important General Rules for Evaluation of the Navel Variants:

- The umbilicus in the infant is much larger in proportion to the body weight than is that of the adult.
- There is no definite relation between the size of the adult and the size of his umbilicus. A small person may have a large umbilicus and vice versa.
- In the adult the depressed umbilicus is far more frequent than the elevated or button-shaped type.
- The button umbilicus is an infantile form.
- A large umbilicus of the horizontal type is associated with a wide linea alba, also with diastasis of the recti abdominis muscles.
- Obesity has a tendency to produce the funnel-shaped umbilicus [2].

There were a variety of umbilical shapes encountered in literatures, including crescent, round, triangular and oval (vertical, transverse or oblique). The most common umbilical shape noted in a Japanese study was the round shape in both men and women, with the oval shape being the second most common [3].

As mentioned before the umbilicus had four main structures—mamelon, cicatrix, farrows and cushion. The combination of these items results in a very wide anatomical variants:

- Absent farrows will result in projection of mamelon, with cicatrix at its dome without folding, and of course no cushion will be appreciated, this usually called as *outie* or button-like umbilicus (Fig. 22.1). Outies are often mistaken for umbilical hernias but are actually a completely different condition affecting only the shape, with a normal umbilical ring, unlike an umbilical hernia.

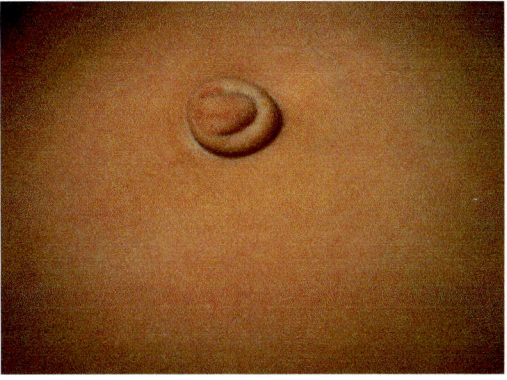

Fig. 22.1 Protrusion (outie) umbilicus

© Springer International Publishing AG 2018
M. Fahmy, *Umbilicus and Umbilical Cord*, https://doi.org/10.1007/978-3-319-62383-2_22

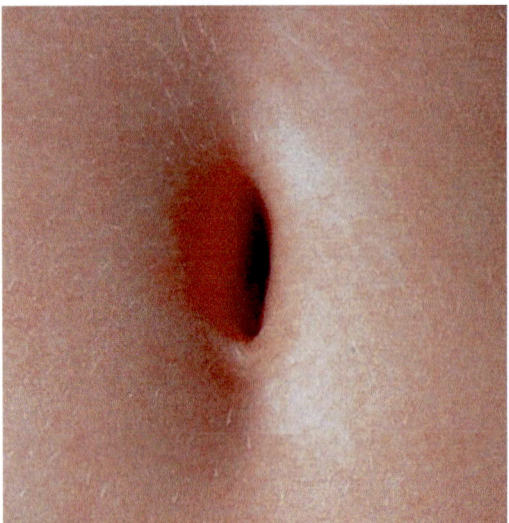

Fig. 22.2 Absent or concealed cicatrix and mamelon and shallow cushion, ended with an innie umbilicus

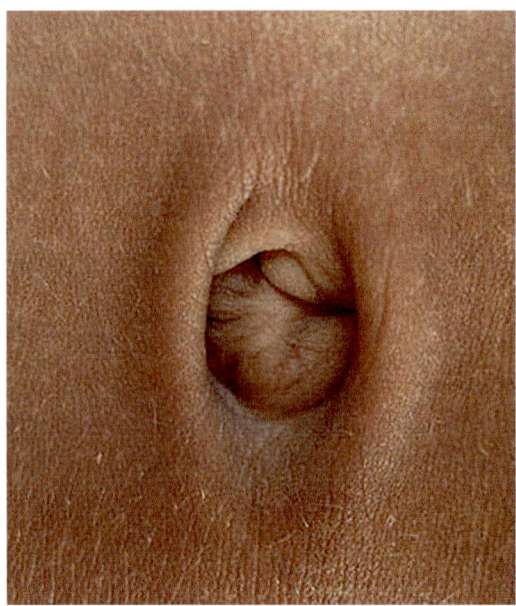

Fig. 22.3 Verticle umbilical cushions

- Absent or concealed cicatrix and mamelon and shallow cushion will end with a different grades of umbilici look like a dimple or pit, and this called *innie* umbilicus. About 90% of the people have an innie, with the other 10% being outies. The reason for the occurrence of an outie versus an innie is a matter of some dispute (Fig. 22.2).
- Distribution of cushion with normal cicatrix and mamelon in the form of two horizontal or transverse folds will give raise to a two distinct umbilical types: vertical and horizontal umbilici (Figs. 22.3 and 22.4), the vertical navel may be either slit like or oval.
- In cases of incomplete cushion; the umbilicus will present as a crescent or horseshoe fold. If the cushion has been padded with adipose tissue, a funnel-shaped umbilicus will result.
- The umbilicus with two vertical primary folds may have another transverse small horizontal one which gives raise to T-shaped umbilicus (Fig. 22.5).

The T- or vertically shaped umbilicus with superior hooding consistently scored the highest in aesthetic appeal [4].

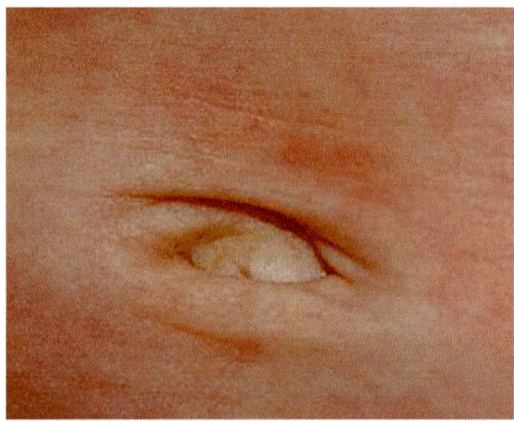

Fig. 22.4 Horizontal umbilicus

The ideal umbilicus should have a natural contour, prominent depth, minimal additional scars and proper superior hooding. Shinohara et al. [5] emphasized that an umbilicus with a natural appearance consists of a ring, a tubular wall, a sulcus, and a bottom, without any excess skin that would interfere with the aesthetic aspect of the umbilicus.

In addition, Lee et al. [6] suggested that an aesthetically optimal female umbilicus must

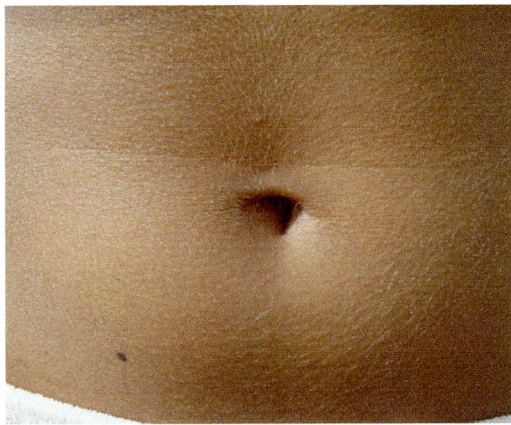

Fig. 22.5 T-shaped umbilicus

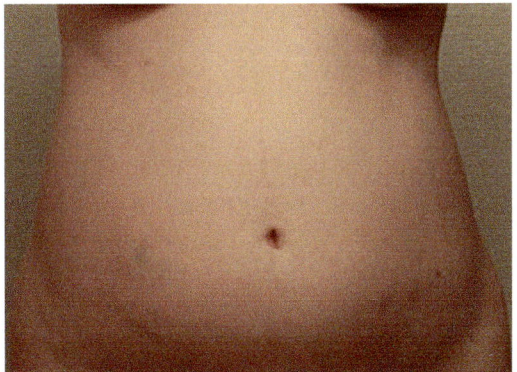

Fig. 22.6 Abnormally small tiny umbilicus

possess the following properties: a vertical ratio of 46:54 (with respect to the xiphoid process and the lower limit of the vulvar cleft), a midline horizontal position, and an oval shape with no hooding or superior hooding. Abnormal smaller umbilicus, without any cushions or mamelon is not acceptable aesthetically (Fig. 22.6).

A flat umbilicus is a rare clinical finding. It can be an isolated anomaly or a component manifestation of Aarskog syndrome [7].

During pregnancy, the uterus presses the navel of the pregnant woman outward, and it usually retracts after birth (Fig. 22.7).

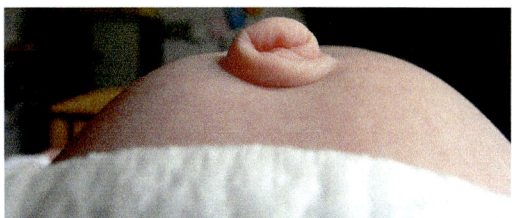

Fig. 22.7 Outie during pregnancy

22.1 Ugly Umbilical Scar

Umbilical reconstruction after exampholas, umbilical hernia repair (specially proboscoid and large one) and after abdominoplasty may end with a non acceptable ugly scar.

Rarely the normal umbilical cord may end with unappealing umbilicus in terms of size, shape, depth/length and overall appearance; many factors may contribute to give raise this defacement:

- Simply outie umbilicus are the result, of individual variations in the anatomy. So the baby's delivery, the cutting, clamping and aftercare of the umbilical cord; none of that affects the navel's final appearance. The navel's shape has nothing to do with anything the physician does or subsequent care from the nurses. It's an anatomical wild card. Having the 'other' kind of navel can take a psychic toll [8].
- Long umbilical stump with a different length of abdominal wall skin creeping over the membranous covering of the cord may result in outie umbilicus; significant long skin covering the umbilical cord is called 'cutis navel', which was discussed in Chap. 31; such cases are usually had no abdominal wall defect and have to be distinguished from umbilical hernia (Fig. 22.8).
- Presence of abnormal structure within the umbilical stump like cases of vitellointestinal or urachal remnant will result in a disfigured large umbilicus, and sometimes the contents of the stump, i.e. arteries and veins, form separate scars within the umbilicus and lead to formation of double mamelons (Fig. 22.9).

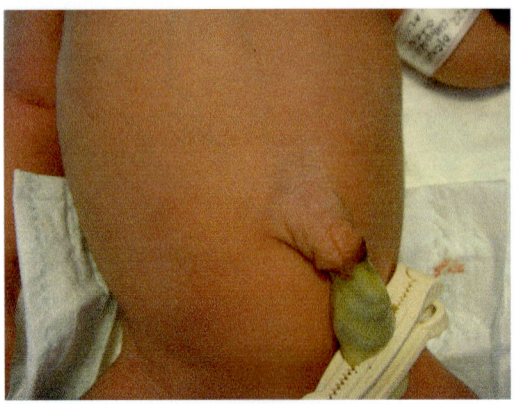

Fig. 22.8 Long umbilical skin creeping over the distal cord may end with an outie umbilicus

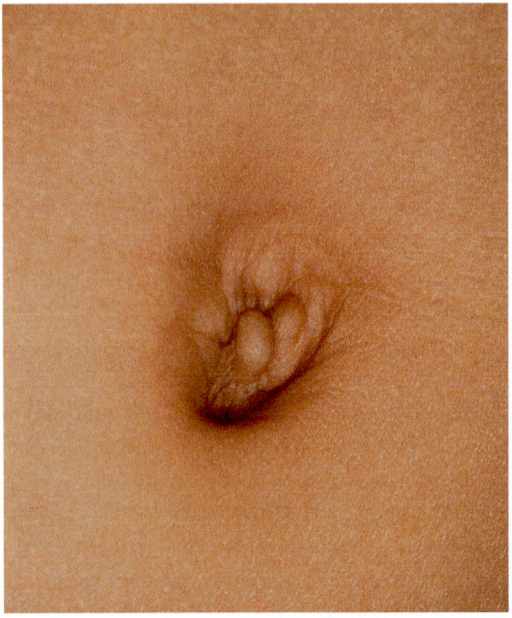

Fig. 22.9 Umbilicus with a two separate scars of obliterated umbilical arteries

- Omphalitis, umbilical granuloma and progressive abdominal distension at early life may contribute to the formation of an ugly umbilicus.

References

1. Bert A, Charles Y. Etude sur la morphologic de l'ombilic. Compt. rend, de l'assoc. des anatomistes. 104, vi, 116.
2. Cullen TS. Anatomy of the umbilical region. In: Cullen TS, editor. Embryology, anatomy, and disease of the umbilicus together with diseases of the Urachus. Philadelphia: WB Saunders; 1916. p. 34–89.
3. Yu D, Novicoff WM, Gampper TJ. The average size and position of the umbilicus in young men and women. Ann Plast Surg. 2016;76(3):346–8.
4. Abbas H, Guneren E, Eroglu LO, Uysal A. A natural looking umbilicus as an important part of abdominoplasty. Aesthet Plast Surg. 2003;27:139.
5. Shinohara H, Matsuo K, Kikuchi N. Umbilical reconstruction with an inverted C-V flap. Plast Reconstr Surg. 2000;105:703–5.
6. Lee SL, DuBois JJ, Greenholz SK, et al. Advancement flap umbilicoplasty after abdominal wall closure: postoperative results compared with normal umbilical anatomy. J Pediatr Surg. 2001;36:1168–70.
7. Tsukahara M, Fernandez GI. Umbilical findings in Aarskog syndrome. Clin Genet. 1994;45:260–5.
8. Shephard BD, Shephard CA. The complete guide to Women's health. Tampa: Mariner Publishing; 1982. p. 419. http://hdl.handle.net/10822/792311

Umbilical Landmark

23

The umbilicus is an important landmark on the abdomen since its position is relatively consistent among humans. The umbilicus is also used to visually separate the abdomen into quadrants.

The umbilical region, in the anatomists abdominal pelvic nine-region scheme, is the area surrounding the umbilicus (navel). This region of the abdomen contains part of the stomach, the head of the pancreas, the duodenum, a section of the transverse colon and the lower aspects of the left and right kidney (Fig. 23.1).

The navel comes in the centre of the circle enclosing the spread-eagle figure in Leonardo da Vinci's 'Vitruvian Man'. The Vitruvian Man is a world-renowned drawing with accompanying notes created by Leonardo da Vinci around the year 1487 as recorded in one of his journals. It depicts a nude male figure in two superimposed positions with his arms and legs apart and simultaneously inscribed in a circle and square. The drawing and text are sometimes called the Canon of Proportions or, less often, Proportions of Man. It is stored in the Gallerie dell'Accademia in Venice, Italy, but is only displayed on special occasions his famous drawing on human proportions. This illustrates the principle that in the shift between the spread-eagle pose and the straight pose, the apparent centre of the figure seems to move, but in reality, the navel of the figure, which is the true centre of gravity, remains motionless (Fig. 23.2).

The colour of the skin around the umbilicus is crucial for diagnosis of different diseases:

- Yellowish discolouration around the umbilicus could be seen in cases of pancreatitis.

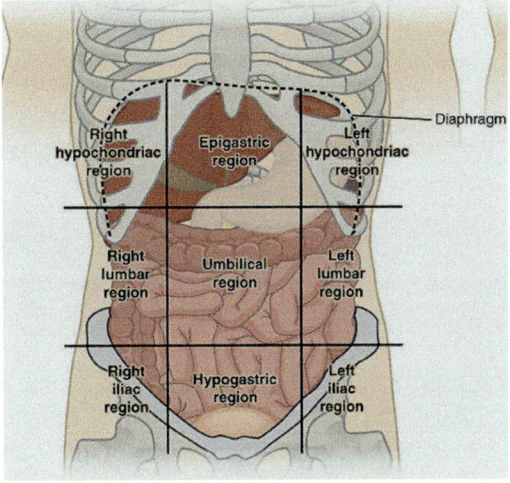

Fig. 23.1 Anatomical abdominal quadrants

M. Fahmy, *Umbilicus and Umbilical Cord*, https://doi.org/10.1007/978-3-319-62383-2_23

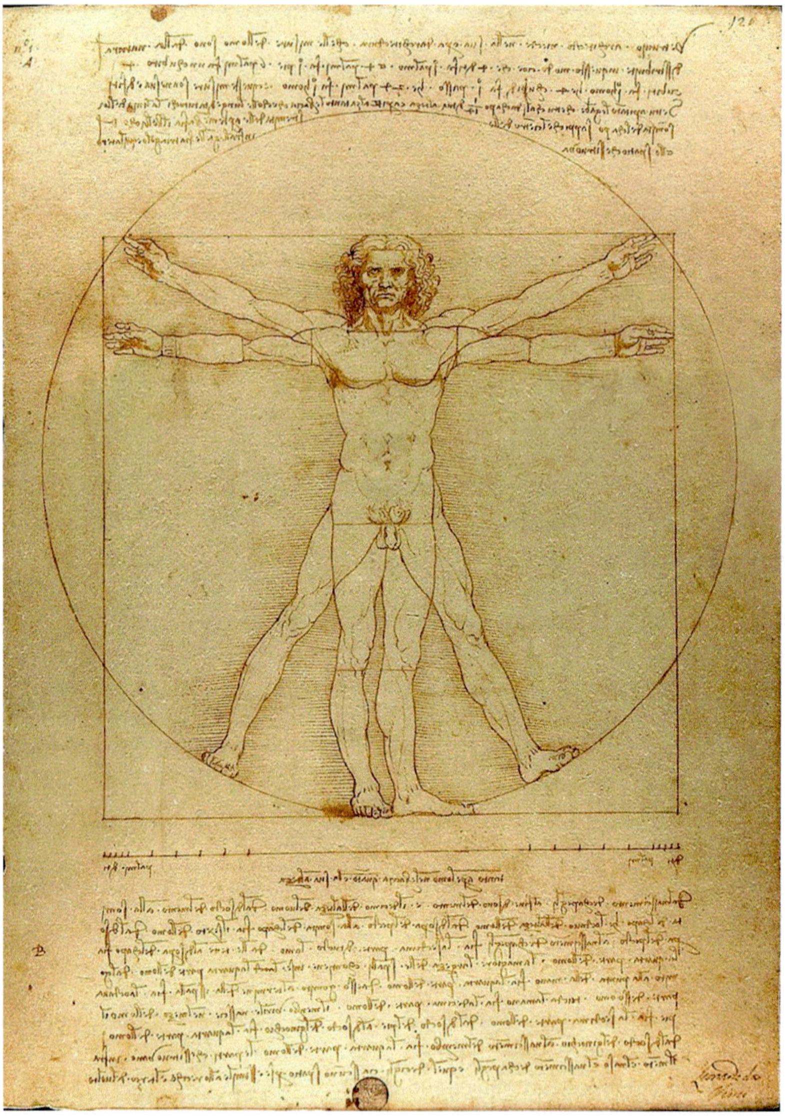

Fig. 23.2 Vitruvian Man, by Leonardo da Vinci

- Bluish umbilical discretion is sometimes diagnostic for cases of ruptured ectopic pregnancy (Cullen's sign), and it arises from the spread of retroperitoneal blood into the falciform ligament and subsequently to sub-cutaneous umbilical tissues through the connective tissue covering of the round liga-ment, so it could be seen also in any case of intraperitoneal haemorrhage (Fig. 23.3).
- Abdominal pain of acute appendicitis starts at the umbilicus and then shift to the right iliac fossa.

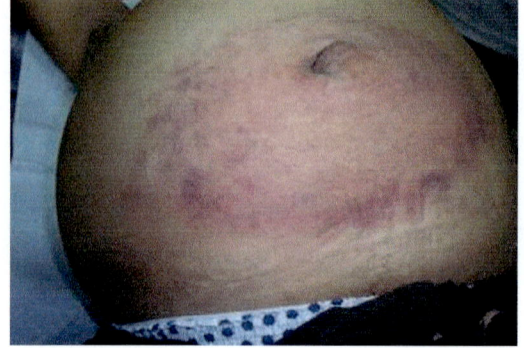

Fig. 23.3 Bluish umbilical discretion (Cullen's sign)

Uses of the Umbilicus

24

Umbilical venous catheterization (UVC): The umbilical vein catheters are a commonly used procedure for intravenous access in neonatal intensive care units. The UVC facilitates the administration of parenteral nutrition and intravenous medication and blood sampling (Fig. 24.1). The use of UVC, however, may cause complications such as infection, thrombus formation and catheter tip migration. Omphalitis is not a rare complication after UVC especially in developing countries but the most serious complication, which is not realized early but had a lethal sequels is portal venous thrombosis and portal hypertension [1]. Also it is claimed that improper placement of UVC may predispose to necrotizing enterocolitis especially in preterm babies [2].

UVC could be done by a closed method as other central line catheterization or through an open operative technique especially in older infants; umbilical vein remains patent and could be cannulated up to the age of 2 months (Fig. 24.2).

Umbilical artery cannulation may be used for blood sampling and invasive monitoring, but the procedure is not innocent. The first cannulation of an umbilical artery is attributed to Dr. Virginia Apgar in the late 1950s. Today, umbilical artery catheterization is a common procedure in the neonatal intensive care unit and has become the

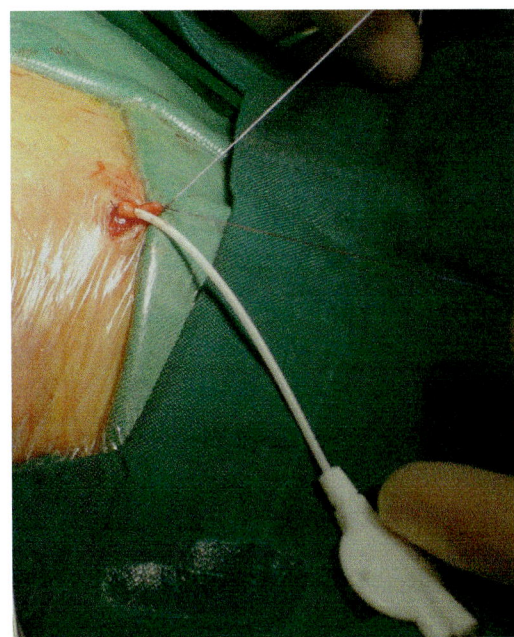

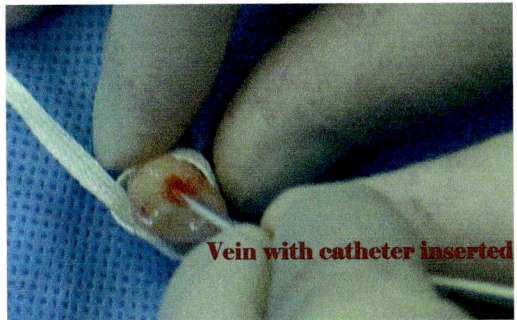

Fig. 24.1 Umbilical venous catheterisation

Fig. 24.2 Open (operative) UVC

© Springer International Publishing AG 2018
M. Fahmy, *Umbilicus and Umbilical Cord*, https://doi.org/10.1007/978-3-319-62383-2_24

Fig. 24.3 Preterm monitoring via umbilical arterial, umbilical venous catheterization and umbilical temperature probe

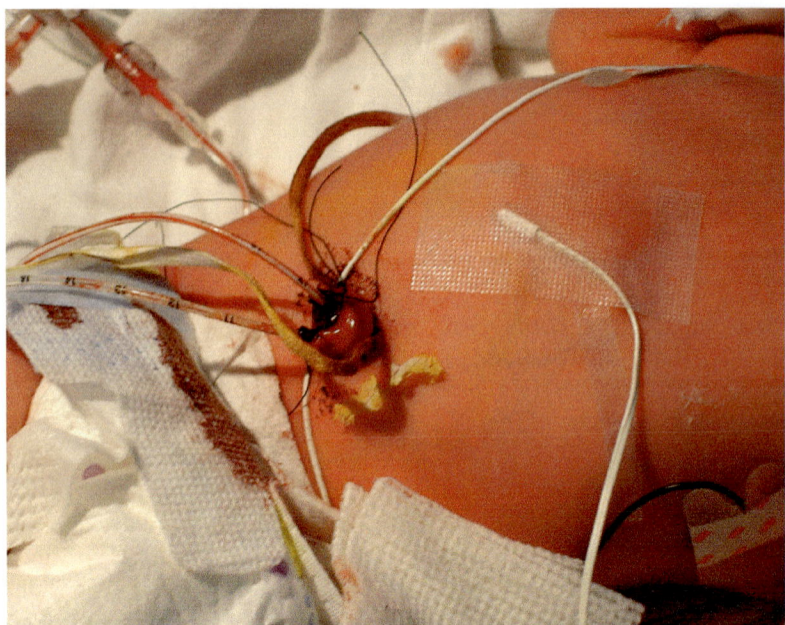

standard of care for arterial access in neonates. The umbilical artery can be used for arterial access during the first 5–7 days of life, but it is rarely used beyond 7–10 days [3].

The umbilicus may be used to measure the body temperature of infants less than 3 months old as an alternative to the rectal route [4] (Fig. 24.3).

Umbilical port (Fig. 24.4): The umbilicus also represents a natural embryonic orifice, and recently it is the preferred site for laparoscopic surgery as it provides a more or less safe site to introduce an instrument, as well as leaves a minimal cosmetic scar after the procedures; umbilicus is the preferable port for cases of single-port laparoscopy with different names: single-port laparoscopy (SPL), one-port umbilical surgery, natural orifice transumbilical surgery, laparoendoscopic single-site surgery (LESS) and embryonic natural orifice transumbilical endoscopic surgery [5].

Umbilical incision: Umbilical incision was used long time ago without resulting in a subsequent obvious scar, not only in paediatric surgery for many operations like Ramstedt's pyloromyotomy for cases of pyloric stenosis but also for many reconstructive surgery like transumbilical breast augmentation.

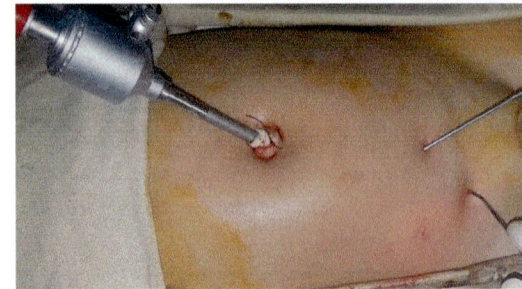

Fig. 24.4 Umbilicus as a port for laparoscopy

Umbilical stoma: The umbilicus could be used as a site for temporary colostomy for infants with imperforate anus or Hirschsprung's disease, some surgeons claiming that this site provides a betterlooking scar than that in other sites (Fig. 24.5).

Also, some surgeons and even patients may prefer the umbilicus as a port for urinary diversions as in cases of ileal conduit and Mitrofanoff procedure (Fig. 24.6).

Belly button used for body fat measurement: By measuring a vertical fold about 2 inches directly right of the belly button by a special clipper (Fig. 24.7).

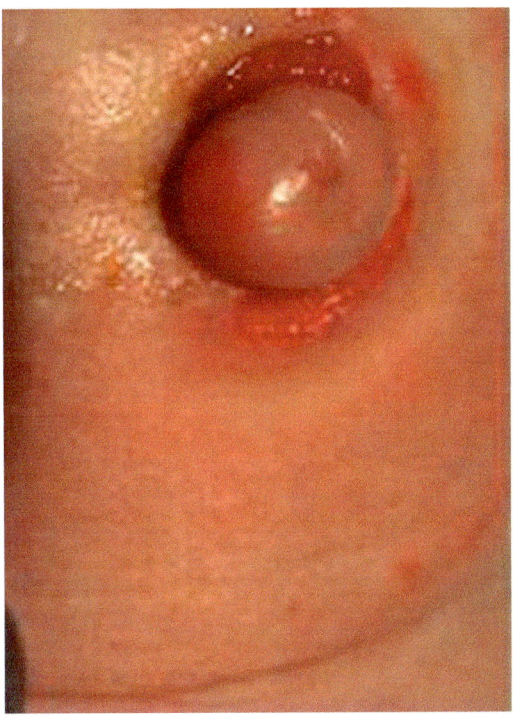

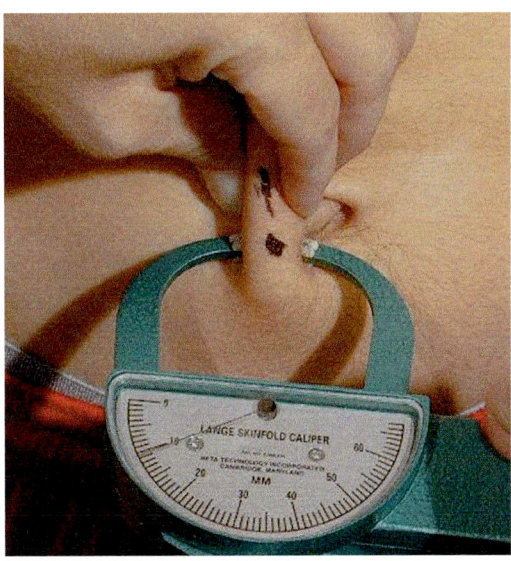

Fig. 24.7 Body fat measurements

Fig. 24.5 Colostomy at the umbilicus

References

1. Butler-O'Hara M, Buzzard CJ, Reubens L, McDermott MP, DiGrazio W, D'Angio CT. A randomized trial comparing long-term and short-term use of umbilical venous catheters in premature infants with birth weights of less than 1251 grams. Pediatrics. 2006;118(1):e25–35.
2. Sulemanji M, Vakili K, Zurakowski D, Tworetzky W, Fishman SJ, Kim HB. Umbilical venous catheter malposition is associated with necrotizing enterocolitis in premature infants. Neonatology. 2017;111(4):337–43. doi:10.1159/000451022.
3. Hermansen MC, Hermansen MG. Intravascular catheter complications in the neonatal intensive care unit. Clin Perinatol. 2005;32(1):141–56.
4. Kravitz H. Temperature of the umbilicus. J Pediatr. 1966;68(3):418–22.
5. Fawkner-Corbett D, Nicholson JA, Bullen T, Cross P, Bailey D, Scott MH. Anatomical variation in the position of the umbilicus and the implications for laparoscopic surgery. Int J Surg. 2010;8(7):540–78.

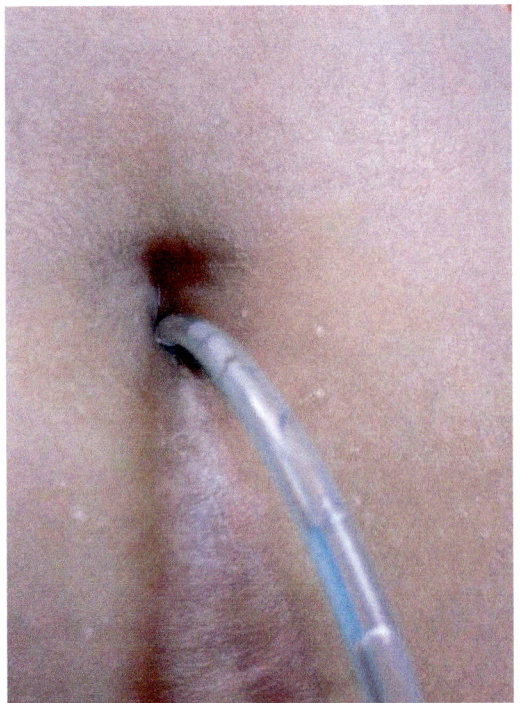

Fig. 24.6 Continent urinary stoma at the umbilicus in Mitrofanoff procedure. This photo reproduced with a kind permission from Prof Yogesh Kumar Sarin, Head of Pediatric Surgery Dept, Maulana Azad Medical College

25

Nomenclatures: Navel gazing, omphaloskepsis also called omphaloscopy, and omphalomancy (Fig. 25.1).

Definition: Omphaloskepsis meaning 'contemplating one's navel as an aid to meditation', sounds like it is thousands of years old. 'Skepsis' is a Greek word meaning 'the act of looking, or inquiry'. The word "omphaloskepsis" was invented only in the 1920s.

Navel Gazing is also related to Omphalopsychite: Hamilton Bailey wrote in his textbook of *Physical Signs in Clinical Surgery*, 'Every time an abdomen is examined, the eyes of the clinician, almost instinctively, rest momentarily upon the umbilicus. How innumerable are the variations of this structure!'[1].

Gerhard Reibmann, a Berlin psychologist, believes that you can diagnose a person's life expectancy, general health and psychological state purely by looking at their belly button: "...." Understanding Yourself Through Your Navel [2].

He reckons that there are six different types of navel, and he claims that each one has a specific personality type and a specific life expectancy associated with it.

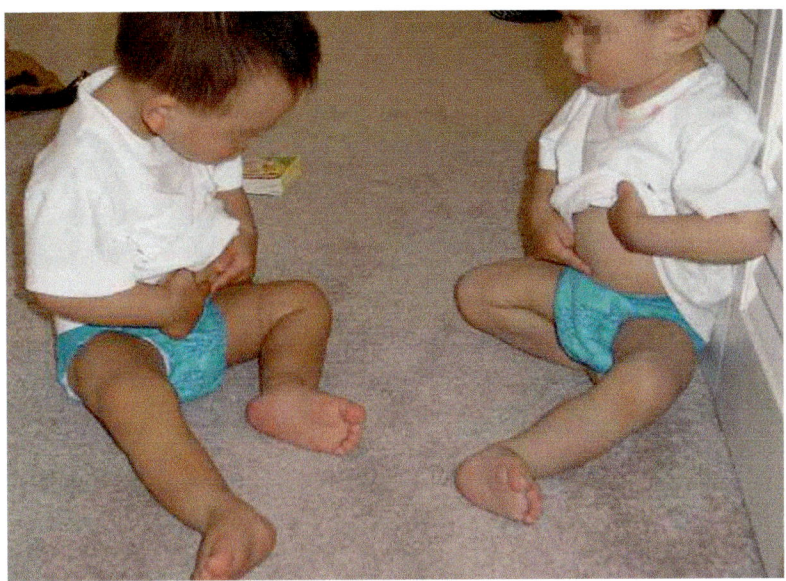

Fig. 25.1 Navel gazing among children

© Springer International Publishing AG 2018
M. Fahmy, *Umbilicus and Umbilical Cord*, https://doi.org/10.1007/978-3-319-62383-2_25

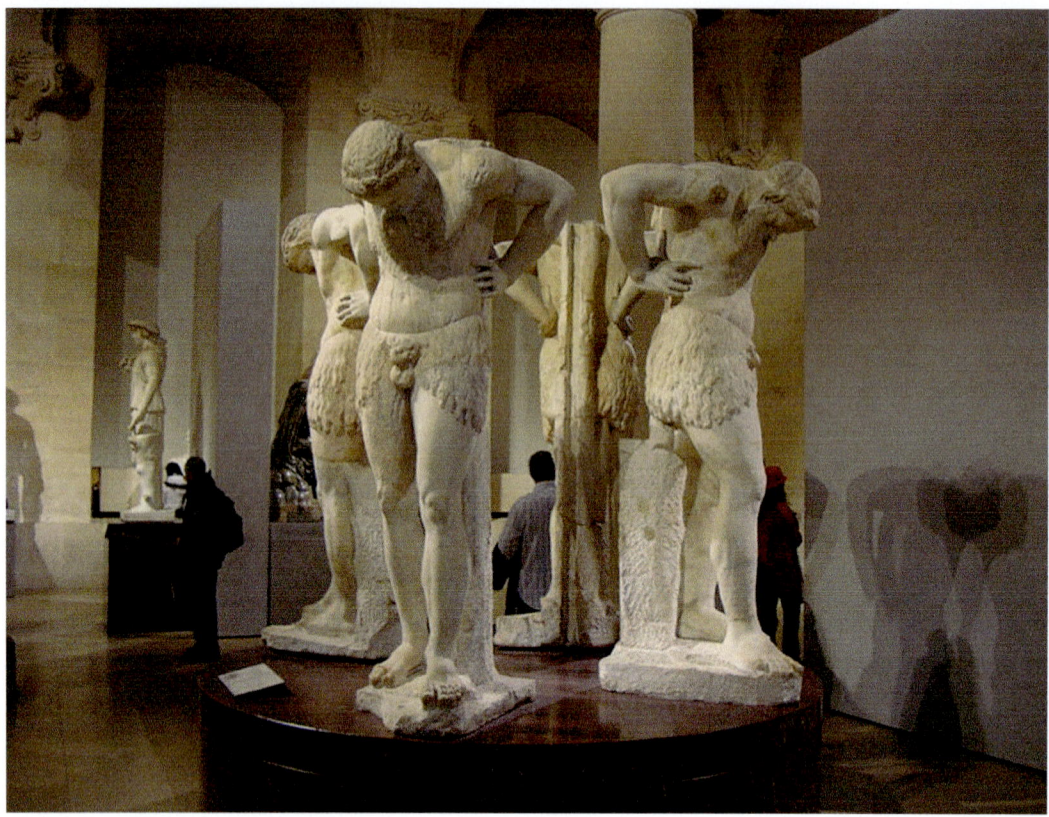

Fig. 25.2 Four large statues of satyrs looking down all standing in a circle at the Louvre, second century after J.C., Rome

Some children and adolescents who had an outies or other forms of ugly umbilicus may had a psychic trauma and exposed to ridicule; the child may recall an extreme measures to avoid public exposure, ducking into a corner of the locker room to change clothes, sucking in his stomach to create the illusion of an innie, tugging the waistband of the swimsuit above the midsection of his exposed body, so nobody could see his supposed damning malformation (Fig. 25.2).

References

1. Clain A. Hamilton Bailey's demonstrations of physical signs in clinical surgery. 14th ed. Bristol: John Wright & Sons Ltd and The English Language Book Society; 1967.
2. Powell FC, Daniel WP. Dermatoses of the umbilicus. Int J Dermatol. 1988;27:150–6. doi:10.1111/j.1365-4362.1988.tb04918.x.

Part IV

Acquired Umbilical Disorders

Omphalitis

Omphalitis will be discussed under the following headings:

- Neonatal omphalitis
- Adult omphalitis
  - Bacterial
  - Non bacterial
- Rare types of omphalitis

Nomenclature: Belly Button Infection of Newborns.

Definition: Omphalitis term usually applied for the bacterial neonatal umbilical stump infection, but other types of specific and non specific umbilical infection are roughly called omphalitis. It is an infection of the umbilicus and/or surrounding tissues, and it is predominantly a disease of the neonate, characterized by discharge from the umbilical cord stump with surrounding induration, erythema, and tenderness (Fig. 26.1).

Omphalitis is not only human-being disease, but it occurs also and commonly in the newborn calf, and chickens, in such cases omphalitis is a condition characterized by infected yolk sacs, often accompanied by unhealed navels in young fowl, and the resulting septicaemia contribute to perinatal mortality in several animal species (Fig. 26.2).

Funisitis (umbilical arteritis, or vasculitis) is an intrauterine inflammation of the connective tissue of the umbilical cord, it is typically preceded by vasculitis of the umbilical artery or veins and may be the result of chorioamnionitis, which may end with abortion. Funisitis may be detected either antenatally or immediately after

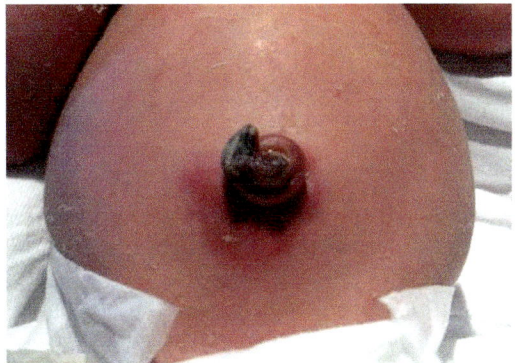

Fig. 26.1 Early bacterial omphalitis of neonate

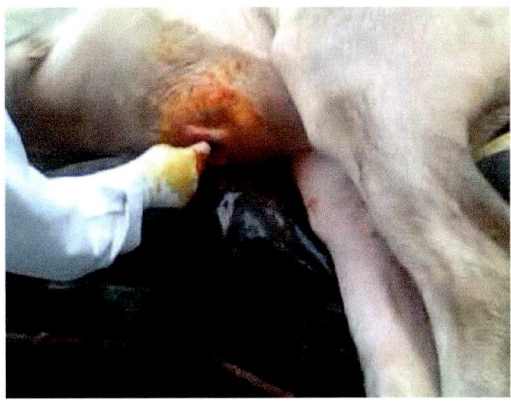

Fig. 26.2 Animal omphalitis, infected umbilical stump of a calf

birth, this usually results in a wet, foul-smelling umbilical stump and is usually caused by inflammation driven by group A strep (Fig. 26.3).

Fig. 26.3 Funisitis characterized by umbilical arterial infiltration of neutrophils

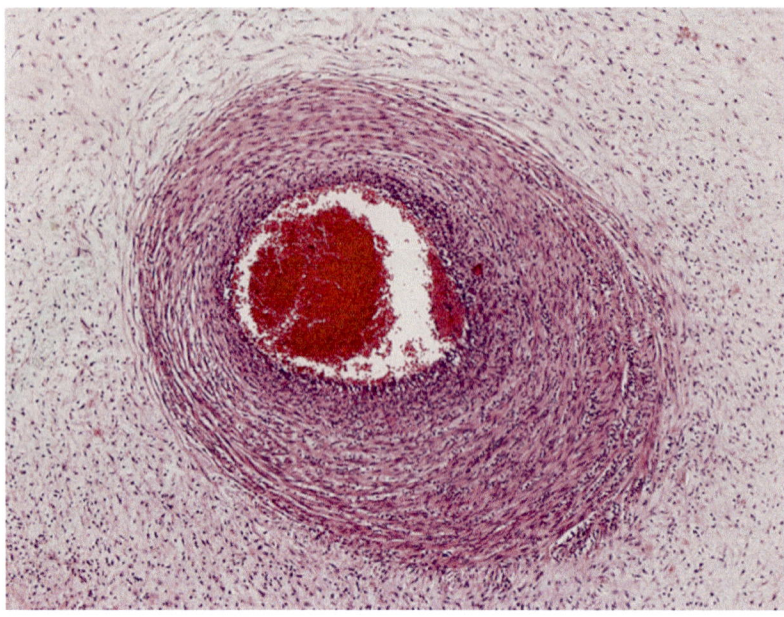

26.1 Neonatal Omphalitis
(Fig. 26.1)

Catarrhal omphalitis: It is also known as the 'weeping navel'.

The clinical signs of catarrhal omphalitis are:

- Serous (transparent) discharge from the umbilical wound.
- Slow healing of the wound.
- Slight reddening of the umbilical ring.
- Normal body temperature.

Sometimes the wound covered with a thick bloody crust under which the discharge accumulates.

In cases when catarrhal omphalitis prolongs for more than 2 weeks (with treatment) it can develop into belly button fungus. Infants with large body mass at birth and those who have a thick cord and a broad umbilical ring are prone to the development of belly button fungal infection.

If left untreated, catarrhal omphalitis develops into purulent omphalitis. If the infection spreads even further, the inflammation goes deeper into the umbilical tissue, which leads to the development of phlegmonous omphalitis.

26.2 Phlegmonous Omphalitis
(Fig. 26.4)

Phlegmon is a spreading diffuse inflammatory process with formation of purulent exudate. The term 'phlegmon' (from Greek 'phlegmone' means inflammation) mostly refers to a walled-off inflammatory mass.

Signs and symptoms: Phlegmonous omphalitis is a bacterial inflammation of the bottom of the umbilical wound, umbilical ring, and of the subcutaneous fat around the umbilical ring. This disease begins much alike catarrhal omphalitis. However, after some days transparent discharge from the wound turns into purulent. The umbilical ring becomes swollen, there is pronounced redness in the umbilical region. The subcutaneous fat becomes dense and starts bulging above the anterior abdominal wall. The skin around the navel is hot. Dilated vessels and sometimes red stripes are seen through the skin. Very often phlegmonous omphalitis is accompanied by an infection of umbilical vessels, which may lead to the development of septicaemia and an infected embolisation may spread to the liver, peritoneal or retroperitoneal spaces.

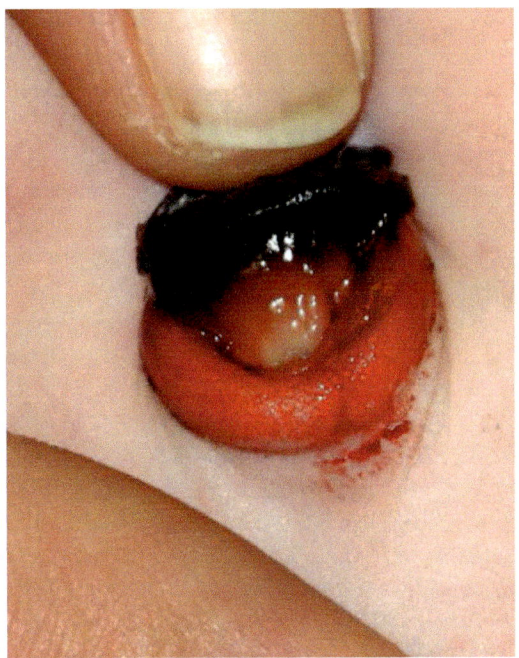

Fig. 26.4 Phlegmonous omphalitis, with purulent discharge beneath umbilical stump

Incidence: The current incidence of omphalitis in the United States is somewhere around 0.5% per year overall, the incidence rate for European countries falls between 0.2 and 0.7% [1]. But the incidence is greater in developing countries where rates are reported to be as high as 40%, although lacking of precise and complete data from many of these countries, the incidence is expected to be more higher and with a wide variance of the presentation and complications [2].

In one study of neonates admitted to an African general paediatric ward, omphalitis accounted for 28% of neonatal admissions. Another hospital study found that, in 47% of infants hospitalized with sepsis, cord infection was the source of the illness, and that 21% of infants admitted for other reasons had omphalitis. A prospective study in urban slums found an incidence for umbilical sepsis of 30/1000 [3]. Many cases are under-reported as babies may be discharged early from hospital and not followed up at home. Cord care after delivery had a crucial role in reducing omphalitis rate, in one large

hospital study of newborns who were routinely bathed with hexachlorophene, the 6-year incidence of cord infections was 0.5% in newborns of normal weight and 2.08% in those born prematurely [4].

Sex: There is no sex predilection has been reported, although males may have a worse prognosis than females, also incidence does not appear to have any racial or ethnic predilection.

Age: In full-term infants, the mean age at onset is 5–9 days. In preterm infants, the mean age at onset is 3–5 days.

Risk Factors: Identified risk factors for neonatal omphalitis may be simply classified to:

- Maternal factors:
  - Intrauterine infection, like placental infection (chorioamnionitis)
  - Uncontrolled mother diabetes
- Delivery situation:
  - Prolonged delivery and early rupture of membranes, nonsterile delivery, and delivery at home.
  - Unsterile cord cutting
- Neonatal factors:
  - Low birth weight, and prematurity
  - Patients who have a weakened or deficient immune system.
  - Neonates who are hospitalized and subject to invasive procedures.
  - Sick babies with other infections such as blood infection (sepsis) or pneumonia.
  - Patients who have had umbilical catheters (Fig. 26.5).

Umbilical catheters have been used in NICUs for drawing blood samples, measuring blood pressure, and administration of fluid and medications for more than 25 years [5]. Catheterization of the umbilical vein is one of the fastest and easiest methods of gaining access to a deep vein. Complications associated with umbilical catheters include thrombosis; embolism; vasospasm; vessel perforation; haemorrhage; infection; gastrointestinal, renal, and limb tissue damage.

Babies with an umbilical catheters may develop omphalitis, due to bacterial colonization, it was found that the umbilical stump is frequently colonised with pathogenic organisms, even when topical antiseptics are regularly applied in the NICU. Also the use of a venous line for infusion of hypertonic or acidic solutions, such as parenteral nutrition solutions, may provide a necrotic focus for abscess formation [6].

Bacteriology: Omphalitis usually caused by *S. aureus*, group A strep (*Streptococcus pyogenes*) and occasionally by gram-negative bacilli like *Pseudomonas aeruginosa* and *E. coli*, also there is a significant role of anaerobes in this infectious disease specially in necrotizing omphalitis [7].

Approximately three fourths of omphalitis cases are polymicrobial in origin, aerobic bacteria are present in approximately 85% of infections, predominated by *Staphylococcus aureus*, group A *Streptococcus*, *Escherichia coli*, *Klebsiella pneumoniae*, and *Proteus mirabilis* [8].

Clinically: It is a rapidly progressive soft tissue infection that arises from the umbilicus and classically spreads along low resistance fascial planes, resulting in tissue necrosis and overwhelming sepsis. Umbilical stump bleeding may occurs with omphalitis as a result of delayed obliteration of the umbilical vessels (Fig. 26.6).

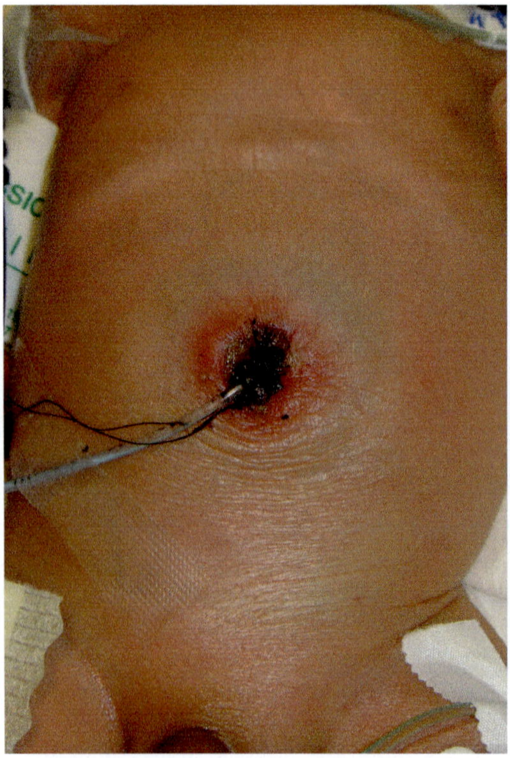

Omphalitis most commonly presents with signs of umbilical inflammation (erythema, induration, and swelling), with or without drainage from the umbilical stalk at the first 2 weeks of life (Fig. 26.7).

Close observation and a high degree of clinical suspicion for the development of localized fluid collections or necrotizing infection are critical and given the potential need for surgical intervention in cases of neonatal omphalitis.

Lack of erythema progression, absence of fever, initial hemodynamic stability and normal activity were falsely reassuring features that delayed operative intervention.

Patients with omphalitis may present with purulent umbilical discharge or periumbilical

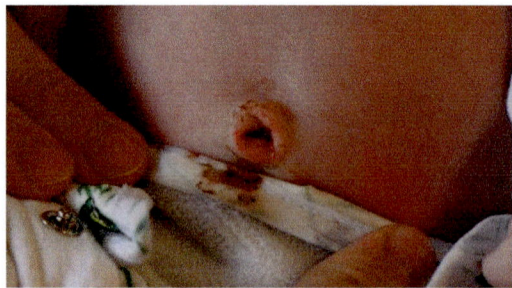

Fig. 26.6 Umbilical stump bleeding as a predictor of omphalitis

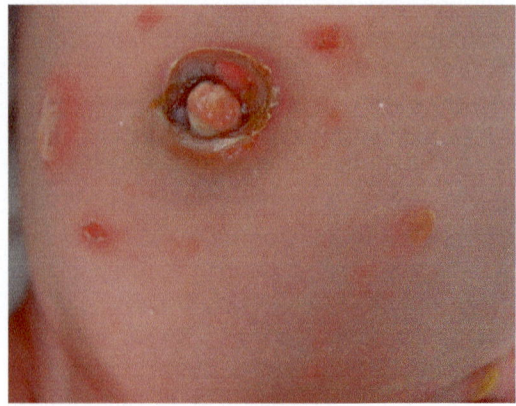

Fig. 26.7 Omphalitis with signs of inflammation (erythema, induration, and swelling)

Fig. 26.5 Omphalitis around an umbilical catheter

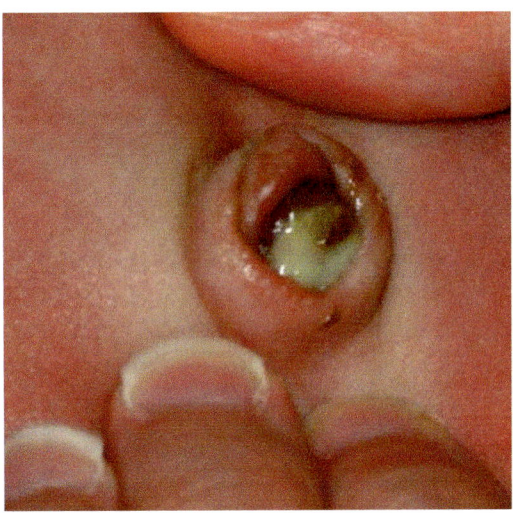

Fig. 26.8 Omphalitis with purulent discharge

cellulitis. Although infections may be associated with retained umbilical cord or ectopic tissue.

Cellulitis may become severe within hours and progress to necrotizing fasciitis and generalized sepsis. Even after the stump falls off, the patient with omphalitis may still present with a malodorous umbilicus with a superficial infection of the skin around the area, somewhat like impetigo (Fig. 26.8).

26.3 Differential Diagnoses

The differential diagnoses of omphalitis include:

- Umbilical granuloma (visible granuloma at the base of umbilicus) (Chap. 27)
- Patent vitellointestinal duct remnants (cystic swelling or fistulous opening with feculent matter discharge) (Chap. 36)
- Patent urachus (fistulous opening with urine discharging) or urachal cyst (Chap. 35)
- Necrotising enterocolitis (abdominal distention, bilious vomiting, bloody and stools)
- General sepsis
- Rarely, appendiculo-omphalic anomalies (Sect. 36.7)

26.4 Investigations

A microbiological swab of the umbilicus should be sent for aerobic and anaerobic cultures. A blood culture should be requested when appropriate. A blood count with differential for white cell counts may show a neutrohilia (or occasionally a neutropaenia).

Other investigations are necessary either to rule out other confusing conditions or to diagnose complications.

- A plain abdominal radiograph is useful if necrotising enterocolitis is suspected, in addition, it may reveal intraperitoneal gas in those cases with peritonitis (caused by gas-producing bacteria).
- Abdominal ultrasonography is useful in imaging the abdominal wall if a cyst is suspected, it is also helpful in the diagnosis of intraperitoneal, retroperitoneal, and hepatic abscesses.
- Doppler ultrasonography is helpful if portal vein thrombosis is suspected.
- In few cases with a suspicious of serious complication, a CT scan may be indicated, specially in cases with suspicious of liver affection (Fig. 26.9).

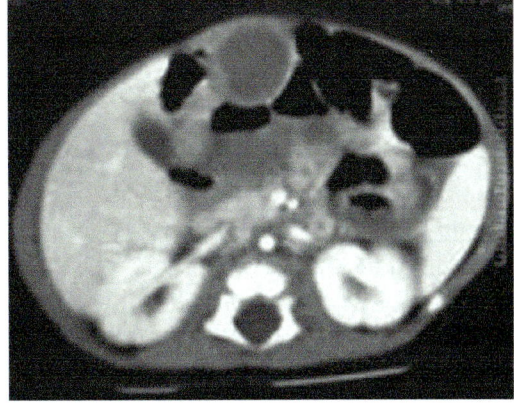

Fig. 26.9 CT scan showing an abscess in falciform ligament secondary to omphalitis

26.5 Complications

Potential sequelae of omphalitis include necrotizing fasciitis, myonecrosis, septicaemia, portal vein thrombosis, septic embolization; particularly, endocarditis and liver abscess, abdominal complications (e.g., spontaneous bowel evisceration, peritonitis, bowel obstruction, abdominal or retroperitoneal abscess), these sequelae are associated with significant morbidity and mortality.

In a retrospective review of 19 neonates and infants treated for major complications of omphalitis: Five (26%) patients presented with spontaneous evisceration of small bowel through the umbilical cicatrix, resulting in intestinal gangrene in one. Necrotizing fasciitis occurred in five (26%) patients involving mainly the scrotum, and in two involving the penis as well. Three (16%) patients had peritonitis, resulting in intra-abdominal abscesses in two. Three (16%) had superficial abscesses, two (11%) had hepatic abscesses resulting in extensive destruction of the left lobe in one, and one (5%) developed an adhesive intestinal obstruction [9].

The mortality rate among all infants with omphalitis, including those who develop complications, is estimated at 7–15%. The mortality rate is significantly higher (38–87%) after the development of necrotizing fasciitis or myonecrosis [10].

26.5.1 Necrotizing Fasciitis (NF) (Fig. 26.10)

Necrotizing omphalitis is a rare disease of the newborn with only few cases reported in the literature.

This is a florid bacterial infection of the skin, subcutaneous fat, superficial and deep fascia that complicates 8–16% of cases of neonatal omphalitis. It is characterized by rapidly spreading infection and severe systemic toxicity. Necrotizing fasciitis typically involves the abdominal wall but may also involve the scrotum or penis [9].

Necrotizing soft-tissue infections are caused by single or multiple organisms, that lead directly to tissue cell death, enzymatic destruction of supporting connective tissue, and destruction of host

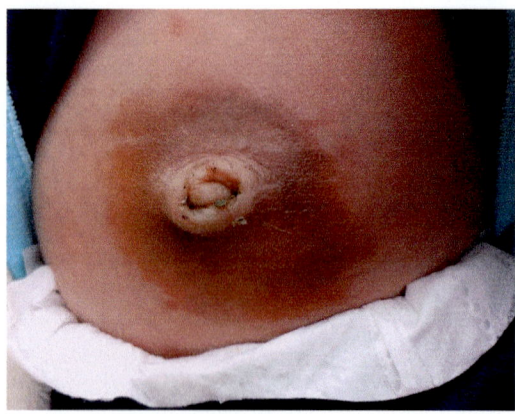

Fig. 26.10 Necrotizing fasciitis with early affection of the deep tissues

humoral and cellular immune responses to infecting organisms.

Certain organisms are well known to invade tissue and proliferate in necrotic areas. Group A *Streptococcus*, *S. aureus*, and *Clostridium* species may elaborate extracellular enzymes and toxins that can damage tissue, and may facilitate movement of organisms through soft-tissue planes, and limit host defences with penetration of systemic antimicrobial agents [11].

Reported survival rates for neonatal necrotizing omphalitis range anywhere from 19 to 40%, reflecting an aggressive disease with significant morbidity and mortality, in most series, omphalitis leading to necrotizing fasciitis is associated with a high mortality rate, up to 80%. Necrotizing fasciitis can also lead to portal venous thrombosis and portal hypertension [12].

Myonecrosis: It generally refers to infectious involvement of muscle in infants with omphalitis, the development of myonecrosis usually depends on conditions that facilitate the growth of anaerobic organisms. These conditions include the presence of necrotic tissue, poor blood supply, foreign material, and established infection by aerobic bacteria such as staphylococci or streptococci, but *C. perfringens*, in particular, does not replicate under conditions of an oxidation-reduction potential. In infections with mixtures of facultative aerobes and anaerobes, the aerobic organisms use oxygen available in tissue, allowing anaerobic bacterial growth (Fig. 26.11).

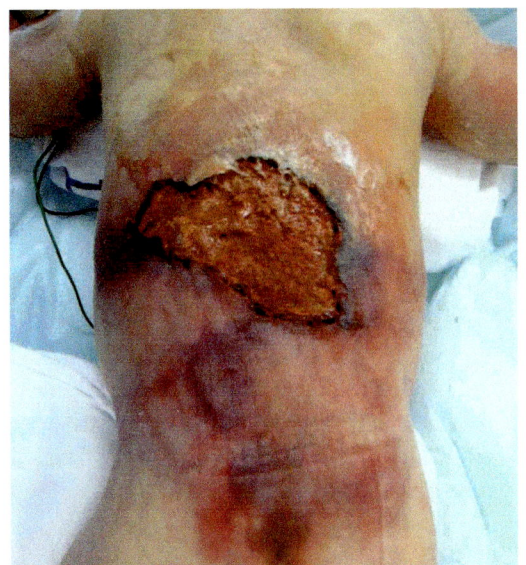

Fig. 26.11 Myonecrosis with extensive erosion of umbilicus and abdominal wall above it

The toxins produced in the anaerobic environment of necrotic tissue allow rapid spread of organisms through tissue planes. Local spread of toxins extends the area of tissue necrosis, allowing continued growth of organisms and increasing elaboration of toxins. Because of progressive deep tissue destruction and subsequent systemic spread of toxins, anaerobic infections, in particular, may be fatal if not treated promptly. In addition, rapid development of edema, which constricts the muscle within its fascia, may lead to ischemic myonecrosis [12].

Sepsis: This is the most common complication of omphalitis. In a study by Mason and colleagues, bacteremia was a complication in 13% of infants with omphalitis. In these infants, disseminated intravascular coagulation (DIC) and multiple organ failure may occur [13].

Septic embolization: Cord infections delay or prevent obliteration of the umbilical vessels, so pathogens are thereby provided a direct access to the systemic circulation.

If septic embolization arises from infected umbilical vessels, it may lead to metastatic foci in various organs, including the heart, liver, lungs, pancreas, kidneys, and skin [14].

Abdominal complications: Abdominal complications include spontaneous evisceration, peritonitis, bowel obstruction, abdominal abscess, retroperitoneal abscess, or liver abscess.

Long-term or late complications of omphalitis: Late complications occur several weeks, months, or years after omphalitis in the neonatal period. These may include nonneoplastic cavernous transformation of the portal vein, portal vein thrombosis, extrahepatic portal hypertension, and biliary obstruction. In one report of 200 patients undergoing portosystemic shunt for portal hypertension due to PVT, 15% of them were suspected to be the result of neonatal omphalitis. A portosystemic shunt may be required if portal hypertension develops [15].

Abscess formation of the falciform ligament in neonates is a known complication of omphalitis, where a soft tissue mass beneath the abdominal wall continuous with a thickened round ligament is a diagnostic feature of a falciform ligament abscess on USG or CT scanning. Many readily accessible abscesses are treated successfully with percutaneous drainage and antibiotics, but a successful treatment of the falciform ligament abscess is rather excision of the ligament itself (Fig. 26.9).

Umbilical Hernia: Umbilical hernia is a common problem in children in Africa, and it may be a result of weakening of the umbilical cicatrix from neonatal omphalitis. This is discussed in Chap. 28.

Umbilical granuloma may follow incompletely eradicated omphalitis due to chronic irritation, this will be discussed in Chap. 27.

Peritoneal adhesions are the result of previous subclinical or treated peritonitis from omphalitis. The adhesions may produce intestinal obstruction, which usually is not amenable to nonoperative measures. Laparotomy and lysis/excision of the adhesions are usually required.

26.6 Treatment of Omphalitis

Medical therapy: Include parenteral antimicrobial coverage for gram-positive and gram-negative organisms. A combination of an antistaphylococcal penicillin, vancomycin and an aminoglycoside antibiotic is recommended. Some believe that anaerobic coverage is important in all patients [16]. Omphalitis complicated by necrotizing fasciitis or myonecrosis requires a more aggressive approach, with antimicrobial therapy directed at anaerobic organisms as well as gram-positive and gram-negative organisms. Metronidazole or clindamycin may provide anaerobic coverage [16]. Medical therapy is indicated only when infection is present. Antibiotics are also administered for acute infection of omphalomesenteric and urachal remnants. Supportive care is essential for survival, these measures include the following:

- Infants should be treated at centers capable of supporting cardiopulmonary function.
- Ventilatory assistance and supplementary oxygen for hypoxemia or apnea unresponsive to stimulation.
- Intravenous fluid, vasoactive agents, or both (as indicated) for hypotension.
- Administration of platelets, fresh frozen plasma, or cryoprecipitate for disseminated intravascular coagulation (DIC) if clinical bleeding is suggested.
- In uncomplicated cases, erythema of the umbilical stump is expected to improve within 12–24 h after the initiation of antimicrobial therapy. Failure to respond may suggest disease progression, presence of an anatomic defect, or an immunodeficiency state.

Surgical Care: Management of necrotizing fasciitis and myonecrosis involves early and complete surgical debridement of the affected tissue and muscle, with the following considerations:

- Early surgical intervention may be lifesaving.
- Delay in diagnosis or surgery allows progression and spread of necrosis, leading to extensive tissue loss and worsening systemic toxicity.
- Although the extent of debridement depends on the viability of tissue and muscle, which is determined at the time of surgery, excision of preperitoneal tissue (including the umbilicus, umbilical vessels, and urachal remnant) is critically important in the eradication of the infection.

- These tissues can harbour an invasive bacteria and provide a route for progressive spread of infection after less extensive debridement.
- Several surgical procedures may be required before all nonviable tissue is removed.
- The mainstays of treatment for necrotizing omphalitis are early initiation of broad-spectrum antibiotics, surgical debridement, large wounds may be sutured later or replaced with skin graft.
- Intraperitoneal abscess or those located in the anterior abdominal wall and other locations should be drained at laparotomy, or accessed extraperitoneally if situated retroperitoneally.

Omphalitis Prevention: Staphylococcal epidemics of pyoderma and omphalitis emerged, the umbilicus was found to be an important reservoir for dissemination of *S. aureus*. Prophylactic routine application of antimicrobial agents to the cord stump helped to control these epidemics. However, successes in preventing colonization by one organism sometimes resulted in colonization by others of equal or greater pathogenicity. The practice of applying, an antiseptic to the cord is now common not only in hospital nurseries but also outside hospitals, yet it has not been thoroughly evaluated. During the 1950s there were outbreaks of omphalitis that then led to anti-bacterial treatment of the umbilical cord stump as the new standard of care. It was later determined that in developed countries keeping the cord dry is sufficient, (known as 'dry cord care') as recommended by the American Academy of Pediatrics. The umbilical cord dries more quickly and separates more readily when exposed to air. However, each hospital/birthing center has its own recommendations for care of the umbilical cord after delivery. Some recommend not using any medicinal washes on the cord. Other popular recommendations include triple dye, betadine, bacitracin, or silver sulfadiazine, there is little data to support any one treatment (or lack thereof) over another. However one recent review of many studies supported the use of chlorhexidine treatment as a way to reduce risk of death by 23% and risk of omphalitis by anywhere between 27 and 56% in underdeveloped countries [16].

26.7   Omphalitis in Adult

- Bacterial
- Non bacterial

Umbilical dermatitis is a common condition, it is usually associated with inadequate hygiene and deepening of umbilicus caused usually by obesity. The condition is really a dermatitis and analogous to intertrigo that often occurs between folds of the skin. Although it is primarily a 'seborrhoeic' dermatitis, but it frequently becomes secondarily infected with skin organisms.

The whole umbilicus may feel hard with dermatitis, especially if the discharge is secondary to another condition such as an ompholith (or, very rarely, a tumour deposit).

If the infection spreads into the subcutaneous tissues and the opening of the umbilicus becomes narrowed by oedema, the whole umbilicus can turn into an abscess.

Cullen described umbilical concretions with local inflammation in the abdominal wall, and in reviewing many cases previously published as tuberculosis and infected dermoids, he considered most of them to be examples of primary umbilical sepsis [17].

Clinical presentation may be obvious with a red, hot, tender swelling with a Peau d'orange appearance in and around the umbilicus (Fig. 26.12). Bacterial omphalitis in adults may be in the form of cellulitis, and if a pus forming organisms (Staphylococci, streptococci, or rarely gram negative organisms) find a way to the deep umbilical tissues an abscess usually formed with exudation of pus (Figs. 26.13 and 26.14).

Recurrent omphalitis at adulthood or older age should arouse the suspicious about the presence of congenital anomalies; like urachal or vitellointestinal remnants (Chaps. 35–36), or rare disorders like pilonidal sinus, omphalolithis or endometriosis in females (Chap. 31).

Recently, omphalitis is a minor postoperative complication after laparoscopic procedures. It is treated quite simply as an outpatient problem, but omphalitis represents discomfort for the patient, and it can cause a delay in the resumption of work. Also, above all, omphalitis is a risk factor for the development of incisional

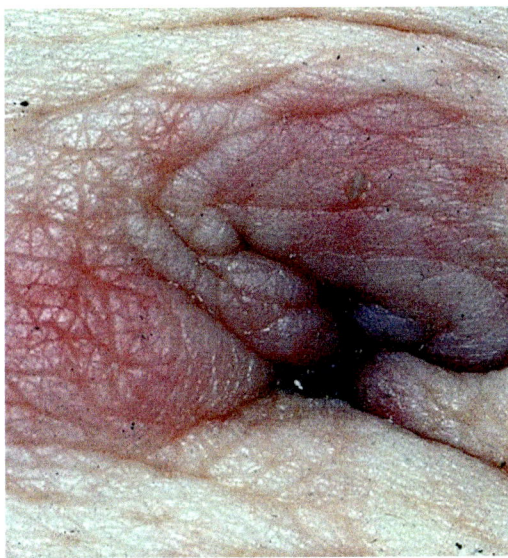

Fig. 26.12 High power magnification of an early adult omphalitis

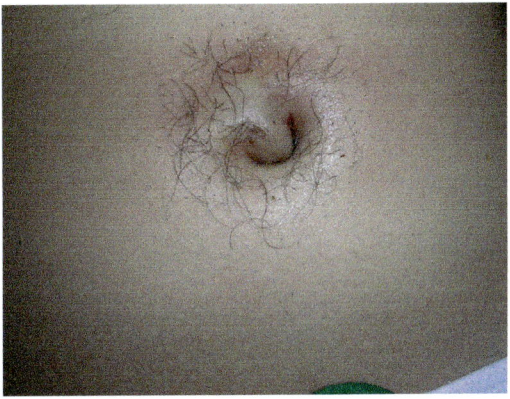

Fig. 26.13 Pyogenic adult omphalitis, with a well formed abscess

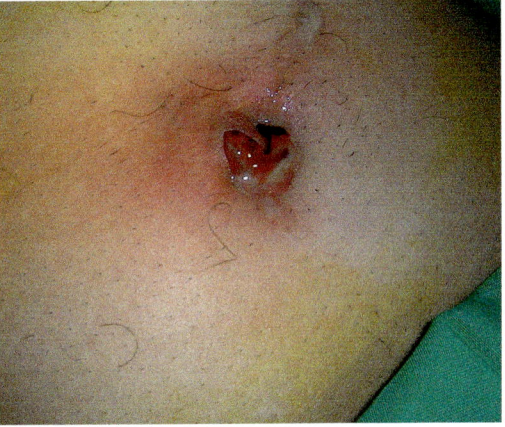

Fig. 26.14 Pus drainage from an umbilical abscess

umbilical hernia, which may occur in greater than 1% of cases [18].

Non bacterial adult omphalitis (Navel dermatitis): Specific and nonspecificic umbilical dermatitis may be a local manifestation of systemic dermatitis; like seborrhoeic dermatitis or psoriasis, but other chronic infection like fungus and tinea may which affect the umbilicus only, with its characteristic features, in many cases the primary focus of fungal infection start at the umbilicus and then spread to the abdominal wall, this commonly affect children and rarely may affect adults (Fig. 26.15), acute viral infection like herpes is not rarely to affect the umbilicus, specially in immunocompromised patients (Fig. 26.16).

Primary irritant dermatitis: It is an exematous reaction of the skin caused by direct contact of toxic irritane substances.

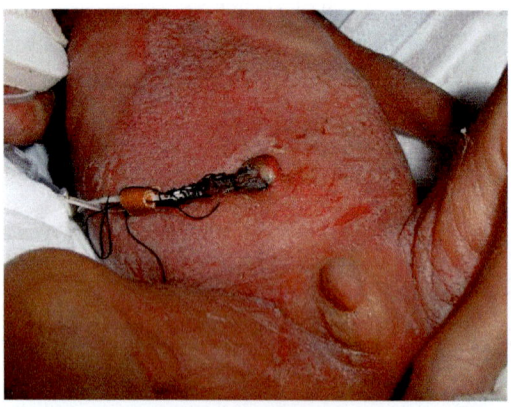

Fig. 26.15 Fungal omphalitis with spreading to the skin around the umbilicus

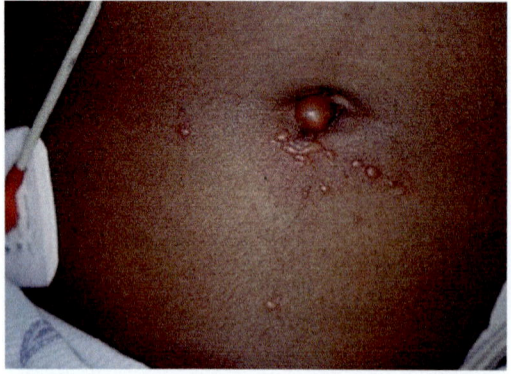

Fig. 26.16 Herpes zoster omphalitis

26.8 Navel Piercing Infection
(Fig. 26.17)

Navel piercing is one of the most common body piercings today. The Egyptian Pharaohs believed that earring at the navel is a sign of ritual transition from the life at the Earth to the eternity, it was popular among ancient Egyptian aristocrats, and was depicted in Egyptian statuary, also navel piercings are said to signify wealth and higher social status back in ancient society. But there is absolutely no proof either in sculptures, drawings, or even mummies that would point to the art of decorating the body with navel piercings during this time [19].

The actual navel is not pierced when a navel piercing is performed, the most common form of navel piercing is through the upper rim of the navel, rarely lateral umbilical rim is used and central piercing of the umbilical cicatrix is called the true navel piercing, which sometimes preferred by those who had a protruded umbilicus (outie).

With the recent wide spread of navel piercing among girls, and sometimes men, by different types of jewellers, which not always done with aseptic techniques and by unqualified personals, there are many possible causes of navel piercing infection, with a wide spectrum of presentations; sometimes only cellulitis, which could be treated and controlled, but an umbilical abscess is not a rare sequel, (Fig. 26.18), other complications like kelloid formation will be discussed later (Sect. 31.6.2).

Piercing omphalitis may be detected early after applying the jewellers if the pathogens find its way to the umbilical tissue from unsterile technique, or latter on due to bad hygiene, and improper care of the pierced navel. Having a tattoo near the pierced area; tight jeans for prolonged periods; carelessness in cleaning the navel; bathing in unclean waters; and frequent touching of the newly pierced navel are a predisposing factors for piercing omphalitis [20].

Umbilical piercing in particular can cause perioperative problems during laparoscopic procedures.

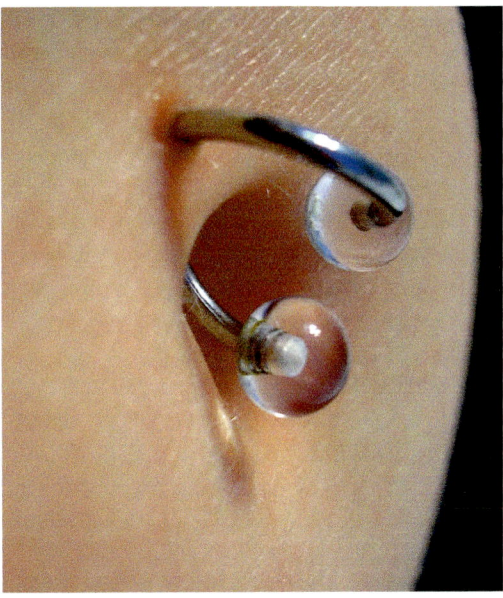

Fig. 26.17 Navel piercing

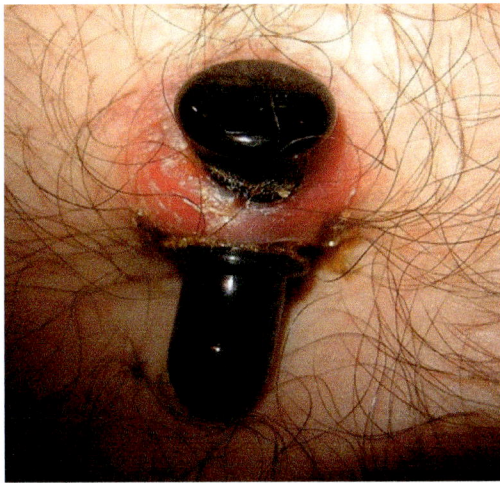

Fig. 26.18 Piercing omphalitis in a male

26.9 Management of Omphalitis in Adults

Early and prompt treatment is mandatory to avoid serious complications; like liver abscess, and to reserve the normal athletic look of the navel.

Mild cases: removal of foreign bodies such as hair-tufts or ompholiths.

Good skin hygiene and topical treatment as for intertrigo.

Moderate/severe cases: as for mild cases, but if significant secondary infection detected then oral antibiotic is indicated to cover Staph aureus, once an abscess is suspected drainage is mandatory to avoid spread of infection to the underlying structures. Specific fungal or viral infection necessitate a specific lines of treatment.

26.10 Rare Types of Omphalitis

Myiasis omphalitis: Myiasis of the neonatal umbilicus is a rare disease with only a few reported cases in the literature, it is defined as the invasion of live mammalian tissue by the immature stage (maggots) of dipteran flies which feed on the host's necrotic or living tissue. Although myiasis is mainly a disease of animals but humans may be affected, sometimes when they are reared in poor hygienic conditions [21]. Unhygienic practices coupled with traditional ways of handling newborn babies and the application of non-sterile instruments during and after delivery at the rural settings are the predisposing factors for myiasis omphalitis (Fig. 26.19).

Medical care and access to maternity, health centres and hospitals will help to reduce home births and traditional handling of neonates. Cord care practices should be taught by qualified medical personnel to mothers and grandmothers who handle babies after birth. This should be practiced as a measure of prophylaxis to prevent the morbidity and mortality associated with myiasis as omphalitis infection persists [22].

Effective treatment of myiasis typically consists of the removal of the larvae, cleaning of the wound and use of local antiseptics and systemic antibiotics to control any possible associated infection.

26.10.1 Umbilical Tetanus Neonatorum (Fig. 26.20)

Tetanus occurs worldwide and it was an important cause of neonatal deaths in developing coun-

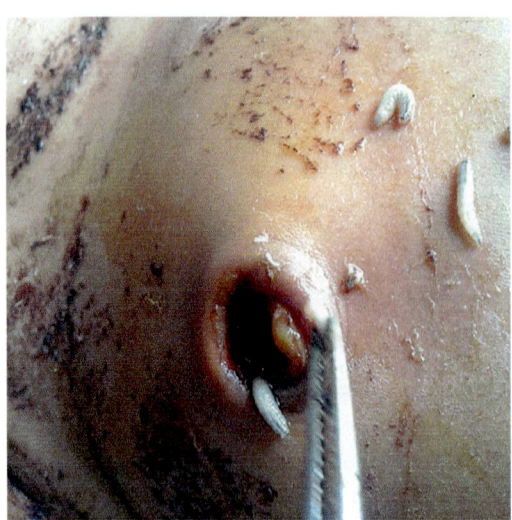

Fig. 26.19 Myiasis omphalitis, with alive larvae retrieved from the umbilicus

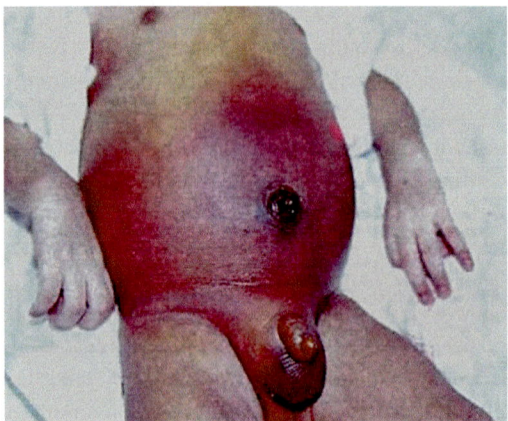

Fig. 26.20 Umbilical tetanus neonatorum, with spread of the infection to the penis and scrotum, a hands clenched to form a fist (claw hand) is noticeable

tries. Tetanus infect an estimated 500,000 neonates each year with about 80% deaths in 12 tropical Asian-African countries alone. Till recently Neonatal tetanus accounted for 6.5% of deaths in infancy in India [23].

It is a rare serious infectious disease characterized by an acute onset of hypertonia, painful muscular contractions, and generalized muscle spasms. It is caused by contamination of umbilical stump with spores of clostrium tetani bacteria present in soil and faces of domestic animal and human, at the time of cutting of cord, and use of unclean sharp weapon to cut the umbilical cord. In all deliveries by untrained person, cord was cut by unsterile instrument in many rural areas in developing countries. Application of ash on umbilical stump and improper maternal immunization during pregnancy are an important factors predisposing to tetanus omphalitis. Tetanic omphalitis is a fatal disease with a very high mortality rate, but it is a vaccine-preventable disease and it is considered as a failure of public health system [24].

Umbilical Tuberculosis: Abdominal tuberculosis also remains relevant in developing countries. It can be responsible for entero-umbilical fistula with purulent secretions and faeces, possibly in connection with a chronic under-umbilical inflammation in peritoneal tuberculosis.

Lint ball omphalitis: 'Belly-button lint 'Foreign body-induced omphalitis'.

Hairball is the most common type of foreign body seen in such cases. Most of the patients are young, hairy male with deep umbilicus with poor personal hygiene. A wide varieties of foreign body may be retrieved from the umbilicus and if it is retained for long time it may induce omphalitis, one interesting report of foreign body-induced umbilical discharge, is due to an old toilet paper ball in the umbilicus. Obesity, deep umbilicus, and poor hygiene may have been the predisposing factors for developing lint accumulation and subsequent omphalitis [25]. Omphalolith will be discussed with rare umbilical disorders in Sect. 31.3.

Different types and lesions of umbilical dermatitis can be launched with photos in this site:

http://medical-photographs.com/251-umbilical-lesions.html

References

1. Bugaje MA, et al. "Omphalitis". Paediatric surgery: a comprehensive text for Africa. Retrieved 23 July 2013.
2. Sawardekar KP. Changing spectrum of neonatal omphalitis. Pediatr Infect Dis J. 2004;23(1):22e6.
3. Simiyu DE. Morbidity and mortality of neonates admitted in general paediatric wards at Kenyatta National Hospital. East Afr Med J. 2003;80:611–6.
4. McKenna H, Johnson D. Bacteria in neonatal omphalitis. Pathology. 1977;9(2):111e3.

5. Schlesinger AE, Braverman RM, DiPietro MA. Neonates and umbilical venous catheters: normal appearance, anomalous positions, complications, and potential aid to diagnosis. Am J Roentgenol. 2003;180:1147–53.

6. Moens E, De Dooy J, Jansens H, Lammens C, de Beeck BO, Mahieu L. Hepatic abscesses associated with umbilical catheterisation in two neonates. Eur J Pediatr. 2003;162(6):406–9.

7. Brook I. Microbiology of necrotizing fasciitis associated with omphalitis in the newborn infant. J Perinatol. 1998;18(1):28–30.

8. Fraser N, Davies BW, Cusack J. Neonatal omphalitis: a review of its serious complications. Acta Paediatr. 2006;95(5):519–22.

9. Sawin RS, Schaller RT, Tapper D, et al. Early recognition of neonatal abdominal wall necrotizing fasciitis. Am J Surg. 1994;167(5):481–4.

10. Bingol-Kologlu M, Yildiz RV, Alper B, et al. Necrotizing fasciitis in children: diagnostic and therapeutic aspects. J Pediatr Surg. 2007;42(11):1892–7.

11. Weber DM, Freeman NV, Elhag KM. Periumbilical necrotizing fasciitis in the newborn. Eur J Pediatr Surg. 2001;11(2):86–91.

12. Samuel M, Freeman NV, Vaishnav A, et al. Necrotizing fasciitis: a serious complication of omphalitis in neonates. J Pediatr Surg. 1994;29(11):1414–6.

13. Mason WH, Andrews R, Ross LA, Wright HT Jr. Omphalitis in the newborn infant. Pediatr Infect Dis J. 1989;8(8):521–5.

14. Moon SB, Lee HW, Park KW, Jung SE. Falciform ligament abscess after omphalitis: report of a case. J Korean Med Sci. 2010;25:1090–2.

15. Orloff MJ, Orloff MS, Girard B, Orloff SL. Bleeding esophageal varices from extrahepatic portal hypertension: 40 years experience with portal-systemic shunt. J Am Coll Surg. 2002;194:717–30.

16. Imdad A, Bautista RM, Senen KA, Uy ME, Mantaring JB, Bhutta ZA. Umbilical cord antiseptics for preventing sepsis and death among newborns. Cochrane Database Syst Rev. 2013;5:CD008635. doi:10.1002/14651858.CD008635.pub2.

17. Vause Greig GW, Shucksmith HS. Primary umbilical sepsis in the adult: report of seven cases. Lancet. 1950;255(6593):4–6.

18. Coda A, Bossotti M, Ferri F, et al. Incisional hernia and fascial defect following laparoscopic surgery. Surg Laparosc Endosc Percutan Tech. 2000;10(1):34–8.

19. Koenig LM, Carnes M. Body piercing, medical concerns with cutting-edge fashion. J Gen Intern Med. 1999;14(6):379–85.

20. Gold MA, et al. Body piercing practices and attitudes among urban adolescents. J Adolesc Health. 2005;36(4):352.e15–352.e2.

21. Ogbalu OK, Eze CN, Manuelrb B. A new trend of Omphalitis complicated with Myiasis in neonates of the Niger Delta, Nigeria. Epidemiology (Sunnyvale). 2016;6:2. doi:10.4172/2161-1165.1000231.

22. Patra S, Purkait R, Basu R, Konar MC, Sarkar D. Umbilical myiasis associated with Staphylococcus Aureus sepsis in a neonate. J Clin Neonatol. 2012; 1:42–3.

23. Thwaites CL, Beeching NJ. CRNewton: maternal and neonatal tetanus. Lancet. 2015;385:362–70.

24. Hatkar N, Shah N, Imran S, Jadhao A. Study of incidence, Mortality & Causes of neonatal tetanus among all neonatal intensive care unit [NICU] admissions in tertiary health care center of SBHGMC, Dhule. J Evol Med Dent Sci. 2015;4(40):6967–73. doi:10.14260/jemds/2015/1012.

25. Steinhauser G. The nature of navel fluff. Med Hypotheses. 2009;72:623–5. doi:10.1016/j.mehy.2009.01.015.

Umbilical Granuloma (UG)

27

Nomenclature: Pyogenic granuloma of umbilicus.

Definition: Granuloma defined as an inflammatory tumor composed of granulation tissue produced in response to chronic infection, inflammation, foreign body irritation or unknown causes. Umbilical granuloma is a bright red stalk of tissue which may persist at the base of the umbilicus after cord separation; this tissue is composed of fibroblasts and capillaries and can grow to different sizes and forms. It has a grainy surface and produces sticky mucus, or bleeding. It is usually visible as friable, wet, pink tissue enlarged into a 'mushroom-like' or small round, cherry-red mass measuring 3–10 mm in diameter. Most fail to epithelialize and persist for more than 2 months (Fig. 27.1).

Historical background: In England attention has been drawn to the granuloma subject by Millar and in Germany by Ledderhose, Pernice and others; in France the subject has been interestingly handled by Lannelongue and Fremont, in the American literature the 1st article on this subject was written in 1897 by Holt and by de Villiers [1].

Incidence: Umbilical granuloma (UG) is the most common umbilical abnormality in neonates, causing inflammation and drainage, it is estimated to occur in 1 in 500 births, and the most common cause of umbilical discharge is umbilical granuloma [2]. Higher rate of incidence (10.5%) was reported from Israel [3]. With the higher incidence of omphalitis in developing and tropical countries, it is expected to have a higher unreported incidence of UG in such countries.

Magnitude of the problem: UG is a minor simple acquired disease commonly affecting neonates, but it carries a great worries to the parents from its look and the bleeding, which may follow irritation by napkin's edge, also its differentiation from other serious congenital anomalies, like a patent vitellointestinal duct, or acquired disease like umbilical polyp is not easy for a paediatrician unexperienced with congenital umbilical anomalies. There are several cases reported with an initial misdiagnosis of umbilical granuloma and treated with silver nitrate and

Electronic Supplementary Material: The online version of this chapter (doi:10.1007/978-3-319-62383-2_27) contains supplementary material, which is available to authorized users.

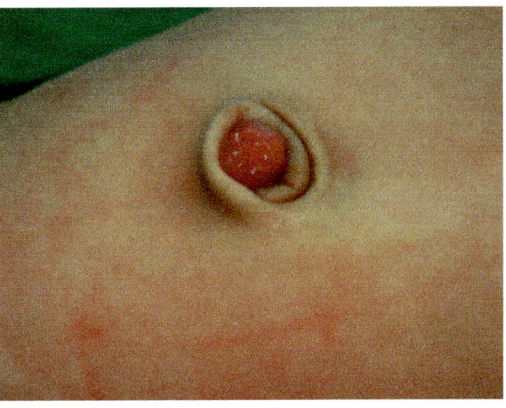

Fig. 27.1 A neonatal granuloma looks like a friable *pink* tissue (a cherry-red mass) inside the umbilical pit

ended with a disastrous complications of bowel evisceration or faecal fistula after cauterization of an umbilical mass Figs. 27.2 and 27.3.

Etiology: The reasons why some children develop an umbilical granuloma, while others do not? have been under recognized, but definitely the formation of a granuloma has to do with how the tissue heals as the umbilical cord separates from the baby. It does not seem to be due to improper care of the remainder of the umbilical cord after the baby is born. In human, the umbilical arteries and vein begin their anatomic obliteration after birth and until about 28 days, this involves a different processes: The inner longitudinal muscular coat contracts and thickens, thus tending to obliterate the lumen of the vessel, proliferation of the intima,

which fills the periphery of the vein with new fibrous tissue, and formation of collagen tissue in the fibromuscular coat of arteries.

The mean time to separation of the umbilical stump is 15.0 ± 7.2 days (range 3 days to 2 months), and the separation site normally heals by 12–15 days. When the fibromuscular ring of the umbilicus closes and the cord sloughs, the ring is covered anteriorly by skin and posteriorly by peritoneum. Pathological lesions of the area may be associated with retained umbilical cord elements [4].

Microscopic examination of the umbilicus after cord sloughing shows emigrating white blood corpuscles in abundant numbers. They soften the dead tissue, which is gradually loosened and falls off, leaving a granulating surface. Occasionally, following separation of the cord, incomplete epithelialization may occur over the ring area, and reddish granulation tissue appears. Granulation tissue is a normal stage in wound healing but it may overgrow and result in the formation of an umbilical granuloma (UG) [5].

UG is called in some references as a pyogenic granuloma, as some believe it may occur as a result of a local secondary infection or previous injury [6].

An umbilical granuloma occurs when there is a delay in the separation of the cord as a result of a low-grade (mild) superficial skin infection in the periumbilical crevasses. The inflammatory process at the umbilicus becomes florid with excess granulation tissue preventing the raw area from developing new epithelial tissue [7].

Irritation of the healing umbilical wound after stump separation before complete epithelization to form a mature scar by any foreign particles may trigger overgrowth of granulation tissue and formation of UG.

Histology: On histologic examination the entire mass is found to consist of young granulation tissue. Its blood capillaries are very abundant and scattered throughout the field with many small round cells. In 4 out of 27 cases collected by Pernice, the surface of the granulation was partly covered over with a delicate epithelium. Millar has pointed out that the superficial cells of the granulation tissue may be so flattened that they fail to epithelialize [1] (Fig. 27.4).

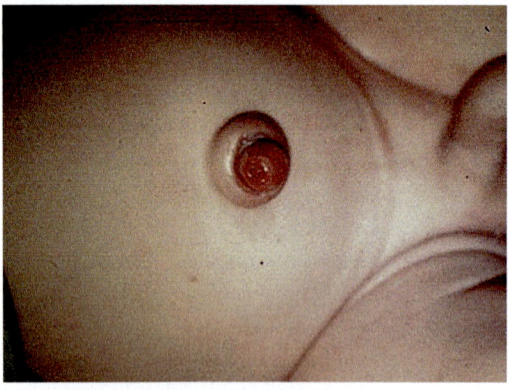

Fig. 27.2 A *red* granular tissue of a neonatal umbilicus with a minute opening at its dome

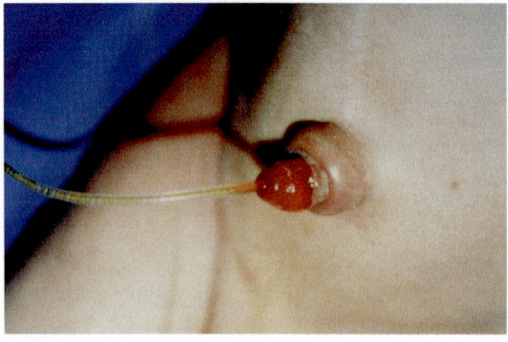

Fig. 27.3 Same case in Fig. 27.2 with a fine catheter inserted in its summit, which revealed an intestinal contents (patent vitellointestinal duct)

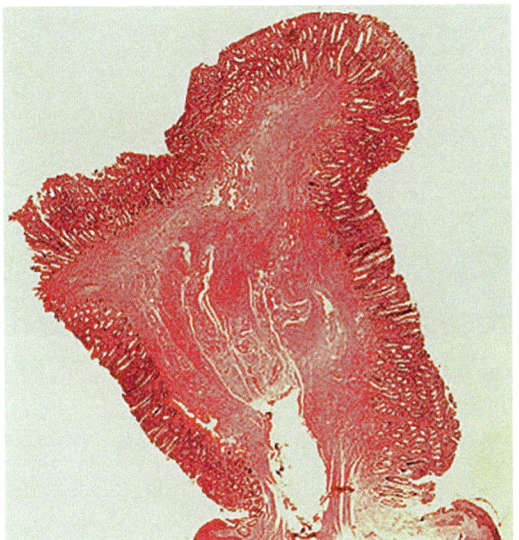

Fig. 27.4 Histopathology of UG

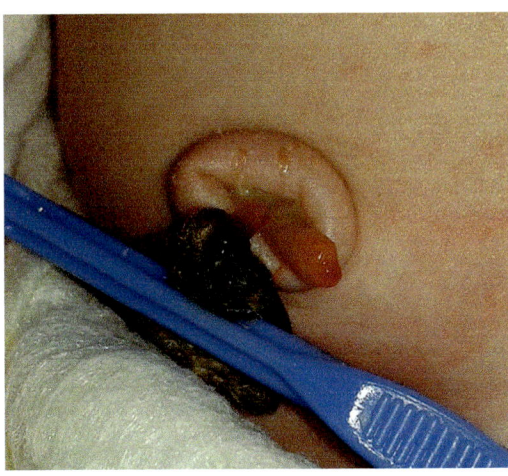

Fig. 27.5 A small *red* swelling at the *left side* of the drying umbilical cord looks like granuloma but proved to be a patent urachus

UG is devoted from any nerve fibres, so it is not painful, and chemical burning, by different modalities, silver nitrate or cryosurgery could be applied safely without any need for local anaesthetics.

27.1 Clinically

Timing of presentation: UG typically forms during the first few weeks of life and should not be present at birth and usually persists for more than 2 months. UG never to appear before falling down of the umbilical stump, the presence of any suspicious tissue at the umbilical base around the drying cord should arouses the possibility of urachal or omphalomesenteric duct remnants (Fig. 27.5).

Types: An umbilical granuloma typically measures 0.1–1 cm in size, at navel bottom separated by a groove of healthy skin, and bleeds easily on contact, and it may be pedunculated, sessile or a fingerlike projection (Figs. 27.6 and 27.7), but rarely it may acquire a larger size (Fig. 27.8).

It is usually visible above the umbilical rims, but in some occasions it may be presented only with bleeding, where the granuloma itself is hidden between umbilical skin folds, and can be seen only after applying a gentle pressure around the umbilicus (Fig. 27.9).

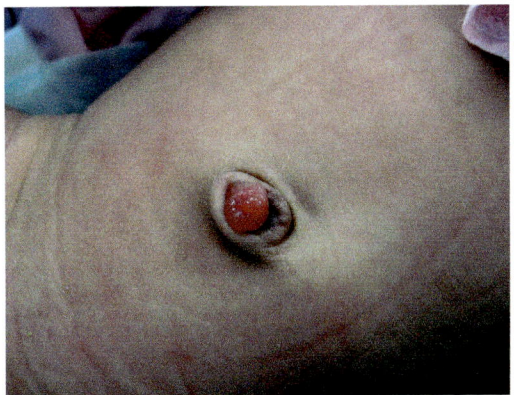

Fig. 27.6 Sessile large umbilical granuloma looks like *red cherry*

It is non-tender (lacking innervation), the tissue is wet, pink, soft, friable with a velvety appearance, and it bleeds easily; it may be enlarged into a mushroom-like or a round cherry-red mass [7] (Fig. 27.10).

Drainage from UG may be clear or have the appearance of a fibrinous exudate or sanguineous or even greenish discharge; bleeding was the first presentation in many occasions; it is very rare to have a frank pus coming from tissue around UG; granuloma exudate should be examined carefully and may be even tested to rule out urine or intestinal contents. A weak umbilical scar in a baby

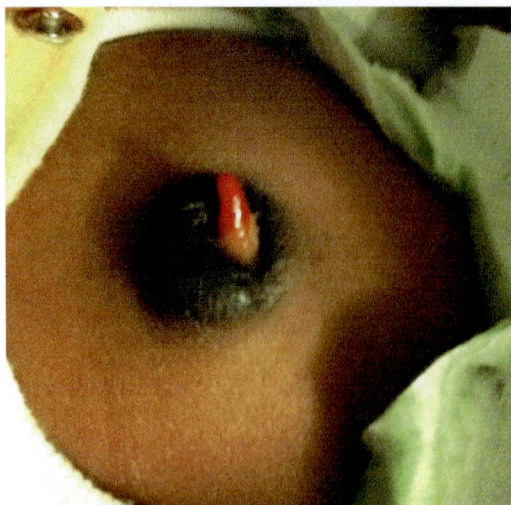

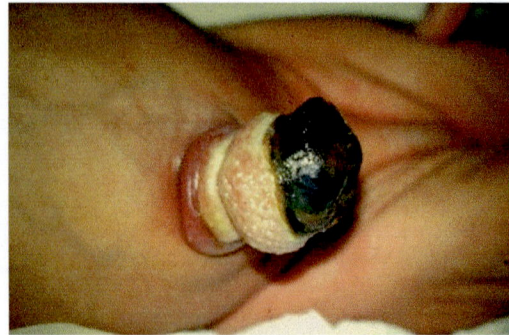

Fig. 27.8 Abnormal huge granuloma with a necrotic tissue covering its dome

Fig. 27.7 UG with a tapered end looks like finger projection

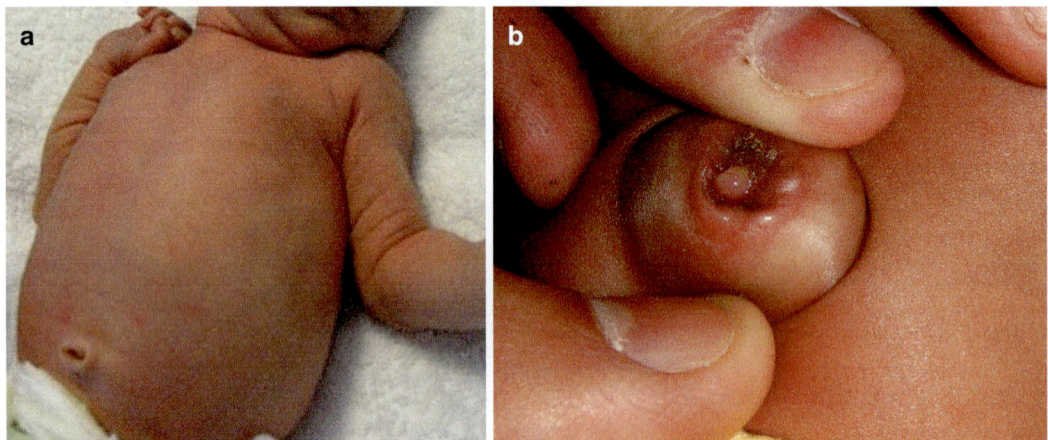

Fig. 27.9 (**a**) A hidden granuloma, (**b**) only visible after gentle pressure over umbilical rims

with abdominal distension and continuous straining may have an UG at the summit of an umbilical hernia (Fig. 27.11).

Diagnosis is mainly clinical, but any doubt about the granuloma discharge should be examined to rule out urine coming from a patent urachus or stool coming from a patent vitellointestinal duct, and any punctum at the dome of UG should be cannulated and investigated with a suitable contrast, to rule out small vitelline or urachal fistulas/sinuses with mucosal protrusion. In case of clinical

suspicion, ultrasonography may be helpful in identifying associated abdominal anomalies. It is advisable to take a bacteriology swab from the UG surface to rule out any specific pathogens.

At the main time, any excised UG should be examined histologically to rule out other rare umbilical swelling, so this justifying surgical excision over other conservative measures used to treat UG (Figs. 27.2 and 27.3).

Differential diagnosis: In rare cases, a piece of tissue that looks like an umbilical granuloma is

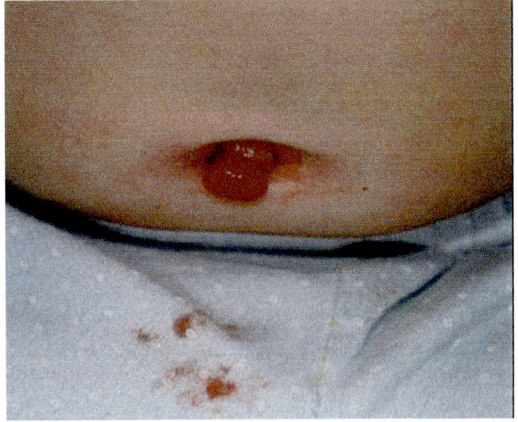

Fig. 27.10 Bleeding from umbilical granuloma

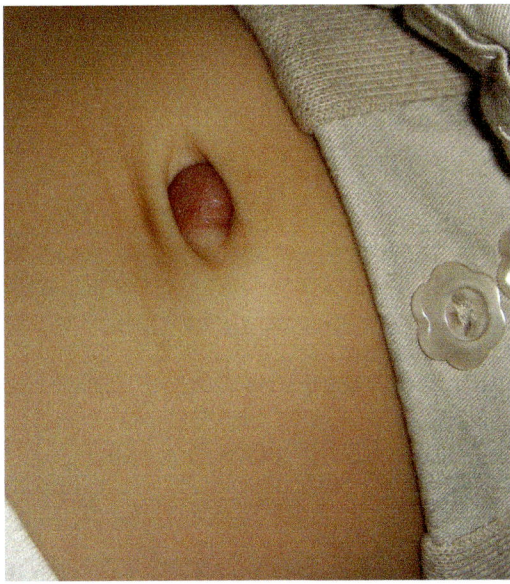

Fig. 27.12 Capillary haemangioma of the umbilicus looks like UG

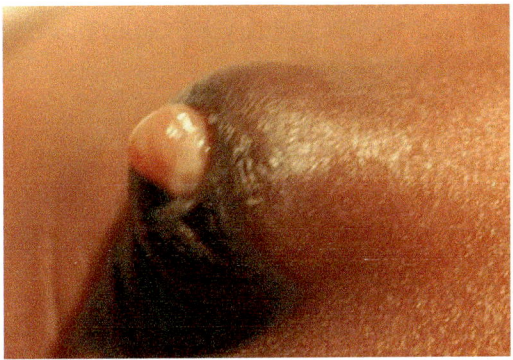

Fig. 27.11 UG at the dome of an umbilical hernia

27.1.1 Management

Prevention: There is no known definitive way that can be applied to prevent the development of a granuloma; although cleaning the umbilical stump will not prevent a granuloma, it is best to keep the area clean and dry around the cord stump until the cord falls off, without omphalitis, as proper cord care, prevention and prompt treatment of omphalitis may be helpful to minimize the incidence of UG [8].

actually connected to the bladder or bowel; it may be difficult to distinguish UG from an umbilical polyp, which is usually brighter red, slightly larger, with a glistening smooth surface and may have a minute opening at its dome; it represents remnant omphalomesenteric duct, urachal tissue or other rare types (Chap. 36) (Figs. 27.2 and 27.3).

UG, especially in older child, should be differentiated from other umbilical swelling as haemangioma (Sect. 30.2), inclusion dermoid cysts, keloid scar and very rarely an ectopic gastric or pancreatic tissue, which may give the same appearance of UG, in adult cases; melanoma, endometriosis and neoplastic lesions should be considered in differential diagnosis (Sect. 30.5) (Fig. 27.12).

As delayed separation of the cord stump may predispose to UG formation, a close observation of cord stump and investigation for immunocompromisation for any delayed or retained stump may help to detect early and manage any granuloma conservatively.

Al Siny et al. recommend proximal clamping of the umbilical cord, which reduced the incidence of UG to 0% in 500 normal neonates, in comparison to 8% incidence in another 500 neonates with classical distal cord clamping [9].

Applying topical antibiotics and eliminating the friction of a wet diaper may allow the granulation tissue to epithelialize [10]. We always advice mothers to use for baby a special napkin with a notch at the umbilicus, especially during the first 2 months (Fig. 27.13).

Spontaneous resolution: There is no definite randomized controlled trial (RCT) that can prove spontaneous resolution of UG without treatment, only a limited trial showed that conservative management is as effective as silver nitrate [8]. Therefore, once the diagnosis is established, proper management is needed for this condition.

Although treatment of umbilical granulomas can be conservative, such as using alcohol, chlorhexidine and many other topical agents, the benefit of excising UG is to have a specimen for histopathological study and to rule out other rare similar lesions.

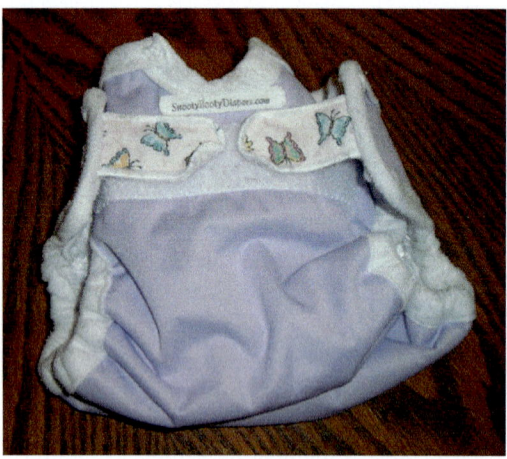

Fig. 27.13 Special napkins for baby with UG

Several noninvasive measures are available to treat umbilical granulomas, which could be categorized as:

Chemical cauterization: A chemical that burns the tissue can be applied directly over the granuloma, to remove the excess tissue and to promote epithelization, because it has no nerves, it does not hurt and repeated applications for several days are usually required:

Silver nitrate: Silver nitrate acts as an antiseptic, astringent or caustic agent, depending on the chemical concentration and duration of application. Standard texts continue to recommend silver nitrate application as the most common treatment for UG, as contact of this substance with the moist granuloma triggers cauterization. Conventional management has been to dry the umbilical stump and carefully cauterize the granuloma with a 75% silver nitrate stick [10] (Fig. 27.14).

Because of the risk of spillage, the granuloma can be dried with gauze to avoid chemical burns or discolouration to the surrounding skin. Furthermore, caution should be exercised if silver nitrate is used for large granulomas because repeated applications can leak onto healthy tissue. Protection can be attained by isolating the skin around the umbilicus with petroleum jelly cream before each application [11].

Silver nitrate application to umbilical granulomas is usually successful. One or more applications may be needed; if the granuloma persists after 3 or 4 applications which are performed at interval of 3–4 days [12].

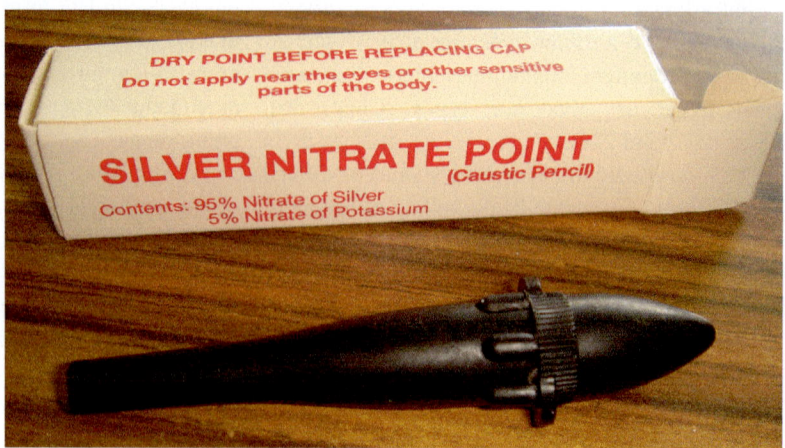

Fig. 27.14 Silver nitrate sticks

Silver nitrate is not innocuous and when applied liberally can cause a minor burn of the periumbilical skin area of the baby (Fig. 27.15). Hypopigmentation and hypomelanosis may complicate a healed skin burn after silver nitrate application, which looks like vitiligo (Fig. 27.16).

In English literature, there are several cases which are initially misdiagnosed as umbilical granuloma and treated with silver nitrate. In this context, Kondrich et al. [13] reported a case of evisceration of the small bowel after cauterization of an umbilical mass, and Montes-Tapia et al. [14] published a case of with appendico-umbilical fistula presenting with umbilical mass and managed with silver nitrate.

Follow-up of few cases of UG managed by silver nitrate revealed an unacceptable unappealing protruding umbilical scar, which may be troublesome for those who are concerned with navel beautification (Fig. 27.17) (Chap. 25).

Common salt has shown to be an effective practice to treat UG. The principle of using this approach is thought to be through its desiccant effect and other biological properties; sodium ion in the area draws water out of the cells and results

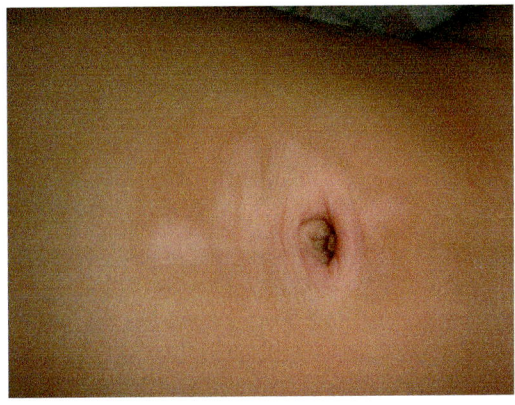

Fig. 27.16 Hypopigmentation secondary to silver nitrate burning, UG remnants still seen at the umbilical base

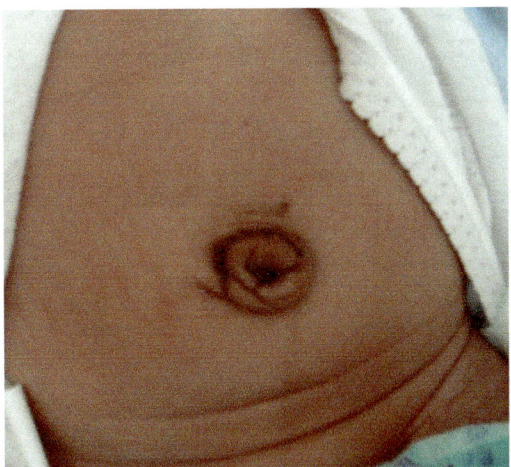

Fig. 27.17 *Brownish* discoloured scar and protrude umbilicus after silver nitrate application

in shrinkage and necrosis of the wet granulomatous tissues. Twice daily application of common table salt to umbilical pyogenic granulomas for 3 days is a simple, cost-effective and claimed to be a curative method that can be performed by parents at home [15].

Many other topical agents were tried and studied in different samples of patients like usage of polyurethane (Lyofoam), topical doxycycline [16] and topical clobetasol propionate cream 0.05% (a European Class IV steroid), which were applied twice a day at home by the parents [17].

Ligature: The granuloma can be tied tight at the base with surgical thread; this will cause the

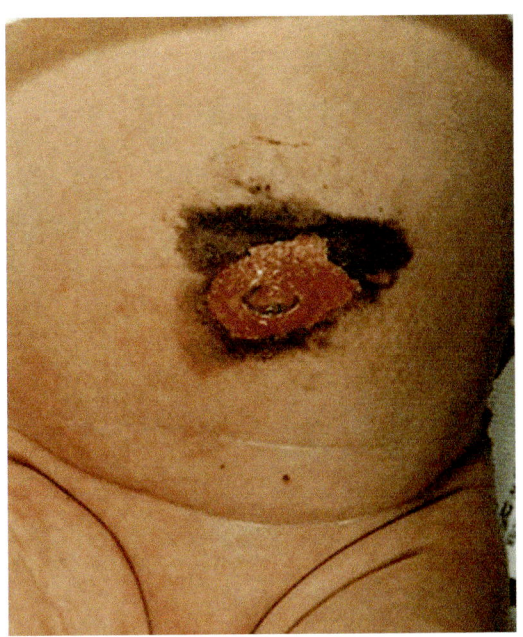

Fig. 27.15 Skin burn around the umbilicus complicating silver nitrate

granuloma tissue to die and eventually fall off; this tying is a traditional domestic practice which was done long time ago by paramedics and barbers in many cultures without medical background (Fig. 27.18). But more recently a double ligature published by Lotan et al. [18] proved tying to be an effective practice in an outpatient clinic. After cleansing and prepping the periumbilical area with a povidone-iodine solution, 3-0 silk sutures are used for ligation. The use of 4-0 silk sutures is only necessary with more delicate and friable umbilical granulomas. The double-ligature technique overcomes the technical difficulty of ligating the granuloma on its base (Fig. 27.19).

The application of a double ligature can be considered for only pedunculated umbilical granulomas, but it is useless in a friable and sessile lesions.

Surgical excision: Surgical excision could be the mainstay of treatment for large or non-resolving UG after chemical cauterization. In this condition, excisional biopsy allows to establish accurate diagnosis as it provides definitive diagnosis (Fig. 27.20).

I recommend the use of electrocautery by bipolar as a treatment of choice for all cases accurately diagnosed as an UG, either with a light anaesthesia or sedation to avoid baby movements; the advantages of this technique include the precise total excision of the annoying granu-

loma in one sitting, with secured haemostats, and to get a tissue sample for histopathological study, which is not possible with chemical cauterization. Also I claim that the surgically excised UG may leave a good umbilical scar behind.

Cryosurgery: Liquid nitrogen (Video 27.1) can be used to freeze the granuloma. In one small study, cryosurgery was associated with skin depigmentation but was favoured because repeat applications were unnecessary. Cryotherapy also offered more rapid healing compared with the use of chemicals and electrocautery [19].

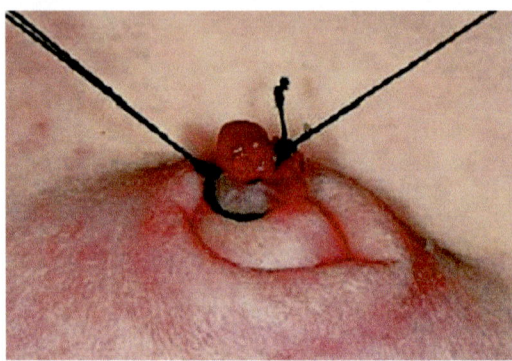

Fig. 27.19 Double ligatures technique

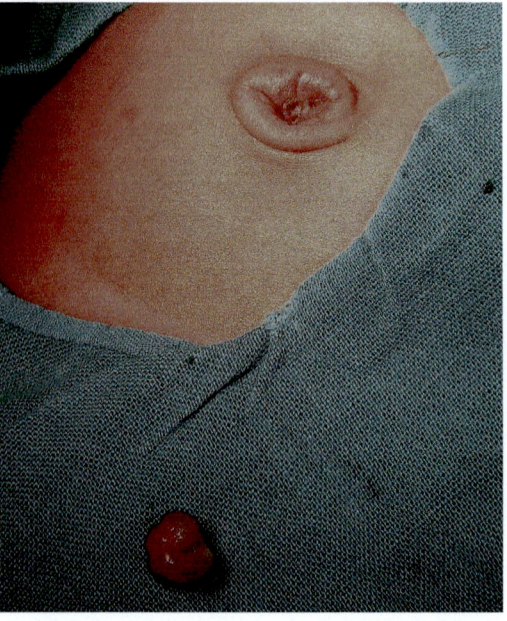

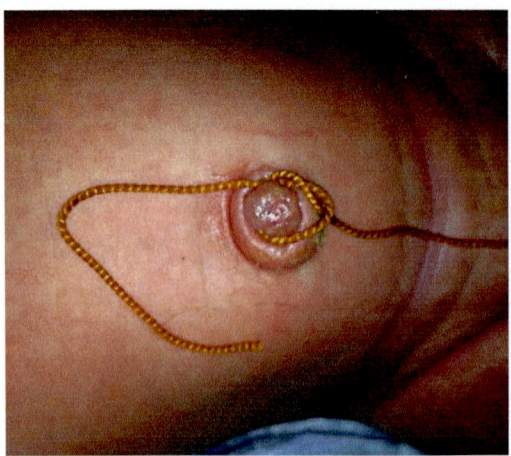

Fig. 27.18 UG tied with a thread

Fig. 27.20 Cauterization excision of UG by bipolar

27.2   Umbilical Granuloma Beyond Neonatal Age

Talc granuloma: A foreign body granuloma may affect the healing umbilical stump in a neonate or an infant, especially in rural areas, where talc powder is still in use for drying the umbilical stump and also as a protection from napkin rashes; McCallum and Hall have criticized the use of such powders, long time ago, on the ground that the application of talc to a raw surface invites the development of a granuloma. In 10 years they have studied 18 of these granulomata; on histological examination these showed inflammatory granulation tissues containing doubly refractile particles and a giant-cell reaction in relation to some of them, with a degree of fibrosis [20].

Older children or adults may develop a granuloma as a reaction secondary to repeated attacks of omphalitis, either bacterial or fungal, especially in immunocompromised patients, and secondary to foreign body in the umbilicus, like hair tuft or omphalolithis; also UG may be seen as a response to irritation induced by umbilical piercing (Fig. 27.21), formed in such cases after removal of the foreign bodies, leaving behind a raw surface. Keloid scar should be differentiated from those granulomas [21] (Sect. 31.6).

Recently with the wide use of laparoscopy, an umbilical granuloma could be detected in a child or adult going for a laparoscopic procedure; also rarely the granuloma may complicate laparoscopic port site at the umbilicus, especially after infection of the port site; in a review of 109 laparoscopic cholecystectomies, only one umbilical granuloma encountered [22].

27.3   Umbilical Lesions Looks Like UG

Healed omphalocele: Conservatively healed omphalocele, especially a minor one, may heal with granulation tissue, with a failure of complete epithelization, and it usually ends with a pigmented weak scar (Fig. 27.22).

Amniotic navel: In rare cases the skin is lacking over the lower part of the cord and the adjacent abdominal wall so that the amnion not only extends over the lowest part of the cord but also spreads out over the abdominal wall skin defect as a delicate, transparent membrane, which will heal by granulation tissue, and may give a picture similar to UG, but the healed amniotic navel is not raised above the skin, not bleed in touch and usually darker in colour (Chap. 34).

Umbilical warts: Different types of viral warts are rarely affecting the umbilical scar, especially at elders and hardly seen at paediatric age; verruca vulgaris is the most common type of wart that may affect the umbilicus. It is a keratotic papilloma of the epidermis that occurs as a result of localized infection by human papillomavirus, usually types 2 and 4; the lesions are of variable duration, eventually undergoing spontaneous regression, but it may need topical management; it is characterized by hyperkeratosis, parakeratosis, hypergranulosis, koilocytosis and papillomatosis. Excision and biopsy may be indicated in some doubtful cases (Fig. 27.23).

Umbilical horn: This condition is evidently very rare in the modern medicine but could be seen in tropical area, the first recorded case in

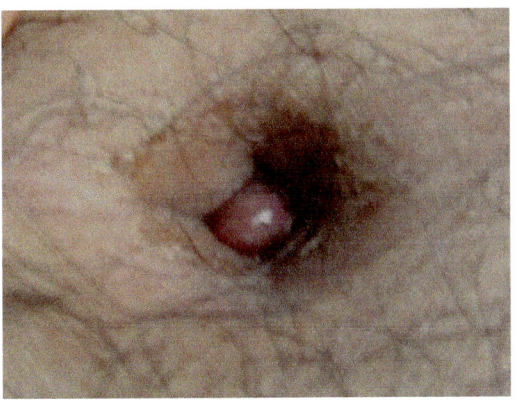

Fig. 27.21   Adult UG complicating navel piercing

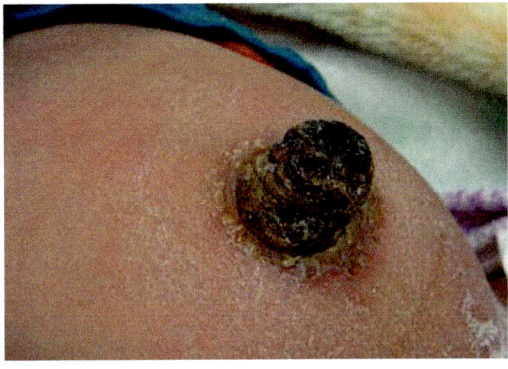

Fig. 27.22   Healed exomphalos minor with a dark protrude scar

literature was in 1890 by Fischer [23]. Cutaneous horn has been noticed on top of many clinical conditions like actinic keratosis, wart molluscum contagiosum, seborrheic keratoses, keratoacanthoma, basal cell carcinoma and squamous cell carcinoma. It is an elongated, keratinous projection from the umbilical skin, ranging in size from a few millimetres to many centimetres that resembles a miniature horn. The base of the horn may be flat, nodular or crateriform. When pressure was made around the umbilicus the small one protruded fully from the level of the abdomen, larger horn may be obvious and usually pointing down. Excision biopsy of the lesion and histopathological examination to rule out malignancy is recommended (Fig. 27.24).

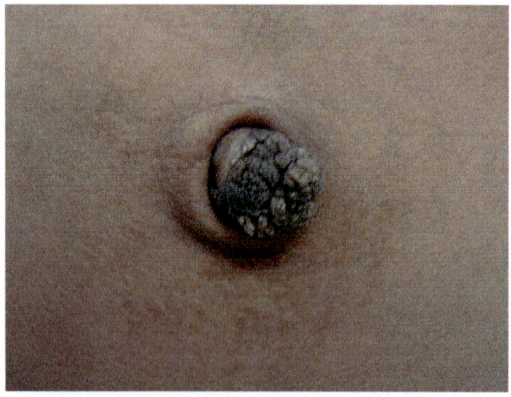

Fig. 27.23 Multiple umbilical warts

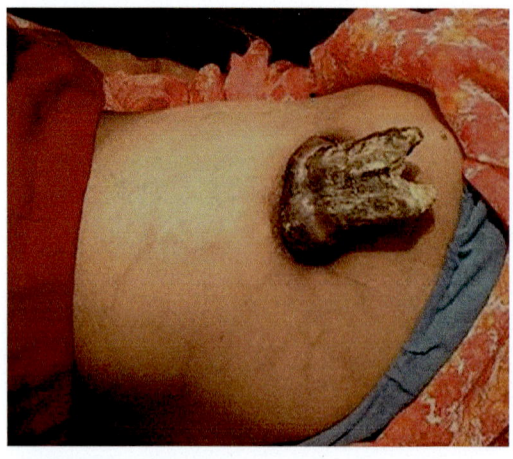

Fig. 27.24 Umbilical horn

References

1. de Villiers JH. The nature of umbilical growths of infants and young children. Pediatrics. 1897;iii:337.
2. Pomeranz A. Anomalies, abnormalities, and care of the umbilicus. Pediatr Clin N Am. 2004;51(3):819–27. doi:10.1016/j.pcl.2004.01.010.
3. Naor N, Merlob P, Litwin A, Wielunksy E. Time of separation of the umbilical cord: a comparative study of treatment with alcohol and Rikospray. Eur J Obstet Gynecol Reprod Biol. 1989;32:89–93.
4. Wilson CB. When is umbilical cord separation delayed? J Pediatr. 1985;107:292.
5. Nagar H. Umbilical granuloma: a new approach to an old problem. Pediatr Surg Int. 2001;17(7):513–4.
6. Yoshida Y, Yamamoto O. Umbilical pyogenic granuloma associated with occult omphalith. Dermatol Surg. 2008;34:1613–4.
7. Campbell J, Beasley SW, McMullin N, Hutson JM. Clinical diagnosis of umbilical swellings and discharges in children. Med J Aust. 1986;145(9):450–3.
8. Daniels J, Craig F, Wajed R, et al. Umbilical granulomas: a randomised controlled trial. Arch Dis Child Fetal Neonatal Ed. 2003;88:F257.
9. Al Siny FI, Al Mansouri NI, Al Zahrani FS. Proximal clamping of umbilical cord and prevention of umbilical granuloma (preliminary results). Med Sci. 2004;11(1):3–7.
10. Snyder CL. Current management of umbilical abnormalities and related anomalies. Semin Pediatr Surg. 2007;16:41–9.
11. Sankar NS, Donaldson D. Lessons to be learned: a case study approach. Finger discolouration due to silver nitrate exposure: review of uses and toxicity of silver in clinical practice. J R Soc Health. 1998;118:371–4.
12. Karagüzel G, et al. Umbilical granuloma: modern understanding of etiopathogenesis, diagnosis, and management. J Pediatr Neonatal Care. 2016;4(3):00136.
13. Kondrich J, Woo T, Ginsburg HB, Levine DA. Evisceration of small bowel after cauterization of an umbilical mass. Pediatrics. 2012;130(6):e1708–10.
14. Montes-Tapia F, Garza-Luna U, Cura-Esquivel I, Gaytan-Saracho D, de la O-Cavazos M. Appendico-umbilical fistula: cause of umbilical mass with drainage. J Pediatr Gastroenterol Nutr. 2012;55(5):e133.
15. Derakhsham Derakhshan MR. Curative effect of common salt on Umbilical Granuloma Department of Paediatrics, Hamadan University of Medical Sciences and Health Services, I R. Iran; 1998. http://www.sums.ac.ir/JMS/9834/derakhshan9834.html.
16. Wang H, Gao Y, Duan Y, Zheng B, Guo X. Dramatic response of topical doxycycline in umbilical granuloma. Glob Pediatr Health. 2015;2:2333794X15607315. doi:10.1177/2333794X15607315.
17. Brødsgaard A, Nielsen T, Mølgaard U, Pryds O, Pedersen P. Treating umbilical granuloma with

topical clobetasol propionate cream. Acta Paediatr. 2015;104(2):e49.

18. Lotan G, Klin B, Efrati Y. Double-ligature: a treatment for pedunculated umbilical granulomas in children. Am Fam Physician. 2002;65:2067.

19. Sheth SS, Malpani A. The management of umbilical granulomas with cryocautery. Am J Dis Child. 1990;144:146–7.

20. McCallum DI, Hall GF. Umbilical granulomata—with particular reference to talc granuloma. Br J Dermatol. 1970;83:151–6.

21. Yoshida YMD, Yamamoto O. Umbilical pyogenic granuloma associated with occult Omphalith. Dermatol Surg. 2008;34(11):1613–4.

22. Esposito C, Alicchio F, Giurin I, et al. Lessons learned from the first 109 laparoscopic cholecystectomies performed in a single pediatric surgery center. World J Surg. 2009;33(9):1842–5.

23. Fischer H. Volkmann's Sammlung klin. Vortrage, Neue Folge, Nr. 89 (Chirurg., Xo. 24), Leipzig, 1890-94, 519.

Umbilical Hernia (UH)

28

Umbilical hernia is the most common type of midline fascial defect and will be discussed as:

- Hernia of the umbilical cord (congenital UH) (Chap. 32)
- Infantile umbilical hernia
- Proboscoid umbilical hernia
- Acquired umbilical hernia (adult UH):
  - Serous umbilical hernia
  - Recurrent UH

Classifications: Richet [1] at 1856 described an umbilical canal for the first time, and he postulated three main types of umbilical hernia: the congenital, the infantile and the adult hernia.

An umbilical canal is formed anteriorly by the linea alba, posteriorly by the umbilical fascia and laterally by the medial edges of the rectus sheaths with an entrance above the site of the obliterated umbilical vessels up to 3.6 cm.

The umbilical canal, like the inguinal canal, traverses obliquely the abdominal parietes from the peritoneum to the skin surfaces, and both have a similar posterior surface of transversalis fascia and peritoneum. It is suggested that herniation down this canal leads to the adult type of umbilical hernia (Fig. 28.1).

Three types of umbilical ring (UR) were identified in the study by Chang-Seok et al. [2]; their classification was based on the presence of the hole of the ring and whether the ring is covered by the ligamentum teres hepatis or not; they concluded that this ligamentum with the umbilical facia had a protective role against formation of UH (Fig. 28.2).

It appears that there are three main types of umbilical hernia in relation to the umbilical canal:

1. A direct umbilical hernia can form through the umbilical orifice when there is an absence or weakness of fascial strengthening. The hernia

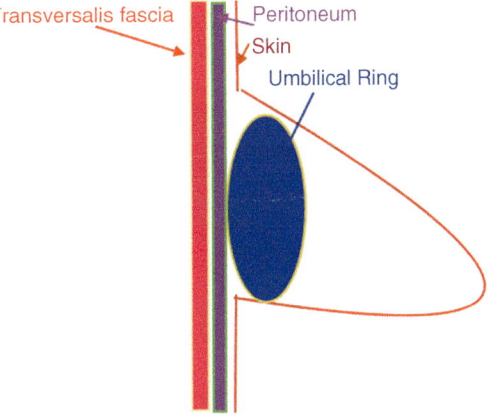

Fig. 28.1 Umbilical canal

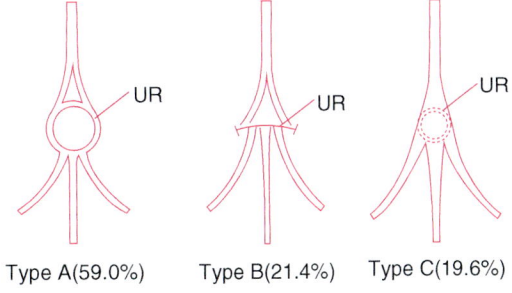

Type A(59.0%)   Type B(21.4%)   Type C(19.6%)

Fig. 28.2 Morphologic variations of the umbilical ring. Redrawn by Springer

© Springer International Publishing AG 2018
M. Fahmy, *Umbilicus and Umbilical Cord*, https://doi.org/10.1007/978-3-319-62383-2_28

tends to 'point' at the superior edge of the umbilical orifice as this area is less strengthened by fibrous tissue. This may be the common type of umbilical hernia seen in infants. It is not affected by the presence or absence of divarication of the recti. The hernia tends to be cured spontaneously when the fascia of the abdominal wall has increased in strength. A fairly wide umbilical orifice does not necessarily mean the presence of a hernia, and a hernia may disappear before the orifice has completely closed (Fig. 28.3).

2. An oblique umbilical hernia may take place through the umbilical canal in later infancy, childhood or adult life. A portion of omentum or bowel passes down the umbilical canal and presents at the upper edge of the umbilicus. This type is more likely to be persistent, and surgical complications might occur. Anatomically this appeared to be of the so-called adult type of hernia in which the hernial protrusion was directed down the umbilical canal and may be an example of the 'semi-

umbilical' hernia mentioned by Browne [3] (Fig. 28.4).

3. Hernias into the umbilical cord: This type is evident at birth, in which a portion of the gut has failed, during embryonic life, to return normally into the abdominal cavity through a narrowed neck. Usually the intestinal wall is firmly adherent to the upper rim of the umbilical orifice, and the 'hernia' cannot be automatically reduced into the peritoneal cavity (Chap. 32).

28.1 Infantile Umbilical Hernia

Historical background: The first references to umbilical hernia were recorded in the Egyptian Papyrus of Ebers (ca. 1552 B.C.). The Ancient Egyptian sculptures and artist were so meticulous to draw a harvester with an aberrant umbilical hernia seen above a truss, which may be an indicator for the failure of this measure in management of UH (Fig. 28.5).

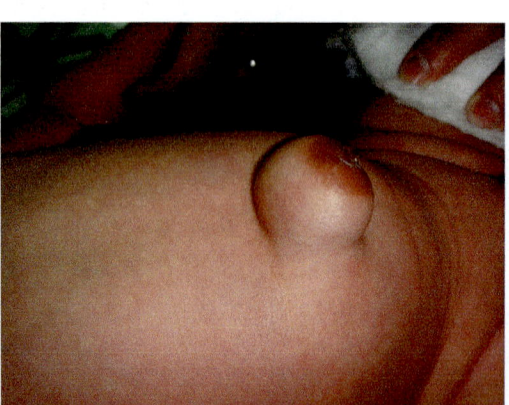

Fig. 28.3 Direct umbilical hernia

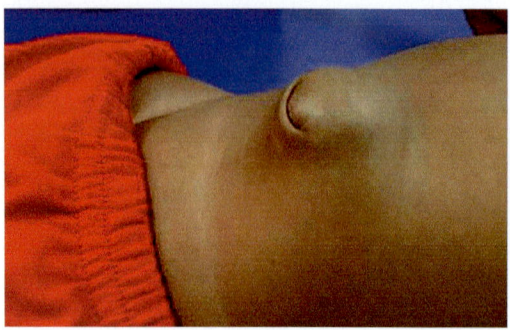

Fig. 28.4 Oblique UH, arising from the superior edge of umbilicus

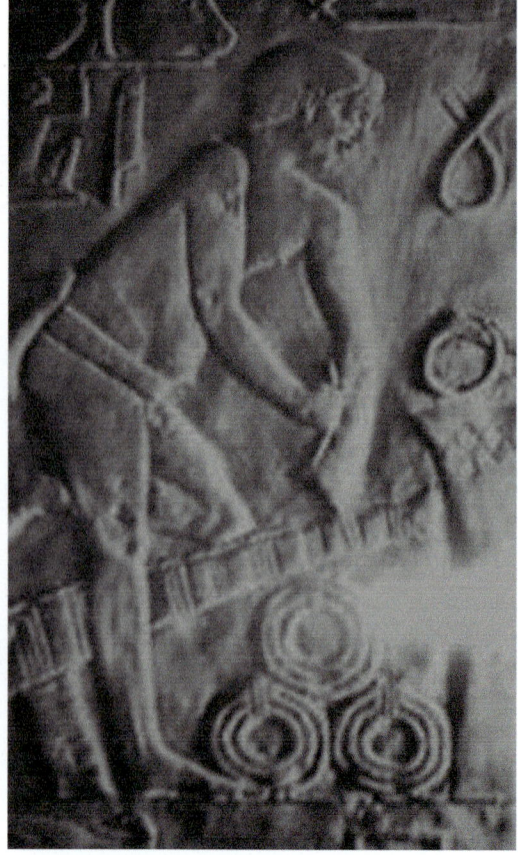

Fig. 28.5 Egyptian Papyrus of Ebers

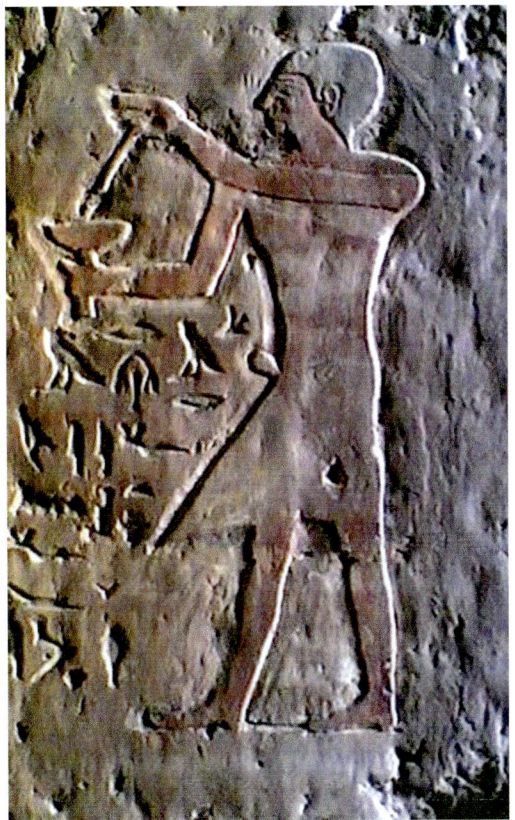

Fig. 28.6 An elderly man suffering from umbilical hernia can be seen in the tomb of Horemheb, at Aswan

An elderly man suffering from umbilical hernia can be seen in the tomb of Horemheb, at Aswan, Egypt (Fig. 28.6).

Also, it is clear from the famous carving of Akhenaten, Nefertiti and their children that both Nefertiti and the child had obvious bulges around the umbilicus with a query umbilical hernias (Fig. 28.7).

The formal description of umbilical hernias comes from the Hindu physician Charaka in his writings dated A.D. one. The ancient Jews also recognized umbilical hernias and treated them conservatively. Celsus, in the first century A.D., treated umbilical hernias with an elastic suture, where an elastic cord of 30–40 cm long is passed around the base of the hernia with a long-curved needle worked through horizontally under the skin. The hernia is then reduced and held in place with the finger, while the elastic cord is drawn tight until the opening is entirely obliterated.

Soranus (A.D. 98–117) was the first one to describe a technique of strapping.

Richet [1] also described an umbilical canal, and he postulated three main types of umbilical hernia: the congenital, the infantile and the adult hernia.

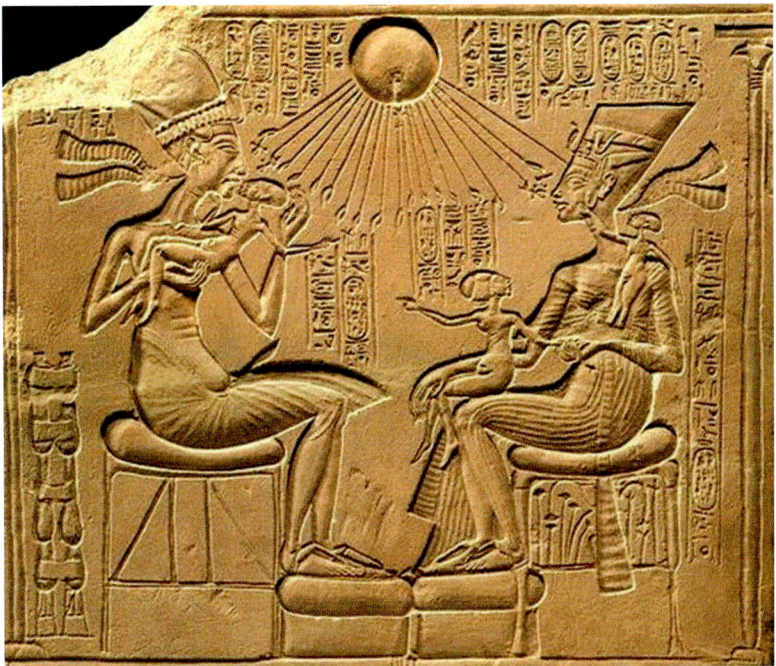

Fig. 28.7 Akhenaten, Nefertiti and their children, that both Nefertiti and the child had obvious bulges around the umbilicus

Erichsen [4] at 1884 declares that these small umbilical hernias are never strangulated and consequently never cause death.

The first recorded description of proper surgical umbilical hernia repair comes from Albucasis, Abul Qasim al-Zahrawi, the great Moorish surgeon (A.D. 1013–1106). But Antonio Benivieni (1443—1502) probably was the first to treat an incarcerated umbilical hernia in a child; he ligated the hernia, and once the mortified flesh fell off, the child regained 'perfect health' [5].

In 1737 Queen Caroline of England had an incarcerated hernia that eventually was lanced to permit drainage of intestinal matter. Surgical treatment had been delayed for 3 days while she was treated with polypharmacy, enemas, aperients and drugs for bleeding, but eventually she died from this hernia complication.

In his *Anatomy of the Human Body*, published in 1750, William Cheselden [6] describes a patient with an incarcerated hernia in whom he amputated the protruding mass of 'mortified bowel and left the end of the sound gut hanging out of the navel to which it afterwards adhered; she recovered and lived many years after, voiding excrement through the intestine at the navel'. Credit for the modern surgical treatment of umbilical hernias is given to Mayo [7], who repaired these defects by overlapping fascia downwards from above ('vest-over-pants').

UH is not only confined to human, but also it is not rare in all mammals, especially dogs and horses (Fig. 28.8).

Definition: Celsus defines a true hernia as a protrusion of loop or knuckle of an organ or tissue through an abnormal opening.

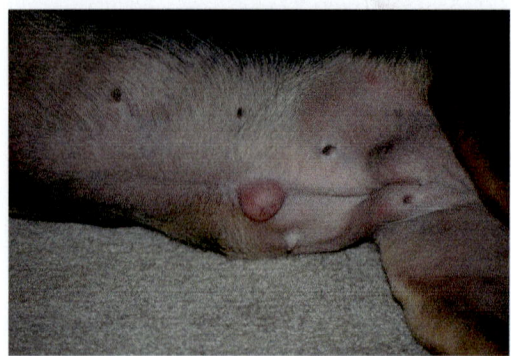

Fig. 28.8 Well-defined UH in a female dog

Umbilical hernia is defined as the presence of a saccular swelling, which protrudes on coughing or crying and can be reduced by simple pressure through a gap in the umbilicus.

Incidence: Is variable in different communities and localities.

UH is a common disorder of the anterior abdominal wall in children (represents >5% of all abdominal hernias). Incidence is estimated approximately 15% with a 10–30% range in white children. Frequency is higher in children of African origin, up to 85% [8].

Etiology: Umbilical hernia is compatible with normal healthy growth, and its occurrence is, in part, dependent on the child's inherited status. The development of the anterior abdominal wall depends on differential growth of embryonic tissues.

Development of the abdominal wall narrows the umbilical ring, which should close before birth. Persistence of the umbilical ring due to persistence of part of omphalomesenteric duct or urachal remnants will result in an umbilical hernia.

Predisposing Factors

- *Breach delivery*: There is a possible tendency of a higher incidence in breach births, and this could be attributed to extensive cord traction in such cases; cord traction either in breach or other modes of delivery increases the incidence of UH [9].
- *Prematurity*: The incidence of herniation after premature or twin births is significantly higher than after a normal birth.
- *Birth weight*: More than 80% of infants weighing less than 1200 g have evidence of an umbilical hernia compared with 21% of infants weighing over 2500 g at birth [8].
- *Length of the cord at birth*: Babies whose cords are of unusual length appear somewhat more predisposed to umbilical hernia.
- *Omphalitis*: A common belief is that sepsis of the umbilicus after separation of the cord tends to induce a hernia. Mild sepsis of the umbilicus after separation of the cord is related to an increased tendency to herniation, but this is not yet proved by a randomized study.
- *Umbilical granuloma*: Woods, in her study of 283 infants with UH, found no relation

between umbilical granuloma and hernia; she followed up 28 cases with granuloma, and no hernia developed, even she claims that treated UG may prevent herniation [9].

- *Size of the umbilical orifice*: It is probable that the palpable size of a gap in the linea alba at the umbilicus in early infancy is not an essential and determining factor as to whether a hernia will develop or not [8].
- *Sex*: UH is ten times more common in females.
- *Family history*: UH diagnosed significantly more frequent in twins. It is a common observation at the clinic that if one infant has a marked hernia, frequently the next baby in the family has one also (Fig. 28.9).
- *Umbilical hernia in coloured children*: There is a widespread opinion that umbilical hernia is an almost a universal condition in coloured children. Cullen in 1916 considered the higher incidence among coloured babies to be due to a thicker cord and a larger umbilicus.
- Mori [10] in 1938 observed a seasonal occurrence of hernia corresponding approximately to the curve for craniotabes and rickets, i.e., the incidence being the highest among babies born in January. I think this finding may have some relationship to

respiratory infection. Bennett-Jones [11] was unconvinced that the high incidence of umbilical hernia in Negro babies was related either to malnutrition, rickets or a large cord. Information received from Nigeria indicates that umbilical hernia is very common among babies there, but they nearly always disappear spontaneously. Probably the higher incidence in coloured babies represents an inherited trait (Fig. 28.10).

- *Umbilical hernia complicating laparoscopic surgery*: With the expansion of the application of different laparoscopic modalities in different surgical practice and with the use of umbilicus as a preferable port, umbilical hernia had been recognized frequently before surgical procedures, and also few cases may complicate laparoscopy. Mayol et al. carried out a prospective trial of 403 patients to assess which factors were predictive of a complication with the placement of trocars, umbilical hernia was found in only 1.5% [12].
- A total of 1071 consecutive patients underwent 1145 transumbilical single-incision laparoscopy (SIL) procedures, followed for 22 months (8–41); 16 (1.4%) developed an incisional umbilical hernia [13].

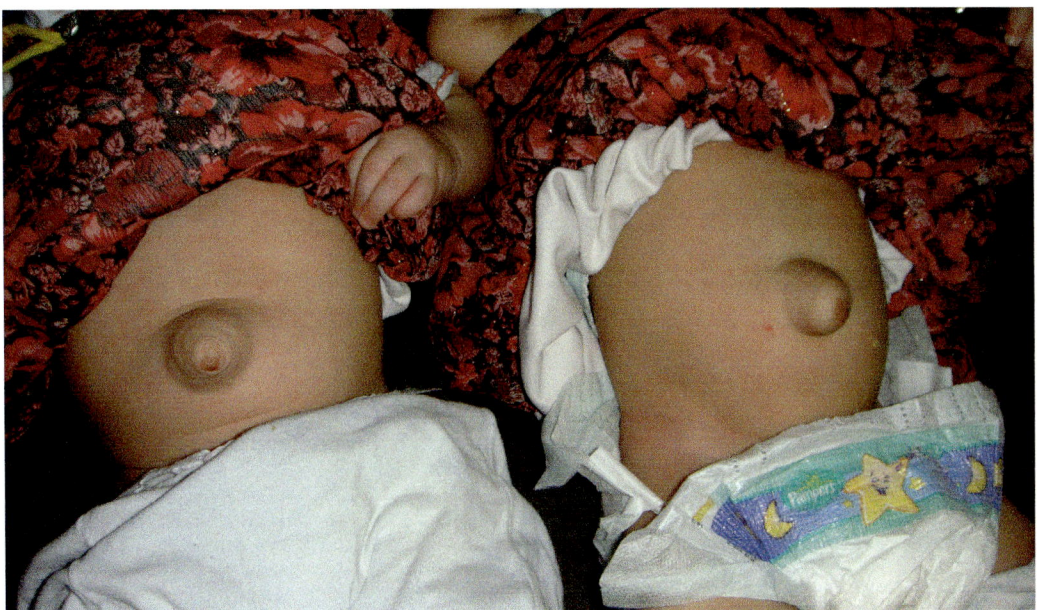

Fig. 28.9 UH in identical twin girls

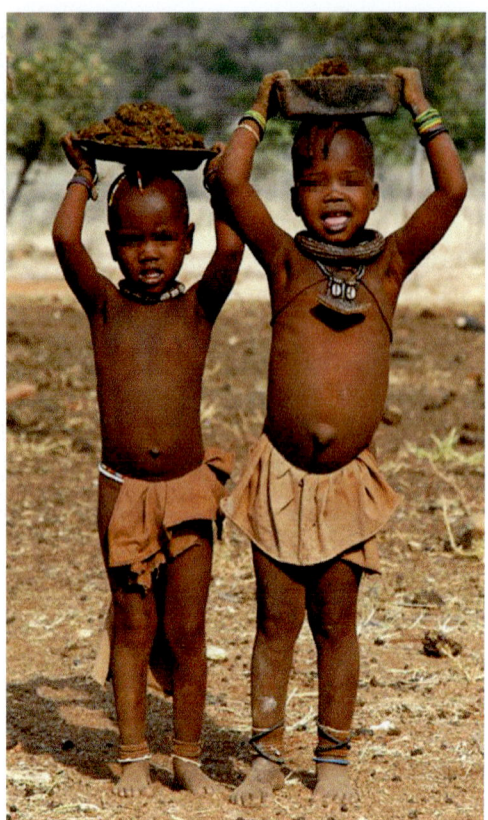

Fig. 28.10 African child with an UH, which is a usual and common condition there

28.2 Immediate Causes Lead to Development of Umbilical Hernia

The preceding observations give a picture of the possible inherent natal and postnatal factors that may influence the later development of an umbilical hernia. However, an immediate physical cause for the occurrence of the hernia, such as chronic constipation, abdominal distension, upper air way obstruction and coughing, excessive crying or repeated vomiting, should be considered, in predisposition of umbilical herniation, and should be managed during the course of conservative measures for management of UH.

28.3 Syndromes Associated with a High Incidence of UH

Generally UH is common to occur in all syndromes and genetic anomalies associated with defective abdominal wall musculature, weak muscle tone and laxity. Constitutional conditions causing either hypotonicity of the abdominal musculature or a rise in the intra-abdominal pressure favour the development of a hernia and aggravate the condition if present. UH in such cases are usually combined with other hernias, commonly a unilateral or even a bilateral inguinal hernia (Fig. 28.11).

Down's syndrome: Umbilical hernia is commonly seen in babies with Down's syndrome, and it may be related to the hypotonicity (Fig. 28.12).

Cretinism: Similarly in cretinism an umbilical hernia is frequently seen and may again be related to severe hypotonia.

Beckwith–Wiedemann syndrome: Is an overgrowth chromosomal disorder usually present at birth, characterized by macroglossia, macrosomia, midline abdominal wall defects (omphalocele/exomphalos, umbilical hernia or diastasis recti), ear creases or ear pits and neonatal hypoglycaemia [14] (Fig. 28.13).

Cutis laxa: Is a disorder of connective tissue, which is often distinguished by the pattern of inheritance, autosomal dominant, autosomal recessive or X-linked; in such cases UH is a common finding.

Hurler's syndrome (mucopolysaccharidosis I): Umbilical hernia in such case may be

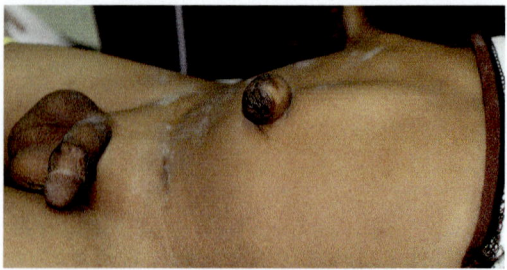

Fig. 28.11 Combined umbilical and right inguinal hernias with a diastasis of recti muscles

Fig. 28.12 Down's syndrome baby with an obvious umbilical hernia

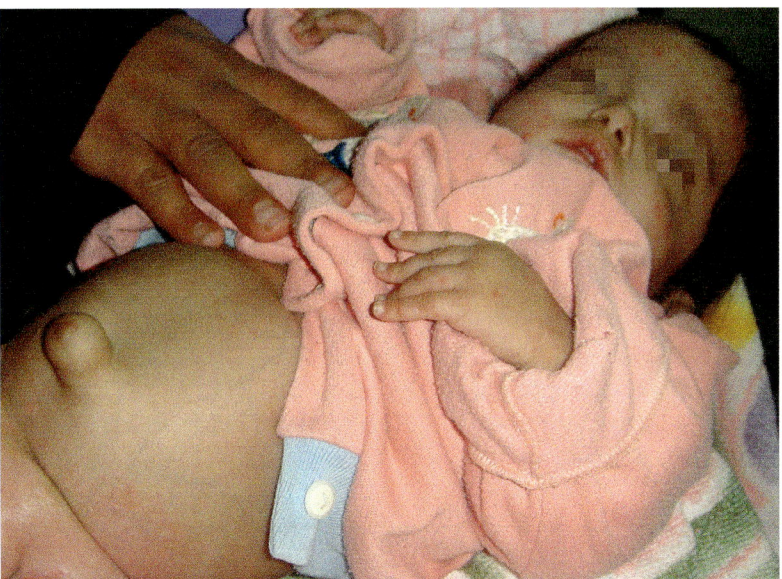

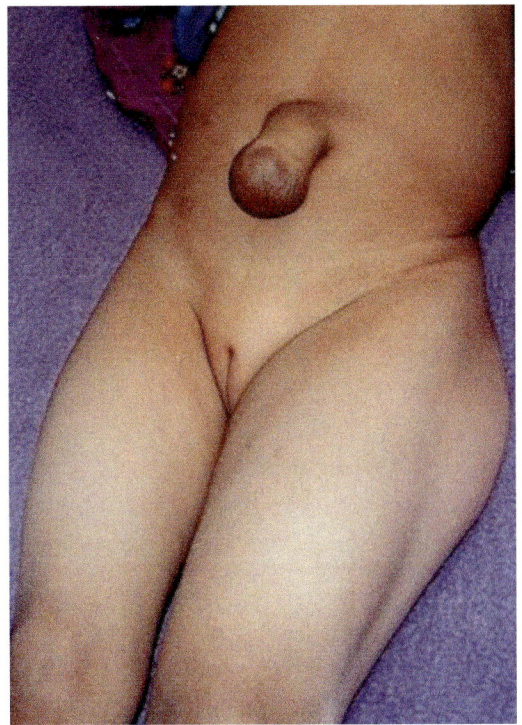

Fig. 28.13 A 5-years-old girl with a Beckwith–Wiedemann syndrome (right-sided hemihypertrophy seen at her thigh) with a protruded UH

secondary to hepatosplenomegaly, with abdominal distension combined with generalized connective tissue weakness [15].

28.4 Pathophysiology of UH

Failure of the normal obliterative processes of the vitelline duct and the urachus leads to abnormal communications or cysts. Retention of components of the umbilical cord can also produce a mass or drainage. A patent umbilical ring at birth is responsible for most umbilical hernias. The umbilical opening is usually reinforced by the attachments of the median umbilical ligament, the obliterated urachus, the paired medial umbilical ligaments and the obliterated umbilical arteries inferiorly and is more weakly reinforced superiorly by the round ligament and the obliterated umbilical vein.

Richet fascia, derived from the transversalis fascia, covers the umbilical ring. The peritoneum covers the innermost portion of the ring. Variability in the attachment of the ligaments and defective Richet fascia may predispose some children to develop umbilical hernias (Fig. 28.2).

However, many children undergo spontaneous closure in the first few years of life. The pressure exerted on the umbilical skin, even when a small umbilical defect is present, can result in marked stretching of the skin and a proboscis appearance.

Proliferation of lateral connective tissue plates passes from the umbilical cord at this point is responsible for closure of the umbilical ring. A failure in the normal growth of the dense connective tissue, which should ultimately occupy the umbilical ring may contribute to local congenital abnormality. In the greater defects like, exomphalos, the supra- and infra-umbilical portions of the abdominal wall have formed, but the intervening area is covered only by amnion, and there is no proper umbilical ring. The ultimate closure of the umbilical ring depends upon the proliferation of encircling mesoderm. When this obliterative proliferation is incomplete, a patent umbilical ring is the result, and hernias through this ring during infancy will be manifested [9].

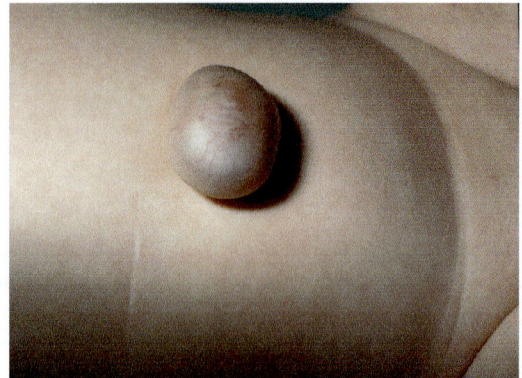

Fig. 28.14 UH with overstretched this skin

28.5   Clinical Picture of UH

Patients with umbilical hernias present early in life with bulging at the umbilicus. The swelling is most prominent when the infant or child is crying or straining. Umbilical hernias usually are asymptomatic and rarely cause pain, but mothers of the baby with such hernia usually attribute any abdominal pain or discomfort to the presence of UH; also parents often mention that the child plays with the redundant skin during swimming and bathing, especially in those with high awareness with their umbilicus. The skin can become severely stretched, which may be alarming to parents and physicians (Fig. 28.14).

Investigations: Diagnosis of UH is usually clinical, but cases suspected to be in association with other specific syndromes will need the congruent investigations; abdominal US will be helpful to rule out any associated abnormalities or related complications. CT scan is helpful to show the exact hernial contents and is indicated especially for complicated or recurrent cases (Fig. 28.15).

Differential diagnosis: UH should be differentiated from other similar umbilical swellings in neonates; an umbilicus cutis (Sect. 32.2) may give the similar look like a hernia, but there is no impulse or expansion on crying and straining; in older children and adults, UH have to be distinguished from other umbilical swellings like malignant nodules, keloid (Chap. 31), haemangioma and papilloma (Chap. 30).

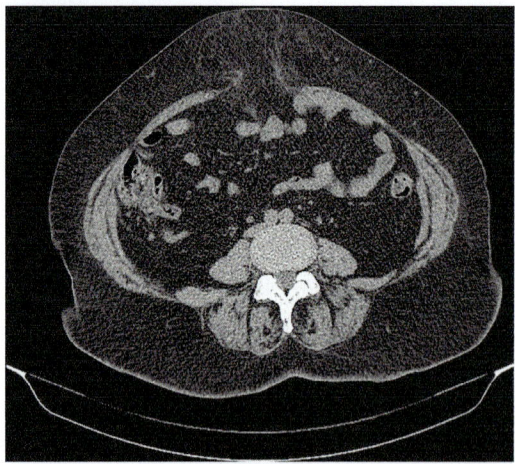

Fig. 28.15 CT scan shows an umbilical herniation of the omentum

28.6   Complications of UH

Adhesion between hernial contents (usually omentum) and the skin is more common than strangulation.

Incarceration of umbilical hernias is rare in the paediatric population, than in adults; over a 15-year period, only 7 children with an incarcerated umbilical hernia were reported at the Johns Hopkins Hospital, in comparison to 101 cases of incarceration that occurred in adults during the 15-year period; this is because of the absence of a muscular ring around UH orifice, whose spasm could provoke this complication, but it is supposed that UH incarceration in children may be much more frequent than it is generally supposed [16] (Fig. 28.16).

Incarceration, strangulation, bowel obstruction, erosion of the overlying skin and bowel perforation are rare events in infants and small children [17] (Fig. 28.16).

The incidence of umbilical hernia incarceration and strangulation has been reported to be 0.07% in 1 of 1500 children and at 0.3% in 1 of 329 children. Worldwide, only 38 descriptions of incarcerated or strangulated umbilical hernias in children were founded [18].

Global morbidity for incarcerated external hernias ranges from 19 to 46%, with major morbidity (pulmonary, cardiac, renal or digestive disease) between 10 and 15% and mortality between 3 and 13% [18].

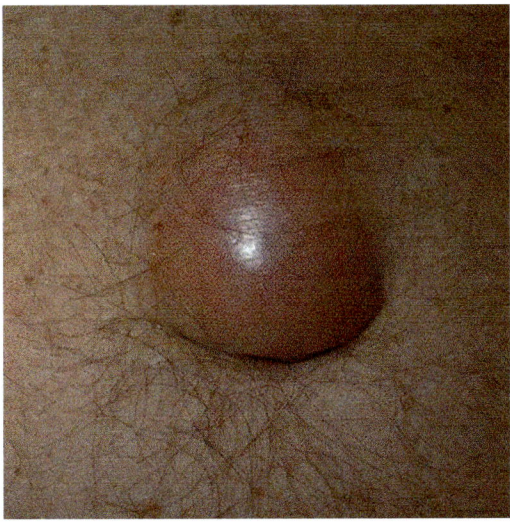

Fig. 28.16 Incarcerated UH in adult

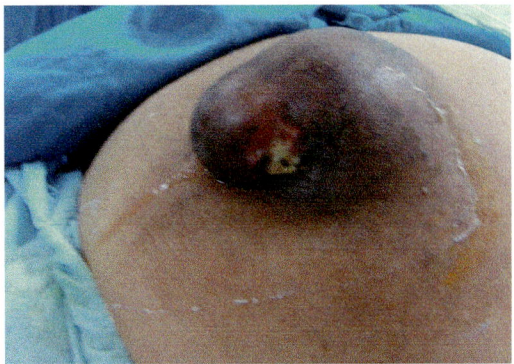

Fig. 28.17 Large UH in a child with incarceration and dusky necrotic skin, a gangrenous bowel detected on exploration

Richter's hernia refers to a condition in which a portion of the bowel wall is entrapped in the hernia sac without symptoms of ileus; this condition tends to occur most frequently in aged patients, particularly elderly females, Richter's hernia is commoner with inguinal than with umbilical hernias.

28.7 Management

Repair can be performed using an open or laparoscopic technique. Laparoscopic repair may be particularly beneficial for patients who are obese and diabetic, have two or more hernias, have diastasis recti or have a defect >2 cm, while open repair may be sufficient for all other patients. Routine mesh placement has been proven to reduce hernia recurrence rates in adult; despite this, half of all umbilical hernias are being repaired with sutures only. In laparoscopic repair, mesh is placed in an underlay (intraperitoneal) position, while in open repair it is placed in the sublay (preperitoneal) position [19].

Nonoperative management may be only considered for high risk or asymptomatic patients.

Regardless of the presence of any predisposing factors, most hernias close spontaneously and do not require operative closure. If not repaired in childhood, 10% of umbilical hernias will persist to adulthood [20].

Debate remains regarding the timing for umbilical hernia repair, and the true instance of complications related to umbilical hernias in adults is not known. Most surgeons agree that, in most cases, small hernias can be monitored safely. Although spontaneous closure does occur, large hernias with large fascial defects are less likely to close on their own, and continued stretching of the umbilical skin may make closure more difficult. Therefore, many surgeons advocate earlier repair in these children. Others argue that umbilical hernias should be monitored until children are aged 5 years.

It is the size of the fascial defect, rather than the size of the external protrusion, that predicts the potential for spontaneous closure. Walker demonstrated that fascial rings measuring less than 1 cm in diameter usually close spontaneously, whereas rings larger than 2 cm seldom do. Accordingly, many paediatric surgeons will repair umbilical hernias with large (>2.5 cm) fascial defects earlier than hernias with smaller fascial defects [21].

The diameter of the umbilical ring defect is predictive of spontaneous closure. The length of the protruding skin is not prognostically significant. Umbilical hernias with ring diameters less than 1 cm are more likely to close spontaneously than those with ring diameters more than 1.5 cm. Surgery is indicated for all symptomatic umbilical hernias. Incarceration, strangulation, skin erosion and bowel perforation are indications for immediate surgery. Similarly, patients presenting with pain should be repaired on an elective basis.

Management of UH in Africa: Most African surgeons do not use the same indications for umbilical hernia repair as are used in developed countries. Instead, they recommend repairing only those umbilical hernias that are symptomatic in children [21].

However, the incidence of incarceration or strangulation seems to be higher in Africa than in developed countries. Because of this, some African surgeons have recommended repairing all umbilical hernias in children. Others, however, continue to recommend conservative treatment in spite of the risk of incarceration. Part of the rationale given is the wide prevalence of umbilical hernias.

Even using selective criteria, Meier et al. [22] have estimated that if all umbilical hernias >1.5 cm were repaired in young children in Africa, about 6–8% of children younger than 4 years of age would require repair; the volume of cases would likely outstrip available surgical resources. The exact criteria for elective repair on which Meier et al. based their estimates were females older than 2 years of age and males older than 4 years of age with a fascial defect ≥1.5 cm in diameter; they estimated that 6% of 2-year-old females and 8% of 4-year-old males would need repair.

If hernias with large (>1.5 cm) fascial defects are indeed the most likely to incarcerate in Africa, as reported by Chirdan et al. [23], one could argue that they should be repaired, as they are the most likely to incarcerate and the least likely to spontaneously close. Consideration should also be given to closing umbilical hernias in patients who live more than 1 h away from surgical resources. More research is necessary to determine the actual incidence of incarceration or strangulation and to clearly define which umbilical hernias are at greatest risk.

For instance, with the wide prevalence of UH in Africa, just as healthcare workers have been specifically trained to suture lacerations or to perform caesarean sections, perhaps consideration should be given to specifically train them to perform simple, straightforward surgical procedures such as umbilical hernia repairs.

Operative details: Umbilical hernias are approached through an incision in the infraumbilical crease. Dissection is carried down to the level of the fascia. Care is taken to avoid injury to contents within the hernia sac and to the umbilical skin. Opening the anterior surface of the sac may help to avoid injury to the bowel. The sac is resected down to the level of the fascia. The umbilical fascia is closed with interrupted absorbable suture. The wound should be inspected and meticulous haemostasis achieved. The umbilicus is tacked down to the fascia with an interrupted suture. The subcutaneous tissue is reapproximated with a few interrupted sutures, and the skin is closed with a subcuticular stitch. Bupivacaine can be injected for postoperative analgesia. The skin is cleaned, and Steri-Strips are applied. A pressure dressing may be used for large hernias to prevent a postoperative haematoma or seroma (Fig. 28.17).

Percutaneous ultrasound-guided (PERC) rectus sheath blocks with a local anaesthetic would result in lower postoperative pain scores following umbilical hernia repair [24].

Umbilicoplasty: Umbilicoplasty is necessary for giant protruding hernias with excess skin. Many

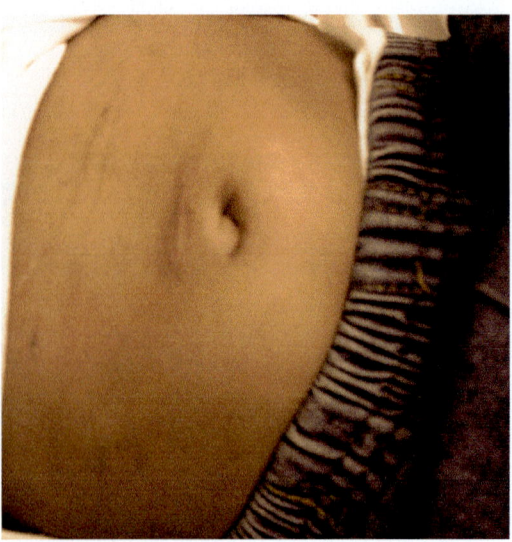

Fig. 28.18 Postoperative UH repair with an acceptable scar and normally looking umbilicus

techniques were described, but the aesthetic results are often unsatisfactory. The number of techniques described in the medical literature for umbilicoplasty in cases of giant umbilical hernias demonstrates that there is no ideal surgical approach for such cases. The difficulty does not lie in the closure of the aponeurosis but in removing the excess skin leading to a satisfactory aesthetic effect.

Routine umbilicoplasty, generally, is not needed. In most cases, a redundant umbilicus appears more natural than a neoumbilicus. Several techniques can be used for extremely protuberant umbilical hernias. A simple technique is to invert the umbilicus over a finger so that the undersurface is exposed. The skin is then incised circumferentially so that a 1- to 2-cm rim of umbilicus remains. The umbilical skin defect is reapproximated from within the umbilicus and tacked down to the fascia [25].

Elective umbilical hernia repair with mesh should be considered in patients with multiple comorbidities given that the use of mesh offers protection from recurrence without major morbidity.

One prospective, randomized, controlled trial reported a reduced recurrence rate of 1% for open repairs with mesh versus 11% in primary suture repairs [26].

Despite this, the trend continues to lean towards primary suture repair, which provides relatively easy access, relatively smaller incision and faster completion and ease of procedure, allowing junior trainees to perform the procedure with less training time compared with the laparoscopic method.

Laparoscopic repair of primary umbilical hernias can be considered as a preferred method of repair where a mesh is indicated and where there is suitable expertise [27].

Follow-up care: Children undergoing umbilical surgery must be seen in the surgery clinic 2–6 weeks following surgery or sooner if problems occur.

Umbilical truss: Truss is well known for UH management since the Ancient Egyptian time and unfortunately is still in use at different developing countries (Fig. 28.5). Different types are still prescribed, and traditional use of strapping with adhesive materials or applying coins is still in use by paramedics inspite of their known complications (Figs. 28.19 and 28.20).

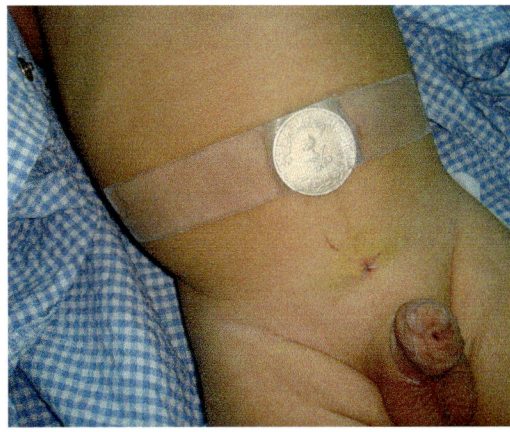

Fig. 28.19 UH in a 2-years-old child managed traditionally by coin and tape

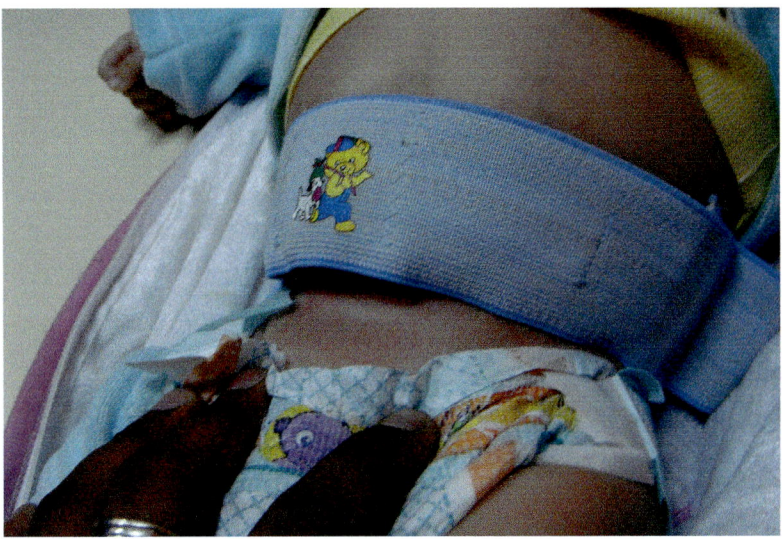

Fig. 28.20 UH truss

Fig. 28.21 Skin excoriation and eczema secondary to umbilical truss

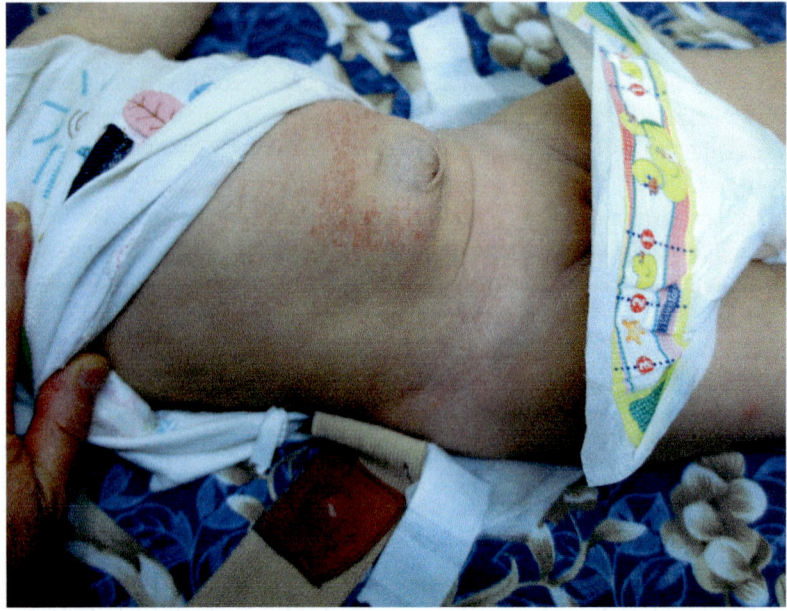

Complications of umbilical truss: Firstly, the truss causes a great deal of irritation ending very frequently in troublesome eczema. Secondly, it is impossible to prevent the truss getting sodden with urine, and it becomes, in consequence, most objectionable and dangerous. Thirdly, the pressure of a truss, strong enough to keep up an ordinary hernia, prevents the muscles from developing in the neighbourhood of the inguinal canal, and consequently the abdominal wall is weakened, and hernia ruptures are liable to occur later in life (Fig. 28.21).

28.8   Proboscoid Umbilical Hernia (PUH)

Umbilical hernia in children had a lot of variabilities from case to case and from locality to another; one of special entities of UH is the proboscoid one.

Definition: A large protuberant umbilical hernia shaped like a proboscis nose, the term derived from the 'Proboscis monkey' with its characteristic nose (Fig. 28.22).

In Africa, proboscoid umbilical hernias are common and may be well accepted and treated conservatively by some surgeons, but this variety

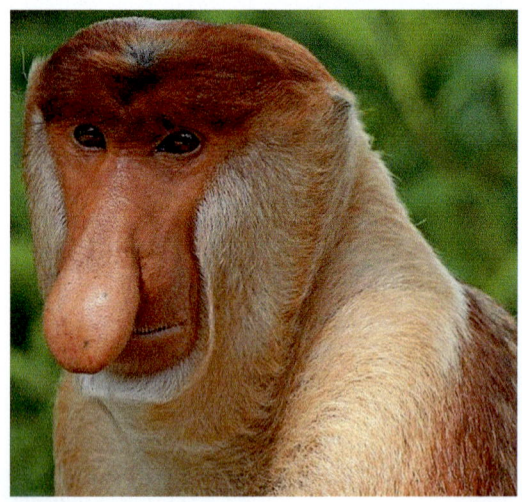

Fig. 28.22 Proboscis monkey, with a characteristic long nose

is not common in Europe, except in association with other syndromes of defective abdominal musculature.

Clinically: In this variety of UH, the facial defect may be not so wide, but there is a large hernial skin with downward displacement of the umbilicus and appearing as descending from above (Fig. 28.23).

Significance: From my follow-up of a considerable number of PUH, this hernia is usually annoying to the family with its large expansile size; it may be difficult for the mother to apply napkins properly without irritation of the redundant hernial skin, which will be liable to contact dermatitis and eczema (Fig. 28.24).

Also in this type of hernia, the older children become anxious with this protruded mass, which is obvious from their cloths and makes the child embarrassed in front of his colleagues during changing cloths throughout sporting (Fig. 28.25).

PUH is more liable for skin necrosis, especially in the contiguous surface with abdominal wall. Incarceration is more common with this variety of UH [23].

Management: PUH has to be operated as early as possible; spontaneous regression is unlikely to occur; follow-up of 13 cases for 3 years results in no regression of size in any, but even the hernial size is progressively increased. The main cause of parental anxiety is the resultant redundant umbilical skin following repair rather than the hernia defect itself, so different types of flaps, with rea-

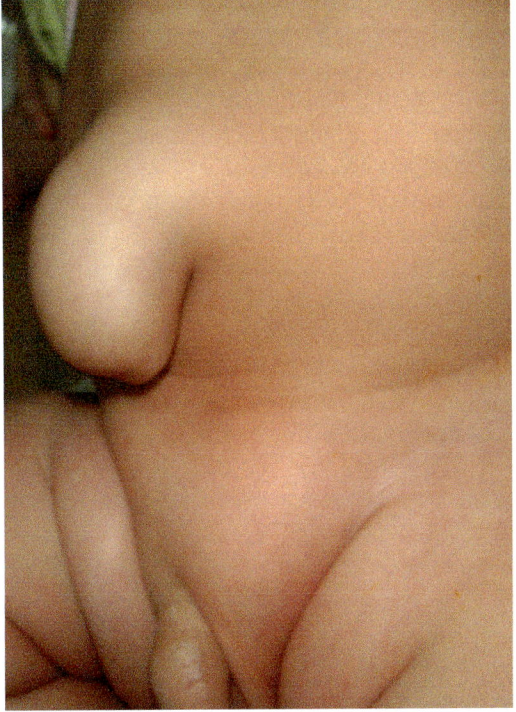

Fig. 28.23 A typical case of proboscoid UH in a 2-year-old boy

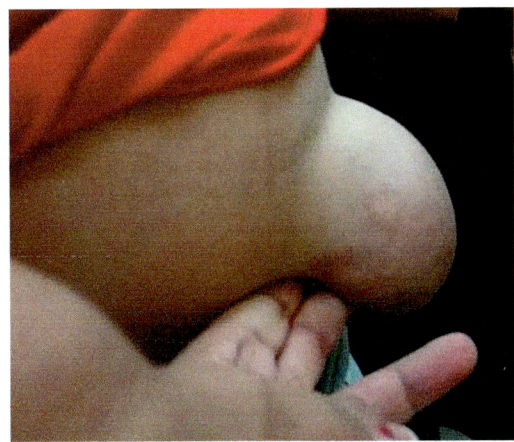

Fig. 28.25 A large proboscoid UH annoying this 4-year-old girl, who is lifting it from her abdominal wall

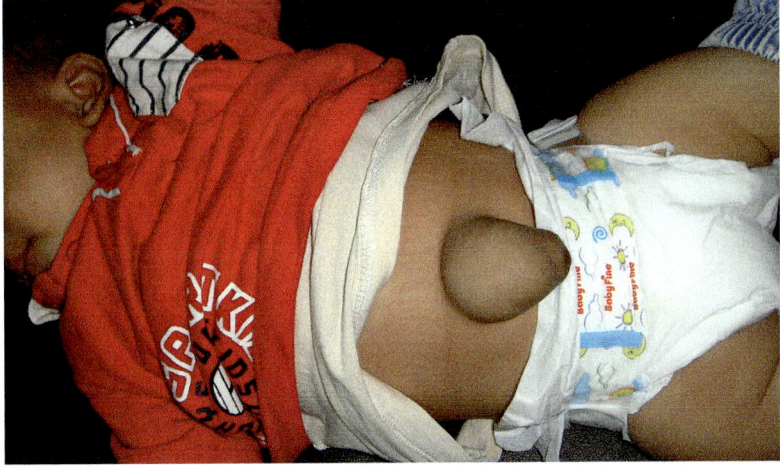

Fig. 28.24 A proboscoid UH interfering with proper placement of napkins

sonable outcome, are recommended for fashioning the umbilicus after repair of the abdominal wall defects in proboscoid hernia [28, 29].

28.9 Acquired Umbilical Hernia

UH in adult may be a concealed congenital UH, which becomes obvious only after increasing abdominal pressure or weakness of the abdominal musculature, or it could be an acquired defect due to same factors; adult hernia is distinguished from paediatric one by more liability for complications and unlikely to close or regress spontaneously. At the same time the recurrence rate is higher especially after open surgery if no mesh is used [26] (Fig. 28.26).

There is no consensus on the best technique for the repair of umbilical hernia in adults. The role of laparoscopic hernioplasty of umbilical hernia remains controversial [30].

28.9.1 Serous Umbilical Hernia

Definition: An umbilical hernia secondary to progressive abdominal distension due to ascites with or without organomegaly. In some instances in which the abdomen contains a large quantity of ascitic fluid, the umbilicus unfolds, as it was, and becomes distended, so as to suggest an umbilical hernia. Indeed, the condition has been termed a serous umbilical hernia. While this unfolding of the umbilicus is not very common, still it is by no means rare. The reason that so little has been written on the subject is evidently due to the fact that the accumulation of ascitic fluid in the umbilical sac has been looked upon as a perfectly natural accompaniment of the abdominal distention associated with a large amount of ascitic fluid [31].

Ascites is usually attributable to nephrotic syndrome, liver cirrhosis, cardiac failure or a combination of one or more of these conditions. Increased intra-abdominal pressure by a large ovarian cyst, either benign or malignant, especially at old age, which may be complicated by a similar umbilical herniation.

Umbilical hernia detected in about 12% of cases of peritoneal dialysis.

Historical background: Perrin [32] in 1910 was the first one to discuss this subject in details, but credit goes to Catteau [33] who was the first one to record such cases.

Ancient Egyptian sculpture demonstrated clearly an umbilical hernia secondary to abdominal distension, either due to ascites or organomegaly (Fig. 28.27).

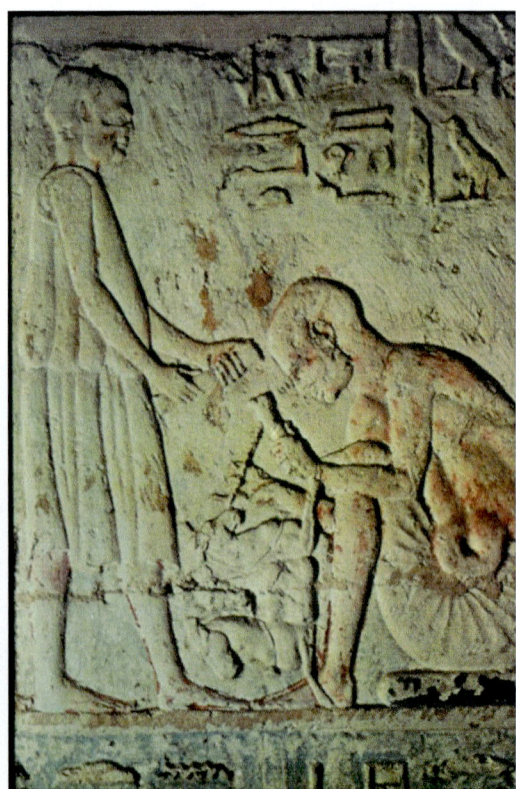

Fig. 28.27 Tuneh el Gebel, Tomb of Petosiris, A sculptor in his workshop with abdominal distension and umbilical hernia

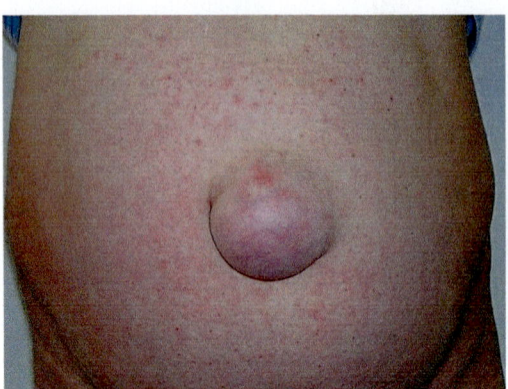

Fig. 28.26 Adult UH

Umbilical hernia with ascites may be presented as:

Slight projection of the umbilicus (Fig. 28.28).
Unfolding of the umbilicus (Fig. 28.29).
True umbilical hernia (Fig. 28.30).

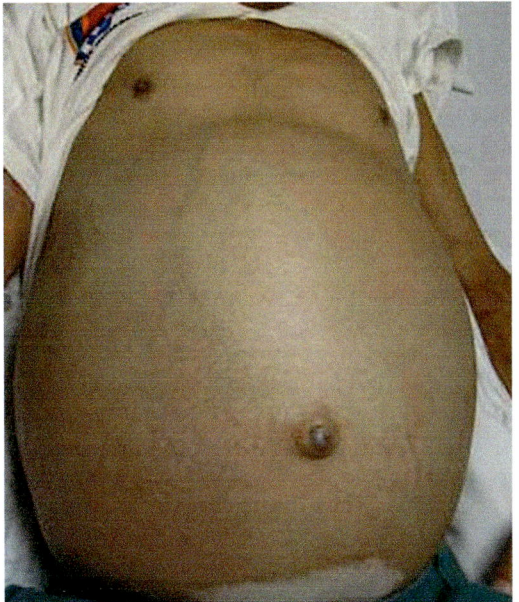

Fig. 28.28 Serous UH with just slight projection of the umbilicus

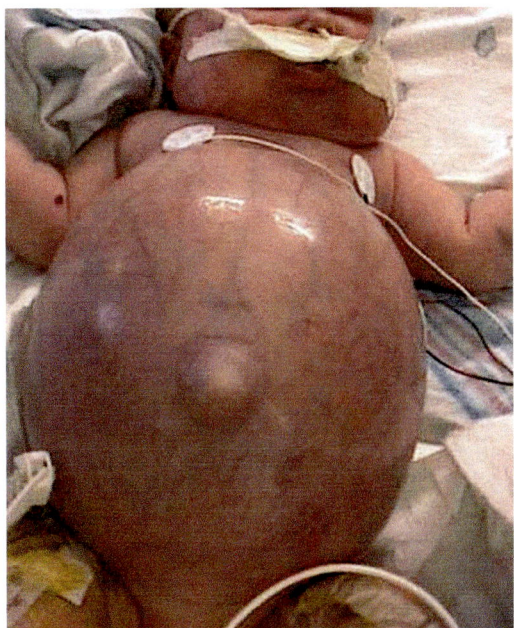

Fig. 28.29 Unfolding of the umbilicus in a neonate with massive abdominal distension with ascites

Hernia may be very small or reaches 2 or 3 cm in diameter. The overhang skin looks normal, and often the sac is seen to contain clear fluid. Sometimes, this can be detected only by transmitted light.

As the intra-abdominal pressure continues, the umbilical tumor may become as large and may be either hemispheric or lobulated. When the hernia reaches such a size, the overlying skin is usually greatly stretched, and the fluid contents of the sac are easily distinguishable.

Serous umbilical hernia in children: Very few cases have been recorded at young age, simply because ascites is much rarer in children than in adults. Larger percentage of serous umbilical hernias in the child, as in early life, are seen in cases of hydrate fettles and in cases of ventriculoperitoneal shunting, especially in cases of high cerebrospinal fluid output (Fig. 28.29).

Bilateral inguinal hernia or hydrocele may be associating the umbilical protrusion in such occasions (Fig. 28.31).

Rupture of the umbilicus distended by ascitic fluid is very rare. The most common complications of umbilical hernias in patients with cirrhosis and ascites include leakage, ulceration, and incarceration. If such a complication is present, there is a high mortality rate after surgical repair.

Managements: Elective repair is the most effective choice, as it prevents complications with a lower mortality; however, the control of ascites before and/or after repair is mandatory but may not always be possible with diuretics and paracentesis.

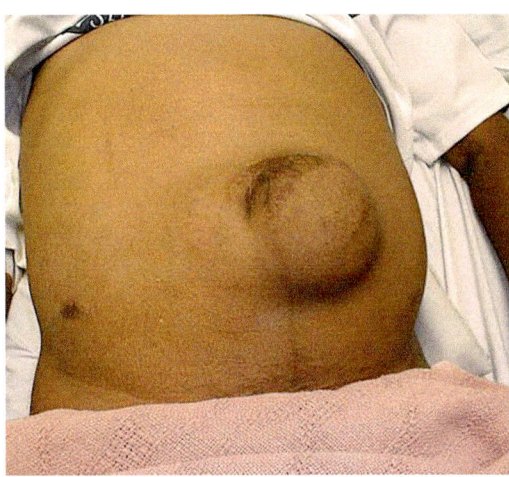

Fig. 28.30 True umbilical hernia with ascites

Fig. 28.31 Combined umbilical hernia and bilateral hydrocele secondary to high CSF output from a ventriculoperitoneal shunting

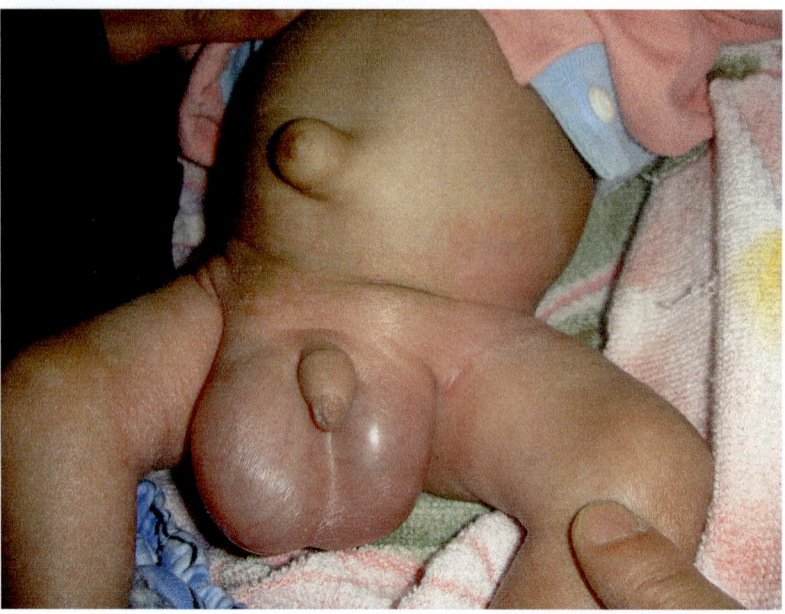

28.10   Recurrent Umbilical Hernias

Ascites, liver disease, diabetes, obesity and primary suture repair without mesh are associated with an increased umbilical hernia recurrence rates (Fig. 28.32).

Umbilical defects following omphalocele or gastroschisis repair are considered as an incisional hernia; even though it is detectable around the umbilicus, such cases are also liable for bowel adhesions. Recurrent hernia patient can be good candidates for laparoscopic hernia repair.

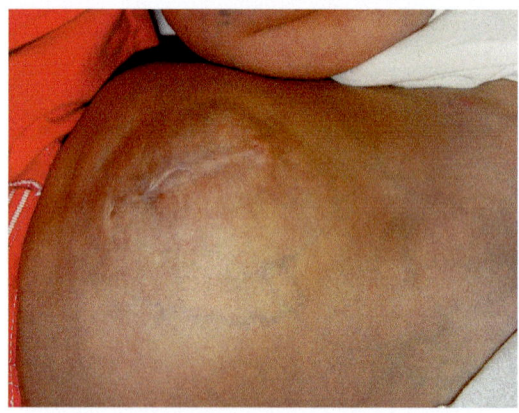

Fig. 28.32 Recurrent UH, with a wide defect and lost umbilical scar, secondary to wound infection

References

1. Richet A. Arch. Gen. Fed. 1856; ser. 5, 8, 641.
2. Chang-Seok O, et al. Morphologic variations of the umbilical ring, umbilical ligaments and ligamentum teres hepatis. Yonsei Med J. 2008;49(6):1004–7.
3. Browne D. Abdominal hernia in childhood. Br Med J. 1952;2:1144.
4. Erichsen JE. The science and art of surgery, vol. 2. 8th ed. London: Longmans, Green & co; 1884. p. 822–3.
5. Brun: treatment of umbilical hernia. Jour. Amer. Med. Assoc, 1912, October 26, 1578. Abstract from Arch, de medecine des enfants, Paris, Sept. xv, No. 9, 641.
6. Cheselden W. The anatomy of the human body. London: C. Hitch & R. Dodsley; 1750.
7. Mayo WJ. Radical cure of umbilical hernia. JAMA. 1907;XLVIII(22):1842–4. doi:10.1001/jama.1907.25220480020002d B.
8. Zendejas B, Kuchena A, Onkendi EO, et al. Fifty-three-year experience with pediatric umbilical hernia repairs. J Pediatr Surg. 2011;46(11):2151–6.
9. Woods GE. Some observations on umbilical hernia of infants. Arch Dis Child. 1953;28:450–62.
10. Mori S. Orient. J Dis Infants. 1938;24:10.
11. Bennett-Jones MJ. Umbilical Hernia in Children. Br Med J. 1944;1:78.
12. Mayol J, Garcia-Aguilar J, Ortiz-Oshiro E, De-Diego CJ, Fernandez-Represa JA. Risks of the minimal access approach for laparoscopic surgery: multivariate analysis of morbidity related to umbilical trocar insertion. World J Surg. 1997;21:529–33.
13. Weiss HG, et al. Wound complications in 1145 consecutive transumbilical single-incision laparoscopic procedures. Ann Surg. 2014;259(1):89–95.
14. Wiedemann HR. Familial malformation complex with umbilical hernia and macroglossia - a "new syndrome"? J Génét Hum. 1964;13:223–32.
15. Hulsebos RG, Zeebregts CJ, de Langen ZJ. Perforation of a congenital umbilical hernia in a patient with Hurler's syndrome. J Pediat Surg. 2004;39(9):1426–7. doi:10.1016/j.jpedsurg.2004.05.024.
16. Ginsburg BY, Sharma AN. Spontaneous rupture of an umbilical hernia with evisceration. J Emerg Med. 2006;30(2):155–7.
17. Okada T, et al. Strangulated umbilical hernia in a child: report of a case. Surg Today. 2001;31:546–9.
18. Hermosa JR, et al. Incarcerated umbilical hernia in a super-super-obese patient. Obes Surg. 2008;18(7):893–5.
19. Hope WW, Cobb WS, Adrales GL. Umbilical hernia in textbook of hernia. New York: Springer; 2017. p. 305–15. doi:10.1007/978-3-319-43045-4_40.
20. Triantos CK, Kehagias I, Nikolopoulou V, Burroughs AK. Surgical repair of umbilical hernias in cirrhosis with ascites. Am J Med Sci. 2011;341(3):222–6. doi:10.1097/MAJ.0b013e3181f31932.
21. Walker SH. The natural history of umbilical hernia. A six-year follow up of 314 negro children with this defect. Clin Pediatr. 1967;6(1):29–32.
22. Meier DE, OlaOlorun DA, Omodele RA, et al. Incidence of umbilical hernia in African children: redefinition of "normal" and reevaluation of indications for repair. World J Surg. 2001;25:645–8.
23. Chirdan LB, Uba AF, Kidmas AT. Incarcerated umbilical hernia in children. Eur J Pediatr Surg. 2006;16:45–8.
24. Litz CN, et al. Percutaneous ultrasound-guided vs. intraoperative rectus sheath block for pediatric umbilical hernia repair: a randomized clinical trial. J Pediatr Surg. 2017;52(6):901–6.
25. Lee SL, DuBois JJ, Greenholz SK, Huffman SG. Advancement flap umbilicoplasty after abdominal wall closure: postoperative results compared with normal umbilical anatomy. J Pediatr Surg. 2001;36(8):1168–70.
26. Arroyo A, García P, Pérez F, Andreu J, Candela F, Calpena R. Randomized clinical trial comparing suture and mesh repair of umbilical hernia in adults. Br J Surg. 2001;88(10):1321–3.
27. Solomon TA, et al. A retrospective audit comparing outcomes of open versus laparoscopic repair of umbilical/paraumbilical herniae. Surg Endosc. 2010;24(12):3109–12.
28. Reyna TM, Hollis HW Jr, Smith SB. Surgical management of proboscoid herniae. J Pediatr Surg. 1987;22(10):911–2.
29. Ikeda H, et al. Umbilicoplasty for large protruding umbilicus accompanying umbilical hernia: a simple and effective technique. Pediatr Surg Int. 2004;20(2):105–7.
30. Lau H, Patil NG. Umbilical hernia in adults. Surg Endosc Interv Tech. 2003;17(12):2016–20.
31. García-Ureña MÁ, et al. Prevalence and management of hernias in peritoneal dialysis patients. Perit Dial Int. 2006;26(2):198–202.
32. Perrin M. An epitome of current medical literature. Br Med J. 1910;1:E21–4.
33. Catteau JF. De l'ombilic et de ses modifications dans les cas de distension de l'abdomen. These de Paris, 1876, obs. 11, 12, 13.

Umbilical Polyp (UP)

Classification: In many textbooks, umbilical polyps are discussed only under the heading of omphalomesenteric one, but from the collection of all reported cases, we are herein classifying this anomaly into:

Congenital polyp:

- Omphalomesenteric duct (OMD) remnant
- Urachal remnant (Chap. 35)
- Ectopic mucosa
- Fibrous umbilical polyp (FUP)

Acquired or neoplastic polyp will be discussed in Chap. 30.

Definition: Generally a polyp is an abnormal growth of tissue projecting from a mucous membrane. If it is attached to the surface by a narrow elongated stalk, it is said to be pedunculated, if no stalk is present, it is said to be sessile. The umbilical one is a red, moist mass, which usually appears since birth and may bleed on touch. During childhood, the umbilicus can be the site of many other lesions; most of them corresponding to inflammatory process, wall defect or neoplastic proliferation [1].

Historical background: Fitz at 1884 [2] described in details the UP related to OMD remnant, but probably the first case of umbilical papilloma was recorded by Fabricius von Hilden (often called the 'Father of German surgery'), which was published at 1526.

Incidence: Remnants of the vitellointestinal duct are said to be present in 2–4% of all routine postmortem examinations, but presumably many people live their allotted span of life despite their presence and at no time have symptoms referable to them [3].

The overall incidence of anomalies of the omphalomesenteric duct is 1 in 15,000 live births, as reported by Kittle. Other cases of UP are only a case report, without any estimated overall incidence in the population [4].

Histology: Histologically umbilical polyp shows branching glandular structures lined by different types of intestinal mucosa, or any other ectopic mucosa, and extensive capillary proliferation with a diffuse chronic inflammatory cells infiltrate in connection with the epidermal surface of the skin.

A study done by Heatley [5] on a total of 19 cases of umbilical mass revealed 16 cases of umbilical polyp, 2 sinuses and 2 patent vitellointestinal ducts. Fourteen cases of umbilical polyp were lined by small intestinal mucosa, and five cases were lined by gastric mucosa in addition to small intestinal mucosa.

Clinical presentation: UP usually presented in the form of a small tumor arising from the bottom of the umbilical depression, measuring a few millimetres, being sessile or pedunculated, and with a bright red, smooth, wet sticky surface, which is sometimes itchy and sensitive or could bleed on contact or it may produces serous secretions staining clothes. A small hole can sometimes cross the lesion (Fig. 29.1).

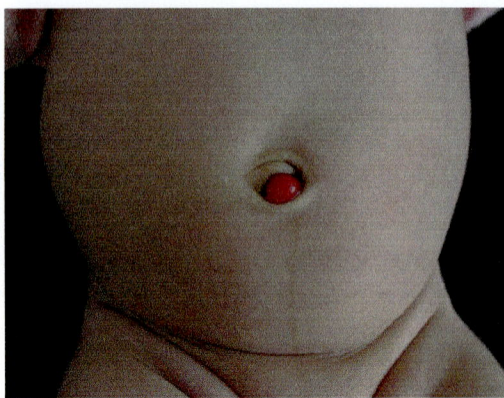

Fig. 29.1 Typical UP with wet, *red* and glistening surface

The lesion is present at birth but the patient may not present until months later having a nonhealing umbilical remnant with persistent drainage or bleeding. Males are affected more often than females.

Diagnosis: Early diagnosis of this lesion can facilitate treatment and lessen the risk from associated congenital anomalies of the primitive vitelline connection and its complications, which may range from intestinal obstruction to intussusception. Diagnosis of an OMD remnant is generally made on physical examination [6].

Currently, there is no established protocol that exists for the workup of umbilical polyps; however, most authors agree that radiographic studies can be useful when suspicious of an underlying abnormality associated with the external lesion; typically, ultrasound is performed first and can evaluate for the presence of a cyst, sinus or deeper tract; if positive or not definitive, this can be followed by a contrast or more detailed study, like CT scan or MRI, which may be indicated in cases with suspicious cyst or swelling in the underlying layers. In few cases the precise diagnosis is often not confirmed until surgery is performed, and the anatomy of the umbilicus is established [7].

Differential diagnosis: It is not acceptable recently to diagnose UP and to differentiate it from the commoner lesions of umbilical granuloma, only after a trial of treatment with silver nitrate, as it was mentioned in many literature. UP should be detected and diagnosed early during neonatal period or immediately after birth, before any attempts of conservative or surgical treatment; the clues for differentiation of UP from granuloma are:

- Granuloma never occurs with the presence of any other umbilical structures; it appears only after falling down of the stump, on the contrary to UP, which could be seen immediately after birth and with the presence of cord stump.
- The presence of any another structure or tissue beside the umbilical cord is definitely going with the diagnosis of UP (Fig. 29.2).
- Presence of any punctum in the umbilical mass is against diagnosis of granuloma (Fig. 29.3), intestinal contents may be appreciated from this punctum when the child cries or coughs (Fig. 29.4) or if a

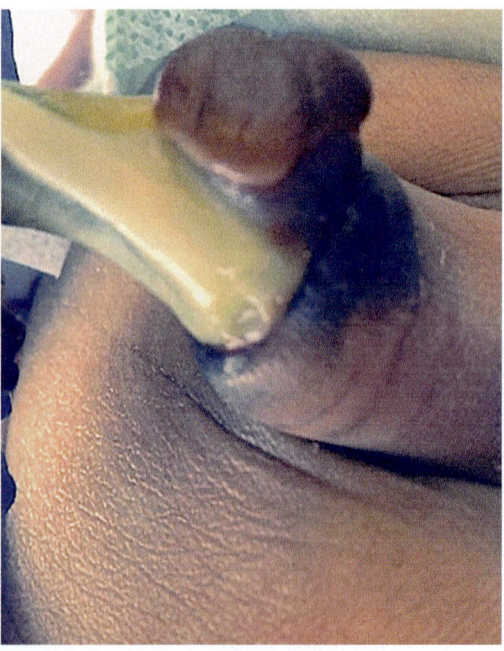

Fig. 29.2 Another outgrowing tissue beside the umbilical cord is diagnostic for UP

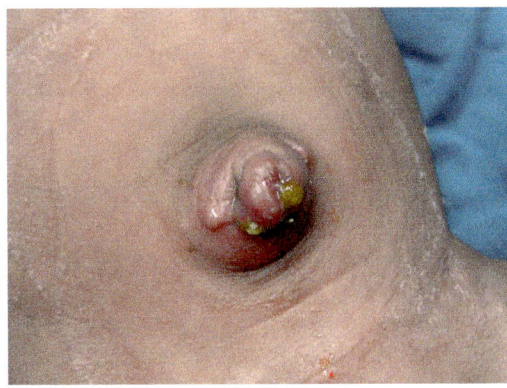

Fig. 29.3 Umbilical swelling with a punctum is diagnostic for UP

UP should be differentiated from rare cases of keloid umbilical scar, haemangioma and the inclusion dermoid cyst (Figs. 29.6 and 29.7) (Chap. 31).

Rarely in an older child or an adult, a prominent abnormal scar at the dome or the bottom of umbilicus may be diagnosed wrongly as an UP, especially if the covering skin is thin and shiny; surgical excision is not needed in such cases, especially if the diagnosis is sure, but in doubtful cases the histopathology may show only an extensive fibrosis of the umbilical scar (Fig. 29.8).

Management: When the umbilical polyp is not associated with any other types of underlying

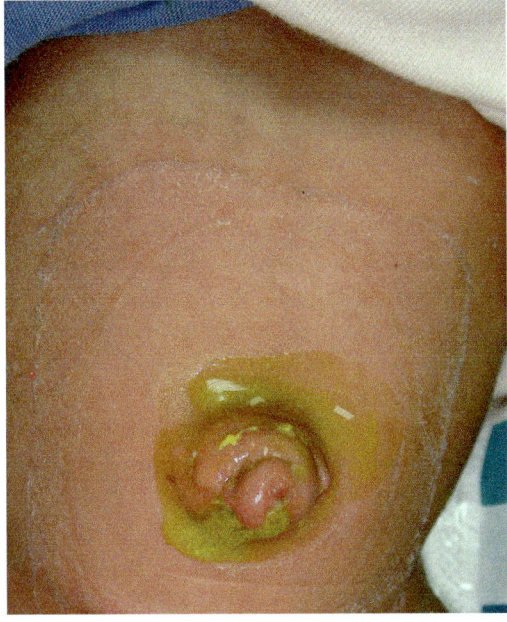

Fig. 29.4 Straining may force intestinal contents to come out from an UP

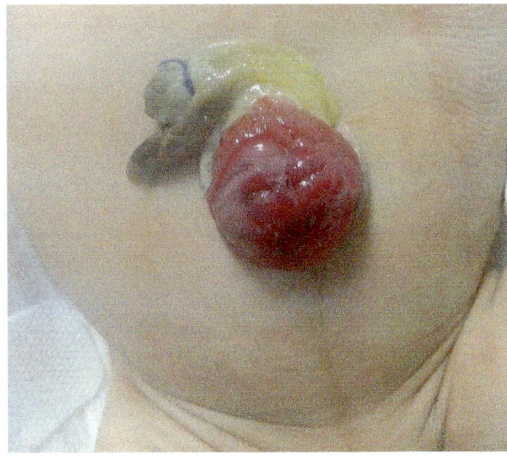

Fig. 29.5 UP formed of intestinal wall with a characteristic corrugations

small feeding tube is cannulated through this opening.
• Relatively glistening wall of the umbilical swelling or corrugations characteristic for intestinal wall is diagnostic for umbilical polyp or remnant of vitellointestinal duct (Fig. 29.5).

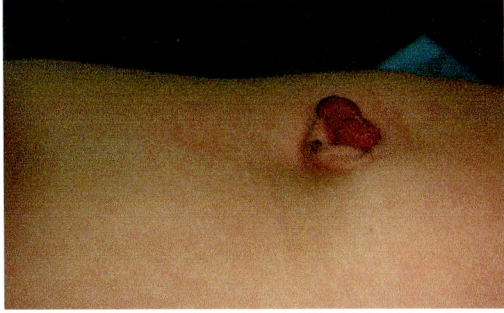

Fig. 29.6 An umbilical haemangioma resembles an UP

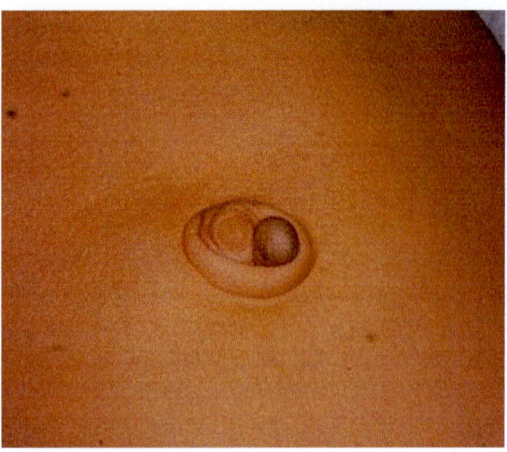

Fig. 29.7 A small inclusion dermoid cyst around the umbilical scar mimicking UP

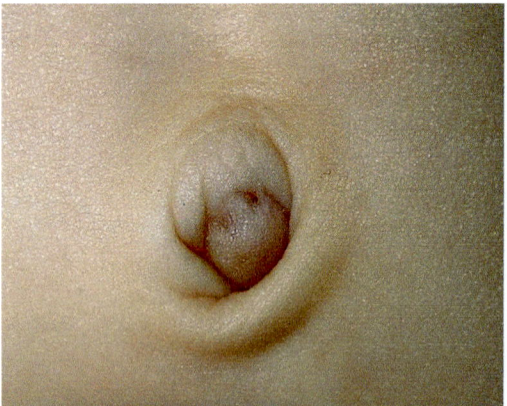

Fig. 29.8 Extensive umbilical scar fibrosis resembling an UP

abnormalities, it may be treated by a simple surgical excision.

29.1   Omphalomesenteric Duct Polyp

It is also called Meckel's polyp or vitellointestinal polyp.

Early in human embryogenesis, the alimentary canal communicates with the yolk sac through the umbilicus. As the embryo grows, the communicating omphalomesenteric duct narrows; by the fifth week of gestation, it is surrounded by the growing umbilical cord. The duct normally loses any vestige of its former existence and disappears by about the sixth week. Under abnormal conditions, part of the OMD persists, resulting in a wide spectrum of anomalies. The most common is Meckel's diverticulum, which occurs in about 2% of the population. This remnant is found at 30–60 cm proximal to the adult ileocecal junction on the anti-mesenteric surface of the small bowel. It may be connected to the umbilicus through a fibrous tract. Other anomalies include a stand-alone fibrous tract, cysts within that tract or within the abdominal wall at the umbilicus, an umbilical sinus or an external polyp at the umbilicus. The total persistence of the OMD (entero-umbilical fistula) is extremely rare, and few cases are documented in the literature. The total persistence of the duct with early manifestations in the neonatal stage, before the cord falls, can be diagnosed by the dilated appearance, which shows a dark swelling of the omphalomesenteric canal. After cord fall, the appearance of this permeable duct is that of a thick umbilical polyp, which can lead to confusion and be interpreted as an umbilical granuloma. However, at some point, and especially with crying or efforts, it will be possible to observe the outflow of gases and intestinal fluid. Partial persistence may also take two aspects: an exudative navel or umbilical swelling. (Details of OMD anomalies will be discussed in Chap. 36)

Omphalomesenteric duct anomalies may be associated with umbilical hernia, intestinal atresias, cardiac malformation, cleft lip and palate and exomphalos; it is also reported in association with trisomy 13 and Down's syndrome. Hence it is important to rule out the presence of other congenital anomalies if a patent vitellointestinal duct has been diagnosed.

Clinically: OMD polyp comes in the form of a small tumor from the bottom of the umbilical depression, measuring a few millimetres to 2 cm, being sessile or pedunculated, with bright red or strawberry colour and smooth, wet surface, which is sometimes itchy and sensitive or could bleed on contact or produce secretions serous staining clothes. A small hole can sometimes cross the lesion.

Although this lesion is noted at birth, some patients may not see that many years later, even in adulthood. Faced with this lesion, the search for a stoma on its surface is required with cannulation by a fine feeding tube or cannula. The diagnosis is confirmed by abdominal ultrasound, which may show the presence of a tubular structure with air that inside connects with the intestine or by means of fistulography.

Contrast radiographic studies or radionuclide studies are useful to rule out other anomalies, but it is difficult to diagnose congenital bands or an umbilical sinus.

Complications that may occur through a patent omphalomesenteric duct include navel infection, periumbilical dermatitis, bleeding of the intestinal mucosa, ileal strangulation, prolapse, bowel infarction and obstruction. More serious complications can lead to up to 18% mortality, especially in the neonatal period.

Thompos [8] has said that 0.5% of patients with Meckel's diverticulum have an associated umbilical polyp. Steck and Helwig [9] reported 31 patients with an umbilical polyp, 19 of whom had a solitary polyp, and 12 had some other anomalies as well.

Treatment: The polyp needs surgical excision, but the degree of surgical exploration required is controversial; some advocate including exploration of the abdominal cavity, but other authors deny any need for such exploration. Early at 1979, Kutin et al. [10] cited a 56% positive yield for an internal remnant in patients with cutaneous umbilical polyps, and they recommend minilaparotomies in all cases of umbilical polyps because underlying anomalies can result in serious complications such as intestinal obstruction. A more recent review by Pacilli et al. [11] suggests the opposite. They present 13 children who underwent surgical excision for umbilical polyps, with inspection and probing of the base of the polyp; 6 of them were suspected of having an underlying OMD anomaly; however, no such anomaly was found in any of the cases after abdominal exploration. In addition, the remaining seven children who did not undergo peritoneal cavity exploration remained asymptomatic after 5.8 years of follow-up. Therefore, they suggest that abdominal exploration may not be necessary, since a polyp can be present alone in the absence of other anomalies. A moderate approach is to perform a simple surgical excision for uncomplicated umbilical polyps, without an evidence of communication to the gut. The rare possibility of another OMD remnant should be discussed with the patient and their family, with thorough education of possible presentations and complications. Peritoneal cavity exploration should be performed if there are pre- or intraoperative concerns of an additional anomaly, either through open minilaparotomy or via a laparoscopic exploration, which is feasible and without any added morbidity even for the young patients; if this is the case, trocar should not be attempted at the umbilicus as usual, instead an upper right quadrant incision could be used for camera and a right lower quadrant port as a working port [12].

29.2 Umbilical Polyp Originating from Urachal Remnants

Umbilical polyp originating from the urachus has been reported occasionally, to stress the possibility that umbilical polyps can originate not only from the omphalomesenteric duct but also from urachal remnants [13]. A urachal polyp may be seen at the dome of a patent urachus, and it is also possible for urachal neoplasm to be presented early as a polypoid mass at the umbilicus in older patients (Chap. 35).

29.3   Ectopic Mucosa Polyp

Ectopic intestinal mucosa may be detected at the base of umbilicus as a polypoid mass in children and also in adult, either alone or sometimes in association with OMD anomalies; the most common mucosa found as polyp in umbilicus is the intestinal one, followed by gastric and pancreatic [14]. Very rarely other tissue types like liver had been reported, such polyps usually had no other associated anomalies, but radiological workup should be considered at least to exclude other OMD anomalies and to delineate exactly the extension of this ectopic tissue; ultrasound may be sufficient to achieve these goals, but CT scan or MRI will give a precise outline [15] (Fig. 29.9).

It is generally agreed that such polyps are a developmental anomaly, with various explanations:

> A totipotent endodermal cells lining the gut or vitel-lointestinal duct may be seeded at the umbilicus and differentiate into colonic, gastric or pancreatic tissue. Another possibility is that ectopic cells may become transplanted or sequestered at heterotopic sites during fetal development.
> Theoretically, they may occur anywhere from the yolk sac to the vitellointestinal junction and result in Meckel's diverticulum, vitelline cyst and umbilical fistula, polyp or cyst.

An ectopic appendicular tissue, with an appendico-umbilical fistula, was reported in few cases and should be considered in the differential diagnosis of an umbilical mass with drainage of a feculent discharge [16].

Surgical excision and histopathology of the excised mass is mandatory and sufficient without any further abdominal exploration if the base of the polyp can be reached without any apparent deep extension [17] (Fig. 29.10).

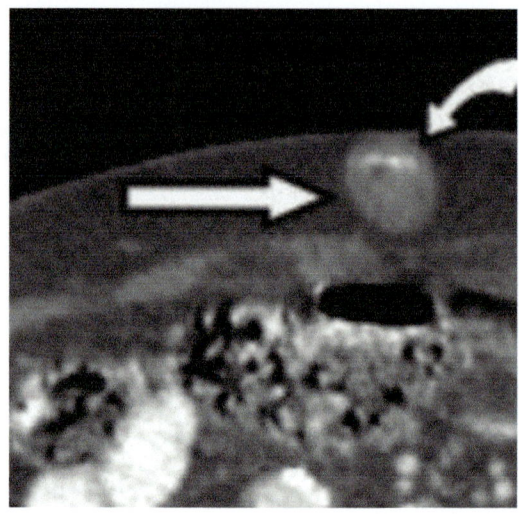

Fig. 29.9 Axial contrast-enhanced CT of an UP shows a rounded non-enhancing soft tissue density with well-defined margins within the subcutaneous tissues of umbilicus (*arrow*)

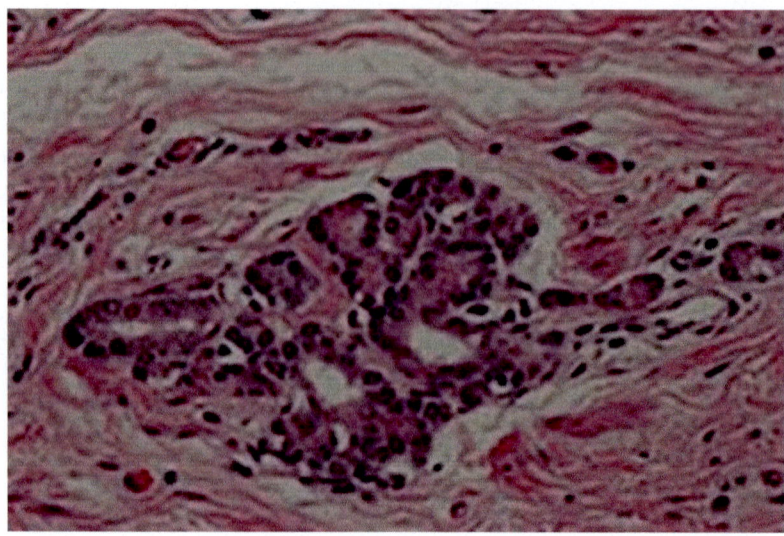

Fig. 29.10 Umbilical polyp composed of an aberrant pancreas (c: ×20)

29.4   Fibrous Umbilical Polyp (FUP)

Fibrous umbilical polyp is a benign myofibro-blastic proliferation, recently described as a defined entity, with only few cases reported, and the largest series of patients published to date came from the United States, (Children's Hospital, Boston, MA) [18], with 14 patients during an 8-year period. The lesion is characterized by a well-circumscribed dome-shaped or pedunculated dermal proliferation of moderately cellular fibrous tissue without significant inflammation (Fig. 29.11).

FUP typically occurs in young children (from 3 to 18 months), and it is rare at older age, most of whom are males, at the site of the umbilical scar, with different sizes according to the age of the patient (Fig. 29.12).

Fibrous umbilical polyp is considered as an acquired benign lesion; to date, the pathogenesis remains unclear, but most authors think it is a reactive process rather than a real neoplasm. In the first case reports, in which FUP was diagnosed as 'umbilical keloid', authors postulated that FUP could represent an overreactive scar process relative to cord section trauma, but the term 'keloid' was a misnomer, because FUP and keloid have a different histology, the latter being composed of a collagen-rich tissue with fibroblasts replacing normal structures, usually with an atrophic epidermis [19]. Keloid of the umbilicus will be demonstrated with rare umbilical problems (Chap. 31).

Perhaps the umbilicus, as a midline defect that is normally filled by dense scar tissue after birth, contains unique fibrogenic factors responsible for the development of this distinct lesion.

Fibroblastic cells were plump to elongate with abundant pale pink cytoplasm. In a subset of lesions, some cells showed atypia or ganglion cell-like morphology. Collagen ranged from sparse to long narrow bundles. Vascularity was sparse and the lesions were nonencapsulated. Immunostaining showed focal staining for muscle-specific actin and desmin in a subset of cases and no staining for cytokeratin [20].

Management is surgical excision, with preservation of normal umbilical look; recurrence was not observed.

Acquired neoplastic polyp will be discussed with cases of umbilical neoplasm (Chap. 30).

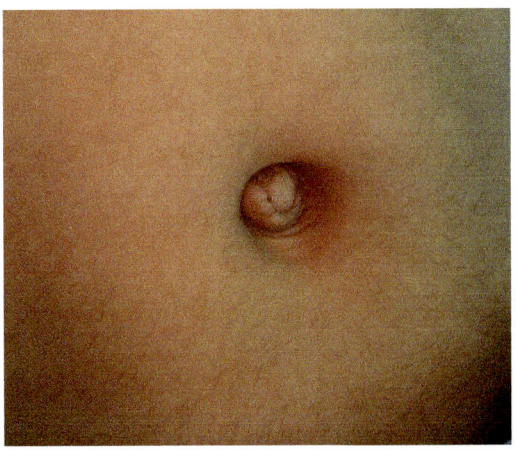

Fig. 29.11 A small sessile fibrous umbilical polyp in a young boy

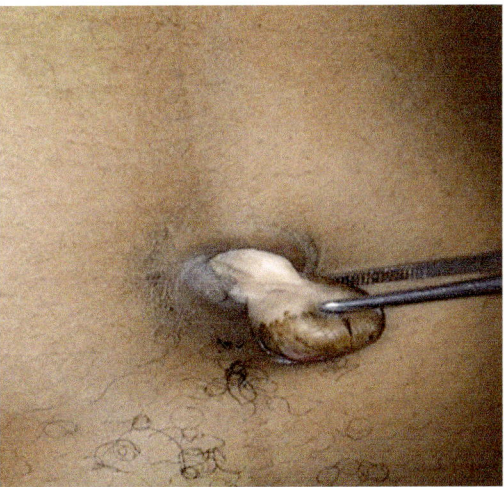

Fig. 29.12 Pedunculated large fibrous umbilical polyp

References

1. Sánchez-Castellanos M, Sandoval-Tress C, Hernández-Torres M. Persistencia del conducto onfalomesentérico: Diagnóstico diferencial de granuloma umbilical en la infancia. Actas Dermosifiliogr. 2006;97:404–5.

2. Fitz R. Persistent omphalomesenteric remains, their importance in the causation of intestinal duplication, cyst formation, and obstruction. Am J Med Sci. 1884;88(175):30–57.

3. Aitken J. Remnants of the vitellointestinal duct a clinical analysis of 88 cases. Arch Dis Child. 1953;28(137):1–7.

4. Kittle CF, Jenkins HP, Dragstedt LR. Patent omphalomesenteric duct and its relation to diverticulum of Meckel. Arch Surg. 1947;54:10–36.

5. Heatly MK, Mirakhur M. Cutaneous remnants of the vitellointestinal duct: a clinic-pathological study of 19 cases. Ulster Med J. 1988;57(2):181–3.

6. Storms P, Pexters J, Vandekerkhof J. Small omphalocele with ileal prolapse through patent omphalomesenteric duct a case report and review of literature. Acta Chil Belg. 1988;88:392–4.

7. Taranath A, Lam A. Ultrasonographic demonstration of a type 1 omphalomesenteric duct remnant. Acta Readiol. 2006;47:100–2.

8. Thomson JE. Perforated peptic ulcer in Meckel's diverticulum. Ann Surg. 1937;105:44.

9. Steck WD, Helwig EB. Cutaneous remnant of the omphalomesenteric duct. Arch Dermatol. 1964;90:463–70.

10. Kutin ND, Allen JE, Jewett TC. The umbilical polyp. J Pediatr Surg. 1979;14(6):741–4.

11. Pacilli M, Sebire NJ, Maritsi D, Kiely EM, Drake DP, Curry J, Pierro A. Umbilical polyp in infants and children. Eur J Pediatr Surg. 2007;17(6):397–9.

12. Jessica W, Hsu BS, Wynnis L. Tom: omphalomesenteric duct remnants: umbilical versus umbilical cord lesions. Pediatr Dermatol. 2011;28(4):404–7.

13. Oğuzkurt P, Kotiloğlu E, Tanyel FC, Hiçsönmez A. Umbilical polyp originating from urachal remnants. Turk J Pediatr. 1996;38(3):371–4.

14. Bambirra EA, Miranda D. Gastric polyp of the umbilicus in an 8-year-old boy. Clin Pediatr. 1980;19(6):430–2. doi:10.1177/000992288001900609.

15. Iwasaki M, Taira K, Kobayashi H, Saiga T. Umbilical cyst containing ectopic gastric mucosa originating from an omphalomesenteric duct remnant. J Pediatr Surg. 2009;44:2399–401.

16. Cevik M, Boleken ME, Kadıoglu E. Appendicoumbilical fistula: a rare reason for neonatal umbilical mass. Case Rep Med. 2011;2011:2. doi:10.1155/2011/835474W.T.

17. Lee WT, Tseng HI, Lin JY, et al. Ectopic pancreatic tissue presenting as an umbilical mass in a newborn: a case report. Kaohsiung J Med Sci. 2005;21(2):84–7.

18. Vargas SO. Fibrous umbilical polyp: a distinct fasciitis-like proliferation of early childhood with a marked male predominance. Am J Surg Pathol. 2001;25:1438–42.

19. Ford T, Widgerow AD. Umbilical keloid: an early start. Ann Plast Surg. 1990;25:214–5.

20. Stock N, et al. Umbilical polyp in an infant. Pediatr Dev Pathol. 2008;11:165–6. doi:10.2350/07-09-0342.1.

Umbilical Neoplasm

30

Generally, umbilical neoplasm classified into: -

A. *Benign*:
1. Endometriosis
2. Haemangioma
3. Dermoid cysts
4. Epithelial inclusion cysts
5. Melanocytic nevi
6. Benign connective tissue growths:
   (a) Fibroepithelial papillomas
   (b) Dermatofibroma

B. *Malignant* (Carcinoma of the umbilicus):
Primary:
1. Squamous cell carcinoma
2. Adenocarcinoma
3. Umbilical melanoma

Secondary:
1. Sister Mary Joseph's nodule

A. Benign Umbilical Tumors:

Benign umbilical nodules are called Pseudo Sister Mary Joseph's nodules [1].

In Barrow's series, primary neoplasms accounted for 38% of all umbilical tumors (78% of these were benign and 22% malignant), and endometriosis represented 32%, while metastatic tumors accounted for 30% of all umbilical tumors [2].

Benign tumors could be detected at any age, but the majority of reported cases were adults.

30.1 Umbilical Endometriosis (UEM)

Although endometriosis is not a neoplastic pathology, we opted to discuss it with other umbilical neoplasm because the lesion clinically may be confusing with other neoplasm, and at the meantime; some cases, specially recurrent one, may as be transformed to other neoplastic pathology; malignant transformation has been reported in 0.3 percent to 1 percent of EM scar and should be suspected in the case of rapidly growing or recurrent lesions.

Nomenclature: Menstruating umbilicus, Villar's umbilical nodule

Historical Background: Endometriosis (EM), a term first used by the German physician Daniel Schroen [3] in 1690, which means the presence of endometrial glands and stroma outside the uterine cavity and musculature. Cutaneous EM of the umbilicus is described for the first time by Villar at 1886, as a nodule in the navel [4].

Definition: Endometriosis is a chronic, mostly benign condition affecting up to 15 percent of reproductive age women, but can occur also in women at menarche and menopause, and exceptionally also in men after long-term hormonal therapy for prostatic tumors [5].

The most common sites of EM are the ovaries, followed by the appendix, intestine, cervix, omentum and the skin. Cutaneous EM (CEM) is

© Springer International Publishing AG 2018
M. Fahmy, *Umbilicus and Umbilical Cord*, https://doi.org/10.1007/978-3-319-62383-2_30

usually secondary, following abdominopelvic surgery, but can rarely appear spontaneously, in the absence of prior surgery; in the latter case it shows predilection for the umbilical region.

Incidence: EM generally affects 7–15% of women in the reproductive age. Extrapelvic presentations in almost all parts of the body have been reported in the literature; however, umbilical endometriosis that is spontaneous or secondary to surgery is uncommon and accounts for only 0.5–1% of all endometriosis cases. Umbilical EM (UEM) accounts for up to 30–40% of all cutaneous EM cases [6].

Presentation: Women with endometriosis often present with dysmenorrhea, menorrhagia, pelvic pain and infertility. Due to its varied presentations, endometriosis remains a difficult condition to diagnose and treat.

UEM presented as a bluish or dark brown nodule, depending on the amount of haemorrhage and the penetration depth of ectopic endometrial tissue. Occasionally, the nodule is flesh coloured, tender, firm or soft in consistency, appears on the umbilicus and is fixed to the underlying tissue; it has bloody or black discharge with cyclic periumbilical pain in active menstrual life [7]. The tumor is variable in size, usually 0.5–9 cm in diameter (mean 2–2.5 cm); the cut surface is greyish white, fibrous with minute cysts (Fig. 30.1). It is usually single and often multilobated, although multiple discrete nodules may be present (Fig. 30.2).

Clinical symptoms include tenderness, pain, bleeding, swelling and growth correlated with the menstrual cycle. However, not all symptoms are present in a given patient, and some patients are totally asymptomatic. UEM may be associated with umbilical hernia; this may be due to weakness of the abdominal wall by the deposited EM nodules. When UEM is associated with pelvic EM, general symptoms such as dysmenorrhea and dyspareunia may be present.

Cutaneous endometriosis may develop spontaneously during pregnancy and is then most often located on the umbilicus.

Etiology: UEM classified to:
- **Primary** or congenital in patients without any previous history of surgery or laparoscopy.

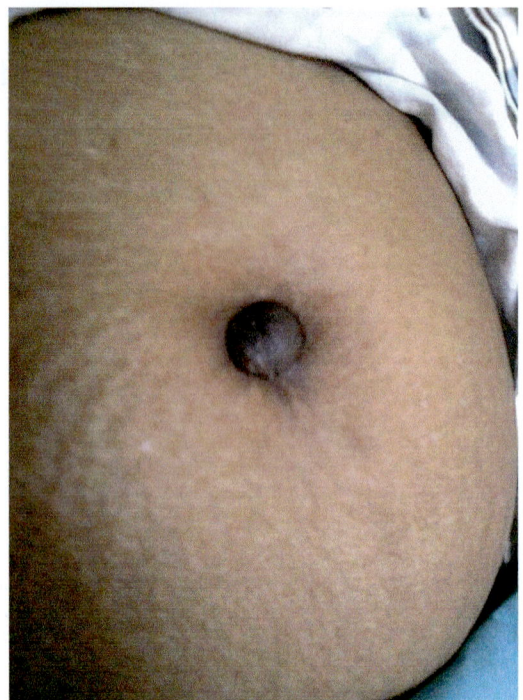

Fig. 30.1 Single nodule of UEM with *bluish* discolouration during the menstruation time

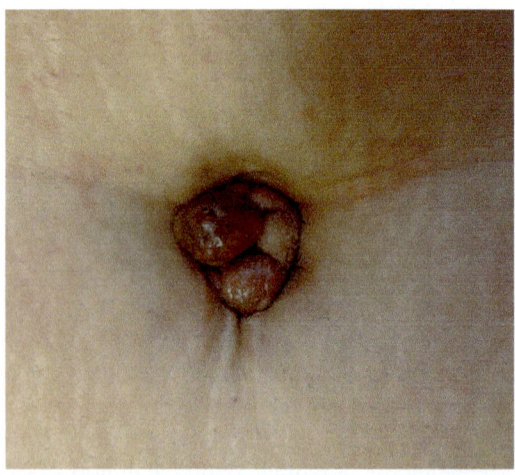

Fig. 30.2 Multiple nodules of UEM showing variable sizes

- **Secondary** due to seeding of the endometrial tissue after surgery for pelvic endometriosis either open or laparoscopic, and it is suspected to see more cases of EM at the umbilicus with the wide use of umbilical port for laparoscopic surgical procedures [8].

There has been great speculation about the pathogenesis of primary UEM, and several theories have been proposed; Latcher [9] has classified these theories into three main categories:

- The embryonal rest theory, which explains endometriosis adjoining the pelvic viscera by Wolffian or Mullerian remnants, during fetal development.
- The coelomic metaplasia theory, which states that the embryonic coelomic mesothelium dedifferentiates into endometrial tissue under stimulus such as inflammation or trauma and becomes manifested latter on due to hormonal affect.
- The migratory pathogenesis theory, which explains the dispersion of endometrial tissue by direct extension, through vascular and lymphatic channels or surgical manipulation.

Still others suggest cellular proliferation of endometrial cells from initial extraperitoneal disease along the urachus. The real mechanism remains a mystery [10].

Diagnosis: A high index of suspicion is the first and foremost tool of the wise diagnostician. Ultrasound may be enough to show the local extension of the umbilical nodule and to detect any other associated pelvic EM (Fig. 30.3); however, many cases may be confused with other lesions and warrant further investigation modalities like MRI, CT scan, dermatoscopy or other lab investigations:

- Magnetic resonance imaging (MRI) can be useful in evaluating patients with suspected endometriosis, where endometriomas appears homogeneously hyperintense on T1-weighted sequences. MRI also has an advantage over laparoscopy for evaluating pelvic and extraperitoneal diseases, as well as lesions concealed by adhesions (Fig. 30.4) [5].
- Computed tomography is more accessible than, but not as sensitive as, MRI (Fig. 30.5).
- Dermatoscopical findings of EM include a homogenous reddish pigmentation with small, well-defined, globular structures of a deeper hue, termed 'red atolls' [11].

- Fine needle aspiration cytology has been used, but its results may be inconclusive [12].
- Serum CA-125 levels may be increased (up to 260 U/mL), but this finding is not specific for EM.
- The usefulness of immunohistochemical marker is limited, as the findings of EM are also present in several fibroblastic cells of the normal dermis [13].

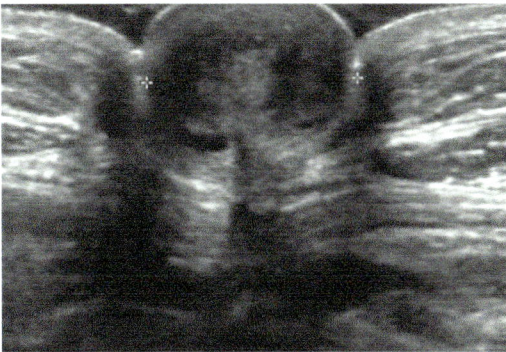

Fig. 30.3 US of the umbilicus demonstrated a hypodense nodule of 1.8 cm in the umbilicus

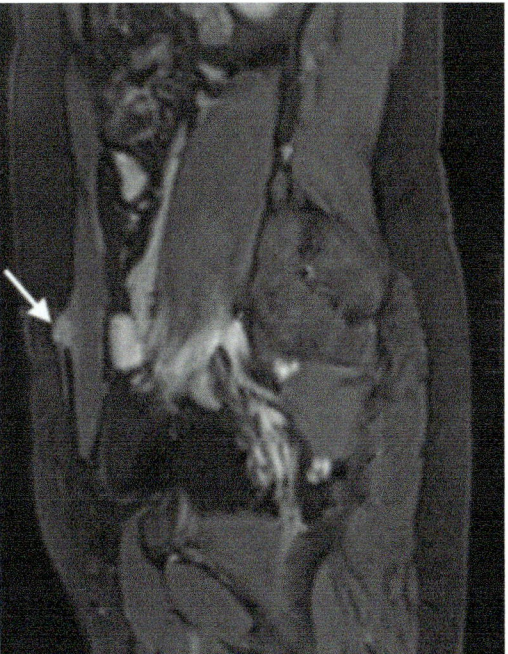

Fig. 30.4 Sagittal fat suppressed T1-WI after administration of gadolinium contrast. There is marked enhancement of the lesion (*arrow*). Notice the intimate relationship with the abdominal wall and surrounding stranding [17]

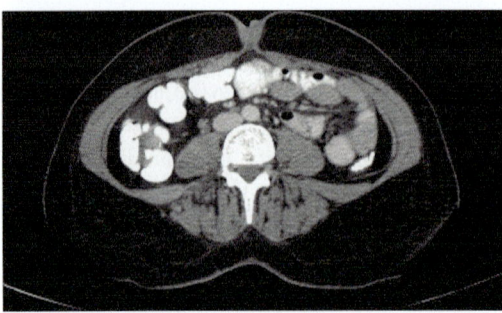

Fig. 30.5 Abdominal CT scan showing an increased density in the subcutaneous tissue of umbilicus, but no intraabdominal extension was observed in UEM

- Laparoscopy: Video-assisted laparoscopy is helpful not only in diagnosis but has also become the standard surgical procedure for excision of the EM with decreased morbidity when compared with modalities other [14].

Histopathology: Histologically, CEM is characterized by the presence of endometrial glands and stroma in the mid- or deep dermis. The endometrial glands are made of tall columnar epithelium with basophilic cytoplasm and basally located nuclei, forming irregular glandular lumina, sometimes with a marked mitotic activity, depending on the phase of the menstrual cycle. The high cellular

and vascular stroma is composed of spindle cells and it is usually oedematous. Menstrual bleeding into the dermis leads to hemosiderin, deposition (which is seen with the Perls stain) scarring and chronic inflammation. Several metaplastic changes can be seen in the glandular epithelium (tubal, oxyphilic, hobnail, mucinous and papillary syncytial) and the stroma (smooth muscle metaplasia, decidualization, stromal endometriosis and elastosis). Atypical changes include reactive atypia and atypical mitoses (Fig. 30.6) [15].

Differential Diagnosis: Differential diagnosis of umbilical endometriosis should include pyogenic granuloma, polyp, residual embryonic tissue (either urachal or vitellointestinal remnants), primary or metastatic adenocarcinoma (Sister Joseph's nodule), nodular melanoma and other neoplasm.

The diagnosis of CEM can be suspected clinically on the basis of the clinical appearance and a good history, but relies mainly on histopathological examination.

The following protocol is suggested in differential diagnosis of an umbilical nodule:

- If a nodule present with discharge, a patent urachus and patent vitellointestinal duct are considered.

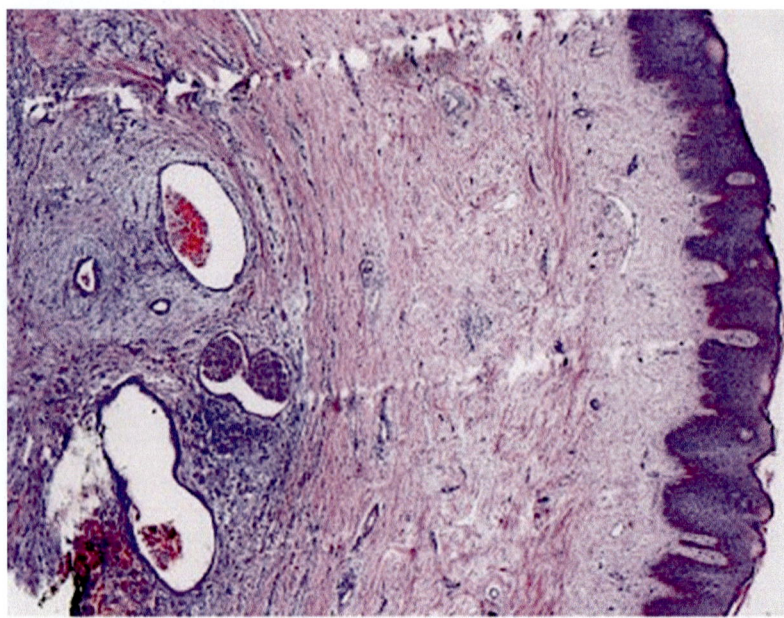

Fig. 30.6 Histological examination of UEM showing a dilated glands lined by columnar cell and localized in the deep dermis (HE × 40)

- If there is no discharge at umbilicus and no signs of infection are present, granuloma, umbilical inclusion cyst, endometriosis or adenoma is considered.
- If there is no discharge but signs of infection are a rare present, consider dermatitis, omphalitis or pilonidal sinus.

Management: Surgical excision of the lesion with sparing of the umbilicus is the preferred treatment of UEM, preferably performed at the end of the menstrual cycle when the lesion is small in order to achieve a minimal excision, although simultaneous laparoscopy has been recommended for pelvic endometriosis (Fig. 30.7) [16].

The technique of removal varies depending on the size and extent of the lesion, from simple excision with wide margins under local anaesthesia to laparoscopic excision en bloc of the umbilicus (Fig. 30.8) [17]. A prolene mesh may be necessary to prevent the development of hernia, if the defect in the rectus sheath is large.

Treatment with gonadotropin-releasing hormone agonists, danazol and contraceptive pills can be given in order to reduce tumor size before but excision or to provide relief from the symptoms; these are insufficient as sole treatments and may lead to incomplete excision. Gynaecologic examination and hormonal evaluation are recommended after excision of CEM in order to detect associated

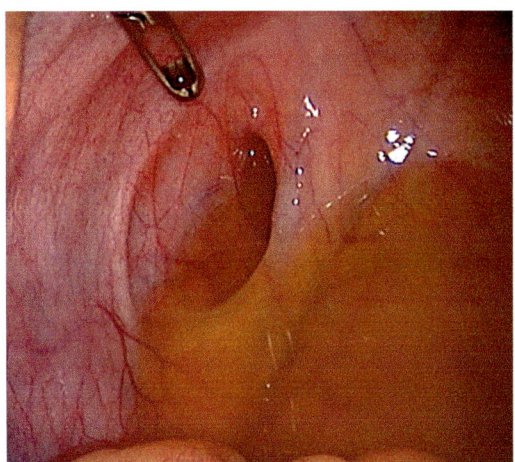

Fig. 30.8 Laparoscopic view of UEM

pelvic lesions. Although local recurrence is uncommon, the patient has been warned of the risk of scar endometriosis and of recurrence [13].

Prognosis: The prognosis of CEM is good; recurrences are uncommon if excision is performed with clean and wide margins. However, malignant transformation has been reported in 0.3–1% of EM scar and should be suspected in the case of rapidly growing or recurrent lesions. The commonest histological subtype is endometrioid carcinoma (69%) followed by clear-cell carcinoma (13.5%), adenosarcomas (11.6%), serous carcinoma and melanoma [18].

In some studies, a statistically significant association between EM and the development of melanoma has been found, with a relative risk of 1.62. It has been speculated that abnormal expression of some tumor suppressor genes (namely, p16Ink4, p53 and PTEN) may favour the development of the two conditions. Long-term hormonal treatment given for EM could also favour the development of melanoma [18, 19].

30.2 Umbilical Haemangioma

The most common tumors of infancy are benign vascular lesions. Before 1982, the term 'haemangioma' was used to encompass a wide range of vascular growths, independent of clinical manifestations, natural history or embryological origin. Subsequently, Mulliken and Glowacki [20]

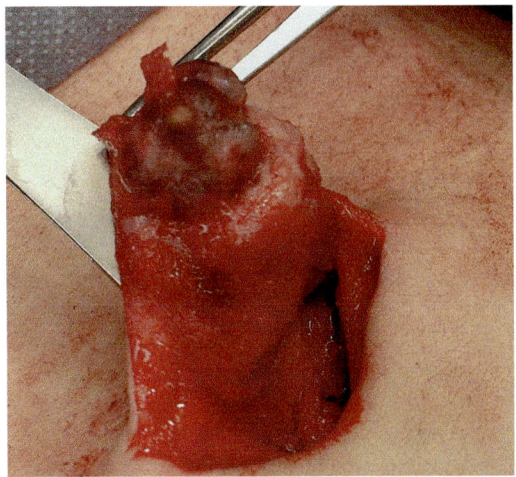

Fig. 30.7 Surgical excision of the UEM, the umbilicus sacrificed to remove the whole endometrial tissues

proposed the first biological classification for vascular birthmarks. Their landmark article was the first to distinguish a haemangioma, characterized by a growth and involutional phase, from a vascular malformation, a structural anomaly derived from arteries, veins or lymphatics.

Recent years have brought new insight into the benign vascular tumors of infancy. While most umbilical haemangiomas remain uncomplicated, certain unique presentations may be a cause for concern; this haemangioma may be seen early after delivery as a presentation of umbilical cord haemangioma, which was discussed in (Sect. 17.2).

Latter on at infancy and childhood, it is very rare to have a haemangioma at the umbilicus, few cases had been reported at older age, umbilical haemangioma may be superficial at the level of skin capillaries and seen as redness of the umbilical mamelon, such cases rarely complicate and may left without treatment, and it could respond to local corticosteroid injection, if it is annoying the patient (Fig. 30.9).

Perlman syndrome (renal hamartomas, nephroblastomatosis and fetal gigantism) is a rare autosomal recessive syndrome and is associated with a cutaneous capillary haemangioma around the umbilicus [21].

Small haemangioma hidden inside the umbilicus may be seen only after eversion of the umbilicus (Fig. 30.10). Umbilical haemangioma may rarely acquire a larger size and becomes pedunculated with surface freckling or ulceration from cloths irritation; such cases have to be differentiated from other similar conditions: umbilical polyp (usually detected since birth with discharge), umbilical keloid (usually following trauma or irritation) and other rare umbilical swellings which will be discussed later on; such anomalies are difficult to differentiate except after excision and biopsy (Fig. 30.11).

Microscopic Findings: The tumor consists of small, arborizing and thin-walled vessels, and tumor cells were small and round to spindle

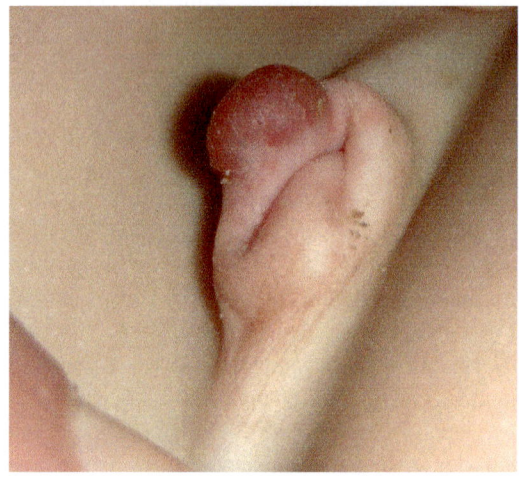

Fig. 30.10 A hidden small haemangioma, only seen after retraction of umbilical cushions

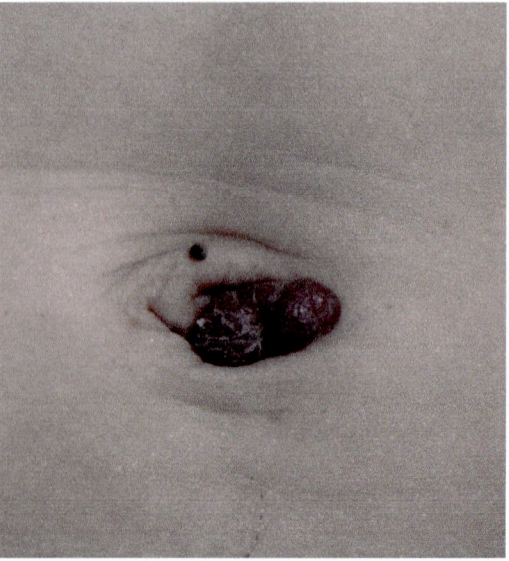

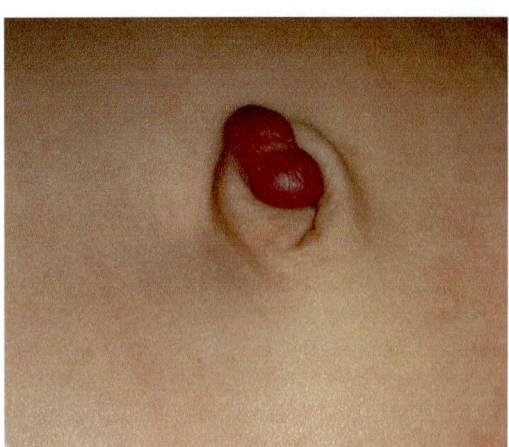

Fig. 30.9 Superficial haemangioma confined to the umbilical mamelon

Fig. 30.11 Large flickered umbilical haemangioma with a small nevus at the supraumbilical region

Fig. 30.12 Histological picture of the Umbilical haemangioma; the tumor consists of small, arborizing and thin-walled vessels (haematoxylin and eosin staining)

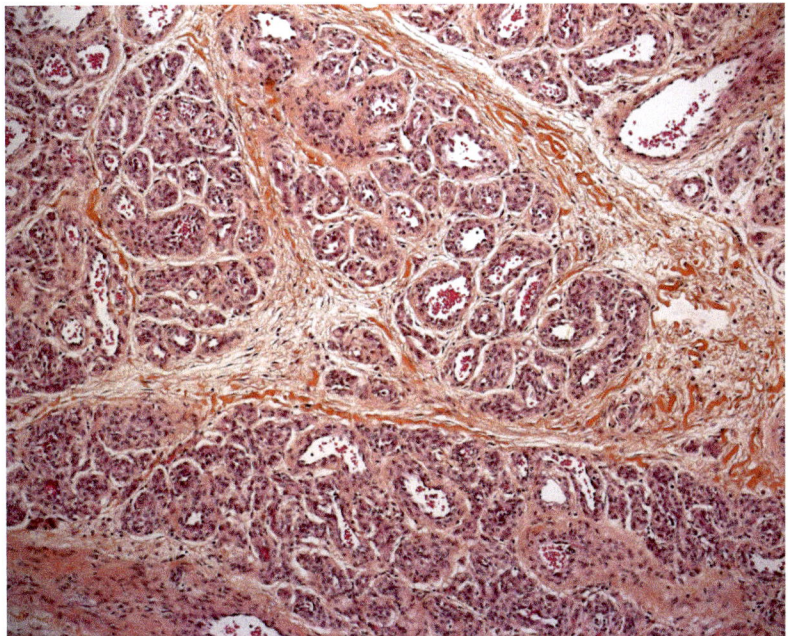

shaped with no significant nuclear atypia. Mitotic figures were seldom seen (Fig. 30.12).

Presence of an umbilical haemangioma warrants the need for screening for other internal visceral or hepatic haemangiomas, at least by abdominal ultrasound.

Treatment: Many treatment options are available for complicated vascular lesions. The mainstay of treatment for ulcerated haemangiomas involves local wound care, which protects against secondary infection and helps to relieve pain. Corticosteroids may be applied topically, intralesionally or systemically, caution must be used when employing intralesional corticosteroids [22], laser could be used for superficial haemangioma, but haemangioma of considerable size can be excised completely with umbilicoplasty.

30.3   Epithelial Inclusion Dermoid Cysts Discussed in Chap. 31

30.4   Melanocytic Nevi

Melanocytic tumours are common lesions of the benign group; the nevi generally had been present for years, and they were excised for diagnosis or because of chronic irritation, growth or increasing pigmentation; the lesions may be polypoid. These were grossly similar to the fibroepithelial papillomas, several of which were also pigmented. The gross distinction between a benign nevus and a malignant melanoma may be impossible and a histopathologic examination is necessary for definitive diagnosis (Fig. 30.11).

30.5   Benign Connective Tissue Growths

30.5.1   Fibroepithelial Papillomas (Umbilical Warts) (Fig. 30.13)

Fabricius von Hilden, in 1526, published the first recorded case of this kind, and since then a few isolated cases only have been published [23].

These soft, fleshy, condylomatous structures ranged from 2 or 3 mm to 1 cm or more in size and were frequently pigmented. The surface typically was thrown into irregular convolutions; down-growing epithelial strands formed an intertwining network within the loose connective tissue of the dermal stroma. Most of the papillomas showed both clinical and histopathologic evidence of the chronic inflammation that was the usual reason for their removal. Similar fibroepi-

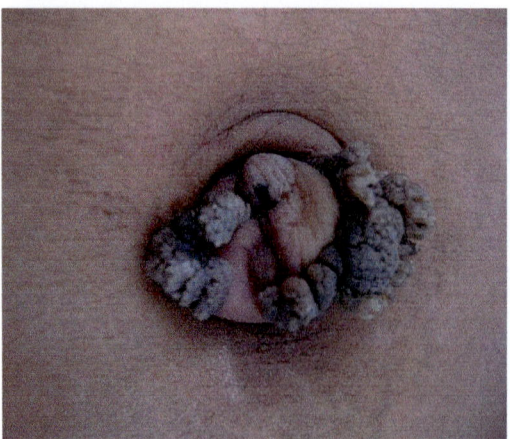

Fig. 30.13 Multiple umbilical warts

thelial proliferations among many patients with cutaneous remnants of the omphalomesenteric duct had been reported [24].

Human papilloma virus which commonly present as cutaneous/genital warts are also implicated as an etiology of the umbilical warts, but minor trauma during activities like bathing and vigorous exercise or the occurrence of superficial infection is discernible. It is suggested that auto-inoculation through bathing or fomites was a likely mode of spread to the umbilicus from the anogenital region [25].

All of the umbilical papillomas had been present for many years, probably from infancy, although this seldom could be determined accurately. Their simple surgical removal revealed no evidence of underlying anomaly, nor was any indicated by follow-up. Most of these tumors have been noted between the 25 and 50 years, although few cases reported in children. Papillomata of the umbilicus occur in about equal frequency in the male and female. As a rule these tumors are pedunculated and localised to its origin, generally of slow growth, but in one reported case, the growth had spread out for a considerable distance into the abdominal wall and is said to occur most frequently in persons with bad personal hygiene [26].

Treatment aims at increasing the clinical disease-free interval and decreasing the bulk of disease, thereby enabling the immune system to act upon the remaining virus-infected cells. Topical applications of caustics, cantharidin and podophyllin are effective in small lesions. Cryotherapy, electrodessication and surgical excision are other treatment options.

30.5.2 Dermatofibroma

Dermatofibroma of the umbilicus may present a problem in clinical differential diagnosis, as keloid, desmoid and granular cell myoblastoma. These are all firm or hard tumors whose gross appearance offers little to distinguish them from cancer. A history of long duration was helpful in several instances, and the microscopic appearance was typical in every case.

Neurofibroma and lipoma, being soft or spongy, are unlikely to be confused with malignant tumors. Umbilical teratoma was an unorganised collection of ectopic tissues, and among them are nerve, muscle, cartilage, vascular structures and epithelium of several types, including columnar and transitional.

30.6   Umbilical Carcinoma (B. Malignant Umbilical Tumors)

There were no gross features to distinguish primary from secondary lesions and none to suggest the site of primary origin. The predominant finding was generally a hard, nodular mass or only ill-defined induration. The lesions occasionally were ulcerated but only rarely painful or tender. Colour varied from that of the normal skin through red, blue, purple, brown and black, evidently depending upon the depth of the growth in the skin, vascularity, secondary inflammation and haemorrhage.

30.6.1 Primary Umbilical Carcinoma

Primary malignant umbilical tumors, which are exceedingly rare, accounting for 17% of the cases of umbilical malignancy and including melanomas, basal cell carcinomas, squamous cell carcinomas, myosarcomas and adenocarcinomas.

It must be assumed to arise in ectopic tissue, such as a remnant of the omphalomesenteric duct and the urachus or possibly in a pre-existing benign endometrioma, and these conditions, themselves, are rare. (Urachal carcinoma is discussed in Chap. 35.)

Historical Background: Cullen collected from the literature a total of 22 cases that purported to be examples of primary umbilical carcinoma. Most of them were recorded around the turn of the century or before. Many of the reports offered little proof that the lesion was primary, or even cancer [27].

Primary Adenocarcinoma of the umbilicus is extremely rare. It must be assumed to arise in ectopic tissue, such as a remnant of the omphalomesenteric duct and the urachus or possibly in a pre-existing benign endometrioma (Fig. 30.14).

Squamous Carcinoma: Basal cell carcinoma (BCC) arising from the umbilicus is extremely rare and only nine cases have been reported [28].

Predisposing Factors: In general, a history of skin trauma, surgical procedure or chronic inflammation can predispose a patient to the development of BCC. The findings for some of the reported umbilical BCC included association of an epidermal inclusion cyst, simultaneous occurrence of lymphoma [29].

Nevertheless, therapeutic management of umbilical BCCs may be difficult if lesions are infiltrative or large in size. In those cases, wide local excision remains the most commonly used treatment [30].

30.6.2 Umbilical Melanoma: Navel Melanoma (Fig. 30.15)

It is well known that melanomas arising in hidden areas such as the umbilicus often suffer from a delayed diagnosis and treatment, and it is located in the vicinity of the umbilicus and does not appear to be very frequent, although its real incidence is difficult to determine due to the lack of statistics about it on the literature, with only 23 cases described in the medical literature since it was first reported in 1916 [31].

Since Cullen reported the first three cases in 1916, 24 cases have been reported in the English literature. Local recurrence was reported due to remaining melanoma cell nests in the omphalomesenteric duct [32].

Management: Primary umbilical melanoma determines a possible early visceral involvement, so it should be approached with a wide excision of the entire umbilical structure,

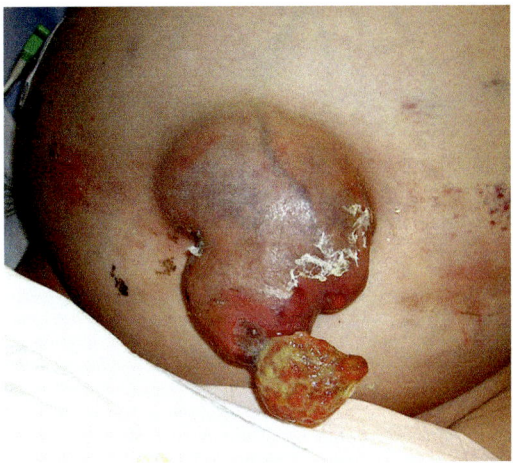

Fig. 30.14 Fungating primary carcinoma of the umbilicus

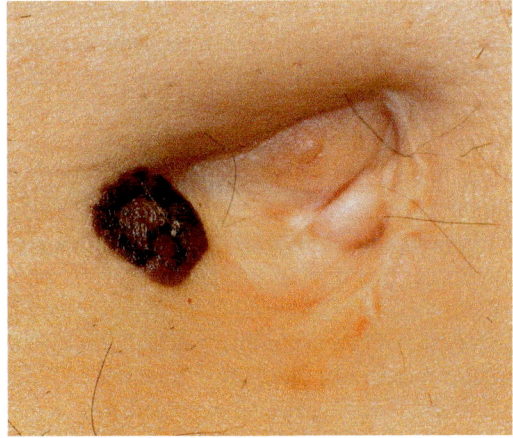

Fig. 30.15 Umbilical melanoma

including the attachment to the underlying peritoneum [33].

Tumor excision en bloc with the underlying peritoneum is required to avoid local relapse. Immediate reconstruction of the neo-umbilicus with local flaps should be carried out at the same time. Several different approaches for reconstruction have been reported to date, based on the use of skin flaps fixed to the rectus aponeurosis in order to obtain a natural appearing deep cavity at an adequate position [34].

Due to its low incidence, the efficacy of sentinel lymph node biopsy in primary malignant umbilical melanoma is still ambiguous. As no suspicious regional lymph node metastasis was detected with ultrasonography, sentinel lymph node biopsy was not routinely performed in all patients [35].

30.6.3 Secondary Umbilical Carcinomas

Sister Mary Joseph's nodule (SMJN) is a metastatic tumor deposit in the umbilicus and often represents advanced intra-abdominal malignancy with a dismal prognosis. The umbilical mass was present prior to the diagnosis of internal malignancy in many patients and was a major diagnostic factor in almost all patients.

Historical Background: The term 'Sister Mary Joseph's nodule' was coined by Sir Hamilton Bailey in his book, *Physical Signs in Clinical Surgery*, in honour of Sister Mary Joseph, Dr. William Mayo's surgical assistant. Sister Mary Joseph identified the relationship between umbilical nodules and advanced intra-abdominal malignancy, from 1890 to 1915; Since then, many cases of have been described in the literature [36].

Significance: An umbilical nodule might represent the first clinical presentation of disseminated malignancy or an indicator of recurrence in a patient with known primary; SMJN should be differentiated early from other common and rare umbilical lesions, especially at older age.

Incidence: The incidence of cutaneous metastases from various malignancies reported is in a range from 1% to 9%, according to autopsy reports. Merely, 10% out of them are presented as an umbilical metastasis [37].

Epidemiological studies revealed that Sister Mary Joseph's nodule predominates in women [38].

The median age of patients at presentation was variable in literatures, it is around 50 years (range, 18–87 years) [39].

A review of the available American literature suggests that it is relatively more common in blacks than in whites [40].

Mode of Extension: The spread of metastatic cancer to the umbilical region has been postulated to occur in several ways:

- Contiguous extension from the anterior peritoneal surface is considered to be the most important route in patients with intra-abdominal malignancy.
- Haematogenous (arterial and/or venous).
- Lymphatic spread.
- Direct extension along the vestigial remnants of embryonal ligaments including the round ligament, the urachus, the vitellointestinal duct remnant and the obliterated vitelline artery.
- In addition, direct implantation following laparoscopy is also implicated.

Primary Site: SMJN can be the first manifestation of an underlying malignancy or an indication of a recurrence in a patient with a previous malignancy.

In male, the commonest primary site is the gastrointestinal tract (35–65%), of which the stomach is the single most common entity, whereas gynaecological malignancies (12–35%), particularly epithelial ovarian tumors, are the most common primary sites in women [41].

The common sites in decreasing order of frequency are:

Stomach (25%)

Colorectal (10%)

Pancreas (7%)

Primary tumors in many other sites have been reported to lead to SMJN, including gallbladder, liver, breast, lung, prostate, penis, peritoneum,

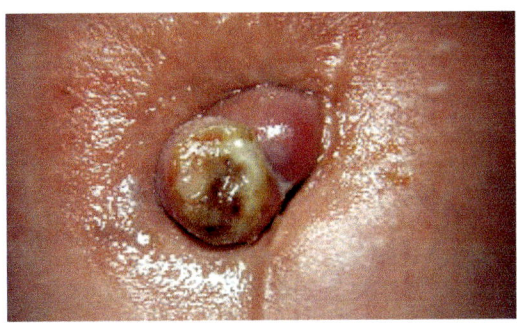

Fig. 30.16 Secondary umbilical nodule with advanced ovarian carcinoma

lymphoma, bladder, kidney, endometrium, cervix, vagina, vulva and fallopian tube [42]. In 15–30% of the cases, the source of the primary site of the tumor is unknown [43] (Fig. 30.16).

Histopathology: The most common histological type is adenocarcinoma (75%), more rarely squamous cell carcinoma, followed by undifferentiated tumors or carcinoids that can metastasise to the umbilicus. Other histopathological types include non-Hodgkin's lymphoma, squamous cell carcinoma, anaplastic carcinoma and cholangiocarcinoma in which more than 50% of tumors were poorly differentiated [44].

Prognosis: The presence of an umbilical metastasis indicates a poor prognosis and is a sign of advanced malignant disease. The survival of these patients has been reported to range from 2 to 11 months from the time of initial diagnosis [45].

In some patients, however, depending on the state of the primary neoplasm and the patient's general condition, surgery and/or chemotherapy may improve survival [46].

Because Sister Mary Joseph's nodule may sometimes be the first and only sign of an internal neoplasm and prognosis is mostly poor, diagnosis has to be confirmed in the early stages to improve average survival. The delay in diagnosis and, consequently, treatment leads to the extremely poor prognosis associated with this disease.

Clinically: It is prudent to examine the umbilicus in all patients with suspected pelviabdominal malignancies. Umbilical metastasis usually appears as a firm, indurated plaque or nodule, which may be fissured or ulcerated with exudation of serosanguineous or purulent discharge. The clinical appearance of umbilical metastasis must be differentiated from that of other lesions [41] SMJN.

Patients with SMJN often present with a painful lump with irregular margins and hard consistency. The surface may be ulcerated and necrotic with either blood, serous, purulent or mucous discharge from it. The size of the nodule usually ranges from 0.5 to 2 cm, although some nodules may reach up to 10 cm in size. The vast majority of patients (82.4%) presented with large nodule >2 cm in size and more than 70% of nodules were text ulcerated (Fig. 30.17) [44].

Differential Diagnosis: Nonneoplastic lesions should be considered in the differential diagnosis of umbilical metastasis; these lesions include pyogenic granuloma, pilonidal sinus, concretion of the umbilicus with the formation of an omphalith, hypertrophic scar and umbilical hernia in adults. Biopsy should be considered in cases of doubt [47].

The potential differential diagnosis to be considered when evaluating a patient with SMJN includes benign cases such as endometriosis, melanocytic nevi, fibroepithelial papillomas, der-

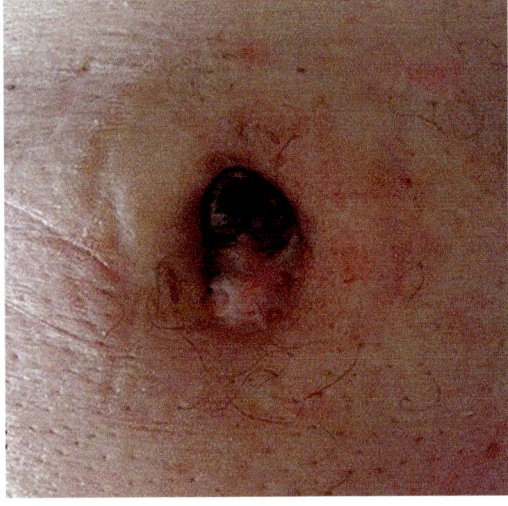

Fig. 30.17 Small blackish umbilical nodule secondary to colonic carcinoma

matofibroma, fibroma, epithelial inclusion cyst, urachal duct cyst, seborrheic keratosis, pilonidal sinus, keloid, foreign body, granuloma, myxoma, omphalitis, polyp, abscess and umbilical hernia [43].

Diagnosis: The diagnosis of SMJN is usually delayed due to nonspecific symptoms that are often misinterpreted as benign umbilical nodules. A high index of suspicion is required in the management and all suspected lesions should be biopsied.

Investigations: Various imaging modalities can aid in establishing the diagnosis, such as ultrasonography, CT, MRI and PET. Once SMJN is discovered, a biopsy—either excisional or fine needle aspiration cytology—is mandatory to establish diagnosis and to find the possible primary site (Fig. 30.18).

The histopathological evaluation may show characteristics of the underlying tumor, or they may have a more anaplastic appearance. In the situation of an anaplastic tumor, immunohistochemical marker studies and ultrastructural examination may help to delineate the tissue of origin.

Dynamic enhanced computer tomography with intraoperative fluorescence imaging using indocyanine green (ICG injection) during open or laparoscopic surgery enables the detection of lymphatic vessel drainage lymph nodes from umbilical tumor to intra-abdominal lymph nodes and these 'secondary' lymph nodes could be detected and resected. This novel method is technically feasible, safe and easy to apply with minimal additional operative time [48].

Management of Sister Mary Joseph's nodule in resource-limited countries poses major therapeutic challenges which need to be addressed. Late presentation with advanced lesions coupled with a lack of therapeutic facilities such as adjuvant therapy services which are among the hallmarks of the disease in developing countries.

Presence of umbilical metastasis usually runs with poor prognosis due to advanced cancer with widespread metastases. However, multimodality therapy including surgery and adjuvant therapy may improve the survival in some patients having good performance status. Rarely, the surgical resection with negative margins with or without reconstruction of abdominal wall defect in isolated umbilical metastatic is a satisfactory curative treatment option, but chemotherapy is usually the mainstay of the treatment. It is dubious to get cured an umbilical metastasis in patients with disseminated cancer. Systemic chemotherapy like FOLFOX (combination of oxaliplatin, fluorouracil and leucovorin) based regimen should be considered as it sometimes gives good response in colorectal cancers. Overall, the prognosis of umbilical metastasis is poor with median survival only about 1 year [49].

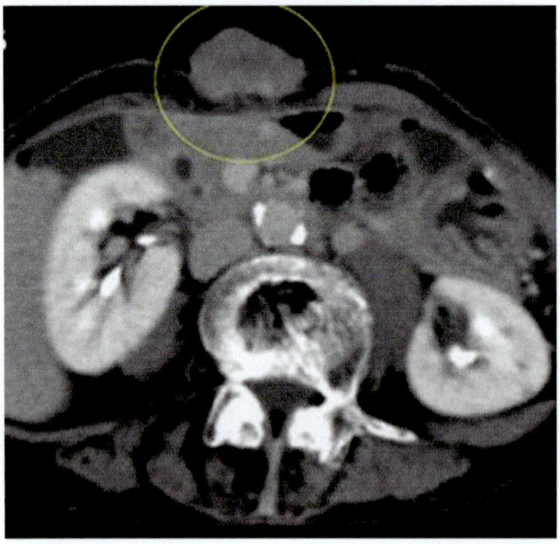

Fig. 30.18 CT scan of umbilical secondary carcinoma

References

1. Amaro R, Goldstein JA, Cely CM. Pseudo Sister Mary Joseph's nodule. Am J Gastroenterolo. 1999;94:1949–50.
2. Barrow MV. Metastasis tumors of the umbilicus. J Chronic Dis. 1966;19:1113–7.
3. Joylene DAlmeida J, Backthan L, Rao SV. Villar's umbilical nodule: a rare case of umbilical endometriosis. JPGO 2015;2(8). http://www.jpgo.org/2015/08/villars-umbilical-nodule-rare-case-of.html.
4. Disputatio SD. Inauguralis. Medica de Uleribus Uteri. Jena: Krebs; 1690. p. 6–17.
5. Hartigan CM, Holloway BJ. MR imaging features of endometriosis at the umbilicus. Br J Radiol. 2005;78(932):755–7.
6. Techapongsatorn S, Techapongsatorn S. Primary umbilical endometriosis. J Med Assoc Thail. 2006;89(10):1753–5.

7. Markham SM, Carpenter SE, Rock JA. Extrapelvic endometriosis. Obstet Gynecol Clin N Am. 1989;16:193–219.

8. Kodandapani S, Pai MV, Mathew M. Umbilical laparoscopic scar endometriosis. J Hum Reprod Sci. 2011;4(3):150–2.

9. Latcher JW. Endometriosis of the umbilicus. Am J Obstet Gynecol. 1953;66:161–8.

10. Ploteau S, Malvaux V, Draguet AP. Primary umbilical adenomyotic lesion presenting as cyclical periumbilical swelling. Fertil Steril. 2007;88(Suppl 6):1674–5.

11. De Giorgi V, Massi D, Mannone F, Stante M, Carli P. Cutaneous endometriosis: noninvasive analysis by epiluminescence microscopy. Clin Exp Dermatol. 2003;28:315–7.

12. Fernandes H, Marla NJ, Pailoor K, Kini R. Primary umbilical endometriosis – diagnosis by fine needle aspiration. J Cytol. 2011;28:214–6.

13. Kyamidis K, Lora V, Kanitakis J. Spontaneous cutaneous umbilical endometriosis: report of a new case with immunohistochemical study and literature review. Dermatol Online J. 2011;17(7):5. http://escholarship.org/uc/item/3mj2444n

14. Schipper E, NezhatInt C. Video-assisted laparoscopy for the detection and diagnosis of endometriosis: safety, reliability, and invasiveness. J Women's Health. 2012;4:383–93.

15. Di Giorgi V, Massi D, Mannone F, Stante M, Carli P. Cutaneous endometriosis: noninvasive analysis by epiluminescence microscopy. Clin Exp Dermatol. 2003;28(3):3157.

16. Fedele L, Frontino G, Biachi S, Borruto F, Ciappina N. Umbilical endometriosis: a radical excision with laparoscopic assistance. Int J Surg. 2010;8(2):10911.

17. Lee H, Kim KR. Intestinal endometriosis: clinicopathologic analysis of 15 cases including a case of endometrioid adenocarcinoma. Korean J Pathol. 2009;43(2):1205.

18. Kvaskoff M, Mesrine S, ClavelChapelon F, BoutronRuault MC. Endometriosis risk in relation to naevi, freckles and skin sensitivity to sun exposure: the French E3N cohort. Int J Epidemiol. 2009;38(4):114353.

19. Case 12190 Abdominal wall endometriosis. https://www.researchgate.net/publication/266318248_Case_12190_Abdominal_wall_endometriosis. Accessed 22 Apr 2017.

20. Mulliken JB, Glowacki J. Hemangiomas and vascular malformations in infants and children: a classification based on endothelial characteristics. Plast Reconstr Surg. 1982;69:412–20.

21. Alessandri JL, et al. Perlman syndrome: report, prenatal findings and review. Am J Med Genet A. 2008;146A:2532–7.

22. Metry DW, Hebert AA. Benign cutaneous vascular when to worry, what to do. Arch Dermatol. 2000;136:905–14.

23. Carson NB. Papilloma of the umbilicus. Ann Surg. 1917;65(2):199–201.

24. Zbid. Cutaneous remnants of the omphalomesenteric duct. Arch Derna. 1964;90:463.

25. Nathan M. Umbilical warts: a new entity? Genitourin Med. 1994;70:49–50.

26. Vijayabhaskar R, Sadasivam OL, Kirushnakumar KS. Papilloma of the umbilicus. Indian J Surg. 2014;76(4):329–30.

27. Cullen TS. Embryology, anatomy and diseases of the umbilicus together with diseases of the Urachus. Philadelphia: W. B. Saunders Co.; 1916.

28. Nakamura Y, et al. Surgical management of umbilical basal cell carcinoma: published work review and the optimal depth of surgical excision. J Dermatol. 2014;41(11):992–5.

29. Ramirez P, et al. Umbilical basal cell carcinoma in a 21 year old man: report of an exceptional case and dermatoscopic evaluation. Dermatol Online J. 2011;17(1):1.

30. Etter L, Cook JL. Basal cell carcinoma of the umbilicus: a case report and literature review. Cutis. 2003;71(2):1236.

31. Zaccagna A, Siatis D, Pisacane A, Giacone E, Picciotto F. Surgical treatment of primary melanoma of the umbilicus with sentinel lymph node biopsy and plastic reconstruction: case report and review of the literature. Eur J Surg Oncol. 2011;37:233–6.

32. Thompson JF, Scoyler RA, Kefford RF. Cutaneous melanoma. Lancet. 2005;365(9460):687701.

33. Di Monta G, et al. Clinicopathologic features and surgical management of primary umbilical melanoma: a case series. BMC Res Notes. 2015;8:147.

34. Kakudo N, Kusumoto K, Fujimori S, Shimotsuma A, Ogawa Y. Reconstruction of a naturalappearing umbilicus using an island flap: case report. J Plast Reconstr Aesthet Surg. 2006;59(9):9991002.

35. Song Y, Xu D, Sun L, Ding K, Hu Y, Yuanb Y. Diagnosis and management of primary umbilical melanoma with omphalitis features. Case Rep Oncol. 2013;6(1):154–7.

36. Trebing D, Göring HD. The umbilical metastasis. Sister Mary Joseph and her time. Hautarzt. 2004;55:186–9.

37. Gabriele R, Conte M, Egidi F, Borghese M. Umbilical metastases: current viewpoint. World J Surg Oncol. 2005;3(1):13.

38. Dubreuil A, Dompmartin A, Barjot P, Louvet S, Leroy D. Umbilical metastasis or Sister Mary Joseph's nodule. Int J Dermatol. 1998;37:70–3.

39. Al-Mashat F, Sibiany AM. Sister Mary Joseph's nodule of the umbilicus: is it always of gastric origin? A review of eight cases at different sites of origin. Indian J Cancer. 2010;47:65–9.

40. Wilson I, Onuigbo B. Metastasis to the umbilicus: possible racial difference. J Natl Med Assoc. 1987;79(2):193–4.

41. Gabriele R, Borghese M, Conte M, Basso L. Sister Mary Joseph's nodule as a first surgery of cancer of the caecum: report of a case. Dis Colon Rectum. 2004;47:115–7.

42. Lombardi LE, Parsons L. Carcinoma of umbilicus metastatic from carcinoma of stomach. Ann Int Med. 1945;22:290.

43. Panaro F, Andorno E, Di Domenico S, Morelli N, Bottino G, Mondello R. Sister Joseph's nodule in a liver transplant recipient: case report and mini-review of literature. World J Surg Oncol. 2005;3:4.

44. Chalya PL, et al. Sister Mary Joseph's nodule at a university teaching hospital in northwestern Tanzania: a retrospective review of 34 cases. World J Surg Oncol. 2013;11:151. http://www.wjso.com/content/11/1/151

45. Rochet F, Francillon M. Cancer of umbilicus: metastasis from biliary tract. Lyon Med. 1942; 167:239.

46. Abdulqawi R, Ahmad S, Ashawesh K. A rare cause of Sister Mary Joseph's nodule. Swiss Med Wkly. 2007;137(39–40):559–60.

47. Powell FC, Cooper AJ, Massa MC, Goellner JR, Daniel Su WP. Sister Mary Joseph's nodule: a clinical and histologic study. J Am Acad Dermatol. 1984;10:610–5.

48. Hori T, et al. Hematogenous umbilical metastasis from colon cancer treated by palliative single-incision laparoscopic surgery. World J Gastrointest Surg. 2013;5(10):272–7.

49. Balakrishnan R, Rahman MA, Das A, Naznin B, Chowdhury Q. Sister Mary Jospeh's nodule as initial presentation of carcinoma caecum-case report and literature review. J Gastrointest Oncol. 2015;6(6):E102–5.

Rare Umbilical Disease

31

31.1 Absent Umbilicus

Congenital absence of navel in a viable newborn obviously does not exist. Abnormalities of the connecting stalk (body stalk anomalies) are lethal in utero or impose a therapeutic abortion before any ultrasound picture can document this anomaly, so few cases had been reported [1]. Very serious malformation detected most often on antenatal ultrasound at the end of the first trimester may be associated with absent or attenuated umbilical cord; like Schisis association (neural tube defects with anencephaly, encephalocele and spina bifida cystica), also cases of defective abdominal wall closure with massive visceral hernia, and anencephaly, of course such cases are associated with a higher miscarriage rate. This will be discussed with cord anomalies (Chap. 34).

The absence of the umbilicus is an aesthetically and psychologically frustrating condition for patients, as many ethnic groups are culturally sensitive to the absence of the navel. Over 60% of children describe psychosocial stress due to the absence of navel.

31.1.1 Congenitally Absent Umbilicus

- Omphalocele, specially large one, may end after repair without a navel, so it is theoretically considered as a congenital absence of umbilicus (Fig. 31.1).

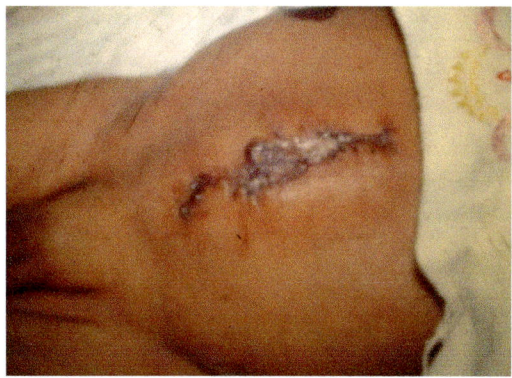

Fig. 31.1 Absent umbilicus after a conservatively managed omphalocele

- Omphalocele-exstrophy-imperforate anus-spinal defects (OEIS) syndrome, which is a rare complex associated with an absent umbilicus.
- Malposition or absence of the umbilicus is encountered frequently in patients with bladder exstrophy, specially in cases with umbilical cord inserted at the dome of exposed bladder (Fig. 31.2).
- Prune belly syndrome with early separation of the umbilical stump and defective abdominal wall musculature may end in survivors without any visible scar for umbilicus (Figs. 31.3 and 31.4).
- Aplasia cutis congenita: Congenital focal absence of epidermis with or without evidence of other layers of the skin, it may show a

© Springer International Publishing AG 2018
M. Fahmy, *Umbilicus and Umbilical Cord*, https://doi.org/10.1007/978-3-319-62383-2_31

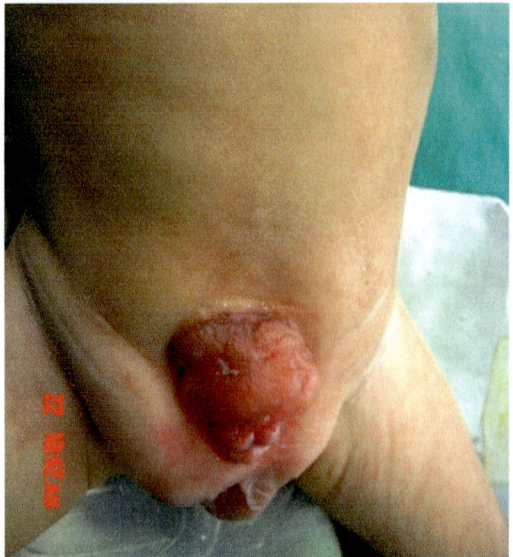

Fig. 31.2 Absent umbilicus is commonly seen with bladder exstrophy

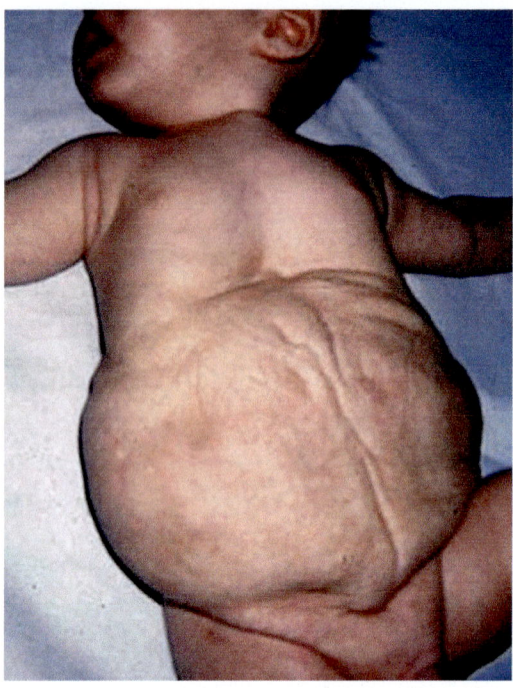

Fig. 31.4 Absent umbilical scar in a case of prune belly syndrome

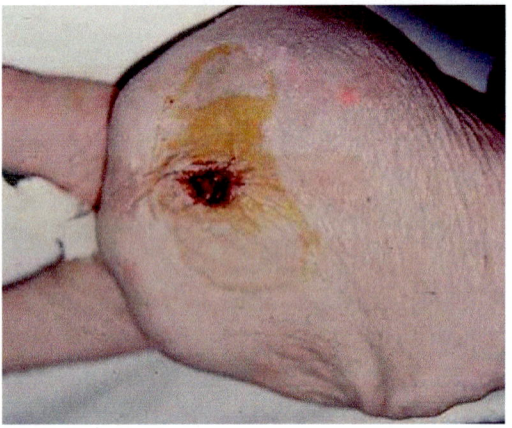

Fig. 31.3 Early avulsed umbilical cord with local haemorrhage in a neonate with prune belly syndrome

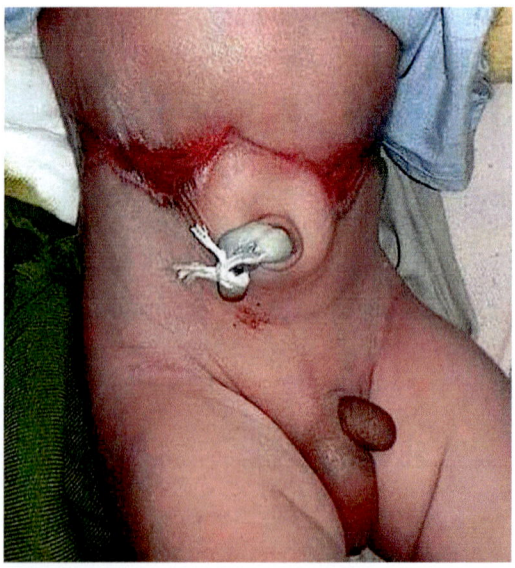

segmental absence of skin dermatome around the umbilicus in few cases [2] (Fig. 31.5).

- Epidermolysis bullosa may be responsible for the disappearance of the navel early after cord separation [3].
- Amniotic band syndrome may result in constricted umbilical cord and cord strangulation, and survived cases may end with an absent umbilical scar.

Fig. 31.5 Segmental skin absence in a case of aplasia cutis congenita; it may result in loss of skin at the umbilicus, but in this case the umbilical skin is preserved

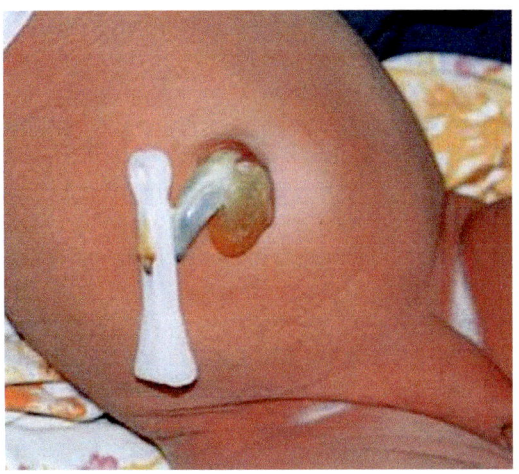

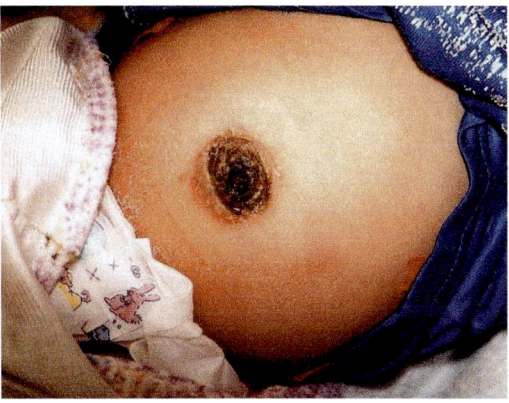

Fig. 31.7 A healed amniotic navel with a darker granulation tissue

Fig. 31.6 Amniotic navel, with a deficient skin replaced by an amniotic membrane at the inferior aspect of the cord

- Abdominal wall dysplasia, which is a condition associated with an increase of apoptotic cell death in the body wall placode, and consequently, the body wall remains very thin, preventing insufficient differentiation of the mesoderm and ectoderm in the abdominal wall musculature [4].

- Focal dermal hypoplasia which was first described by Goltz et al. [5], may be manifested at or around the umbilicus with an absent umbilicus.

- Amniotic Navel: (Fig. 31.6) Normally the skin of the abdominal wall extends for about 1 cm over the umbilical cord, the base of which it cylindrically encircles. In very rare cases the skin is lacking over the lower part of the cord and the adjacent abdominal wall, so that the amnion not only extends over the lowest part of the cord but also spreads out over the abdominal skin defect as a delicate, transparent membrane. The navel ring, the fibrous tissue, abdominal muscles and peritoneum are, however, normally developed. The disc of amnion becomes devitalized and dried like the cord stump, turns dark in colour and separates after a few days [6]. The skin defect either heals by granulation and scar formation, and in such case it may be difficult to differentiate the healed amniotic navel from umbilical

granuloma; but the last is more raised above the skin and bleed on touch (Fig. 31.7), or in other occasions, the transition to the normal abdominal skin is complete and will lead to disappearance of any mark of previous presence of this amniotic membrane.

31.1.2 Acquired Absent Umbilicus

Acquired cases of absent navel is not rare, as the umbilicus may be sacrificed during surgery for a neonate, child or adult, if the surgeon is not enthusiastic enough to recognize the navel importance and to pay a significant attention and talent to preserve navel. Surgery for gastroschisis, omphalocele and bladder exstrophy may naturally end with an abdominal wall devoid of navel, unless the surgeon reconstructs a new one.

The trend of fashioning a bowel stoma through the umbilicus was practised by some surgeons, and I think it should be stopped, as it usually ends with navel scarification (Fig. 31.8).

Umbilicus may be sacrificed in emergency surgery for trauma and internal haemorrhage along the exploratory incisions, where the attempts of reconstruction of the umbilicus, during emergency, usually fail to bring umbilicus back to the normal look (Fig. 31.9).

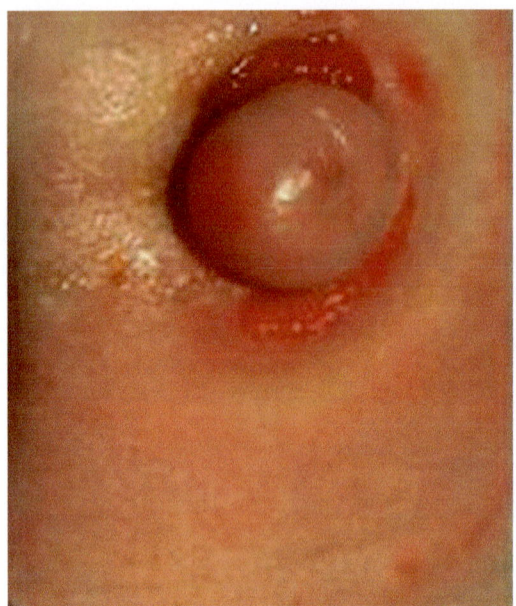

Fig. 31.8 A colostomy fashioned at the umbilicus

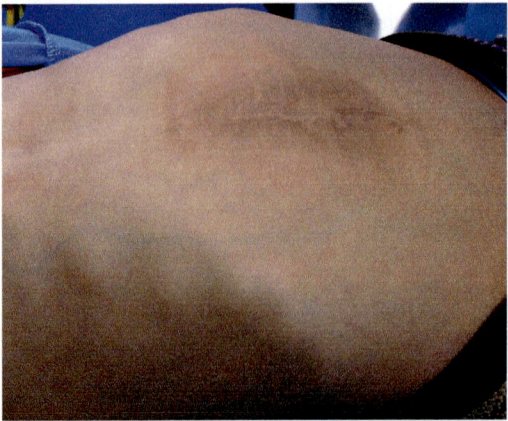

Fig. 31.9 A midline exploration scar, with umbilical scarification

Other causes of navel excision include rare primary tumors, where the umbilicus excised with the tumour eradication [7].

Management: Navel absence is responsible for an unnatural appearance of the abdomen, and an unsightly scar navel is immediately catches the eye. An omphaloplasty may sometimes pose challenges to surgeons; research has been performed to help the reconstructive surgeon locate the umbilicus in an aesthetically pleasing location.

The ideal umbilicus should have a natural contour, prominent depth, minimal additional scars and proper superior hooding. Shinohara et al. [8] emphasized that an umbilicus with a natural appearance consists of a ring, a tubular wall, a sulcus and a bottom, without any excess skin that would interfere with the aesthetic aspect of the umbilicus.

The goal of aesthetically pleasing umbilical reconstruction is to create a neoumbilicus with sufficient depth and good morphology, with natural-looking superior hooding and minimal scarring, [9] although many reports have presented techniques for creating new and attractive umbilici.

Umbilicoplasty is required not only in conditions such as congenital absence due to bladder exstrophy, gastroschisis, omphalocele and cloacal exstrophy but also in cases of a protruding umbilicus and traumatic umbilical malformation. Various methods have been employed in order to reconstruct the umbilicus, including the purse-string method, the use of several local flaps and the use of an ear conchal cartilage graft [10]. Every method has advantages and disadvantages; however, none of the above methods can guarantee optimal results.

31.2 Omphalith

Synonymous and Nomenclature: Umbilical concretions, omphalolith, omphalokeratoliths, umbilical bezoar and umboliths. The term omphalolith comes from the Greek words omphalos (meaning navel) and lithos (meaning stone). Friedman and Liles [11] want to stress the keratin composition of the umbilical mass, so they added 'kerato' from the Greek word 'keras' (meaning horn) to the name of the lesion; they introduced the term omphalokeratolith. However, the term omphalith is most common.

Definition: An omphalith is a hard, smooth, pearly white with a firm, dark brown cap calculus of different sizes and shapes found in the umbilicus. It generally occurs in a deeply retracted umbilicus. It is an umbilical foreign body resulting from the accumulation and concretion of keratinous and amorphous sebaceous material, which collects within an unusually deep umbilical cleft.

Historical Background: The first series of 28 cases was described by Dr. Thomas Cullen in his textbook, *The Umbilicus and Its Diseases*, published in 1916 [12].

Clinically: Umbilical concretions seem to be much more frequent in men than in women and usually occur during the period of life in which the patient is most actively engaged in work, namely, between the twentieth and sixtieth year. They are exceptional in children. Umbilical stones are generally asymptomatic, and presentation is due to complications. Omphalolith may be presented with a firm, black umbilical mass, which is easily removed with a warmed otic glycerin preparation (Fig. 31.10). There may be an accompanying putrid odour or drainage from the moist base of the umbilicus; however, the lesion itself neither drains nor smells.

As a rule, the patient is unaware of any trouble until abdominal pain is felt. This is usually referred to the umbilical region and may be increased on muscular exertion, on defecation or on pressure upon the abdomen. On visual examination sometimes, nothing is detected. Later induration is noted in the umbilical region, the umbilical opening becomes very small, and the surrounding tissue feels hard. The overlying skin may or may not be reddened.

On histopathological examination, umbilical concretions show laminated keratin and somewhat amorphous sebaceous material, as well as hair and often bacteria. Superficial portions of the concretion which are very firm and dark in colour are partially attributable to melanin, likely with a contribution from the oxidation of lipids [13] (Fig. 31.11).

Omphaliths: They are common in the elderly Japanese population, because of a certain superstition that 'touching' umbilical sesame could trigger abdominal pain [14].

Complications: Secondary bacterial infection may leads to omphalitis and abscess formation, very rarely this condition may be presented with secondary peritonitis, if the umbilical stone erodes the abdominal wall and finds its way to peritoneal cavity [15].

Differential Diagnosis: A particular attention has to be paid for differentiating this

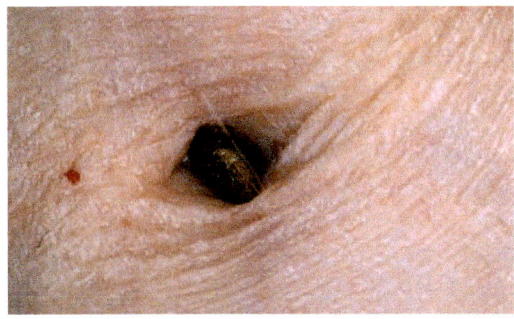

Fig. 31.10 An omphalolith before removal

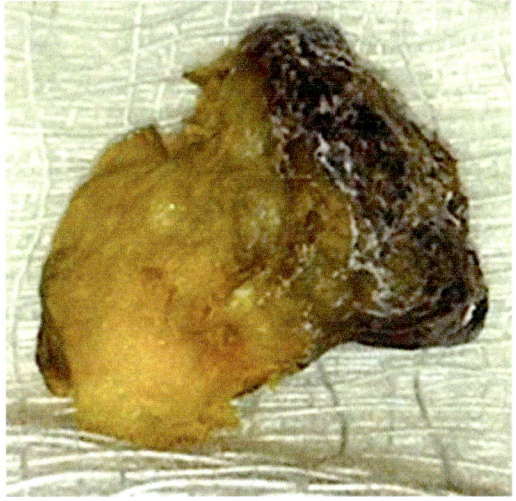

Fig. 31.11 An umbilical stone, with the *brown* uppermost part, owing to oxidized melanin and sebum

condition from other benign and malignant conditions of the umbilicus, including keloid, dermatofibroma, malignant melanoma, umbilical endometriosis, primary umbilical malignancy and umbilical metastasis (Sister Mary Joseph nodule).

Omphalith also should be differentiated from the terra-firma forme dermatosis (TFFD), which is not a commonly known clinical condition resembling dirt on the skin, hence the clinical name. This condition has been predominantly reported in children. Terra firma is a Latin phrase meaning 'solid Earth' (from terra, meaning 'Earth', and firma, meaning 'solid'). The phrase refers to dry land mass on the Earth's surface and is used to differentiate from sea or air [16] (Fig. 31.12).

The correct and timely diagnosis and treatment with either isopropyl or 70% ethyl alcohol swab is still the gold standard in most cases.

Clinical Significance of omphalith Awareness among the clinicians about the existence of omphalolith is essential to save time for the clinician and to reduce the economic burden on the patient by avoiding costly investigations and treatment. Proper counselling regarding the cleansing of the umbilical area is essential before laparoscopic surgery, as this sites may be a source for development of secondary infection at the port sites.

Investigations: The stones could be detected by abdominal plain X-ray, as it is usually radiopaque, ultrasound and rarely abdominal CT scan, may be indicated only in doubtful cases.

Treatment: Miles Porter reported a case of umbilical concretion treated with surgical excision in the *Journal of the American Medical Association* in 1920 [12]. He noted that a noninvasive treatment would likely have been possible if he had been more familiar with the condition. His analysis concludes with a statement that all physicians have become acquainted with in one form or another.

Treatment is noninvasive evacuation of the concretion and cleansing of the umbilicus. It should be noted that the presence of associated inflammation or infection, including granuloma formation, may serve to complicate the appearance of the lesion.

It can be removed by squeezing the stone from the umbilical foramen or through adequate opening of umbilical foramen under local anaesthesia to the periumbilical area. A speedy disappearance of the symptoms usually follows.

31.3   Belly-Button Lint

Nomenclature: Navel Lint, Navel Fluff, Belly Button Fluff, and dip Lint.

Definition: It is an accumulation of fluffy fibres in the navel cavity. Lint is the common name for visible accumulations of textile fibres and other materials, usually found in and around the umbilicus. Many people find that, at the beginning and end of the day, a small lump of fluff has appeared in the navel cavity [17].

Belly button lint is quite common among hairy man (Fig. 31.13). Usually it is washed off during bathing or shower and rarely does it cause any inflammation [17]. Steinhauser has recently suggested that abdominal hair is mainly responsible for directing the fibres from clothes into the navel where they are compacted; shaving abdominal hair can prevent lint accumulation in the umbilicus.

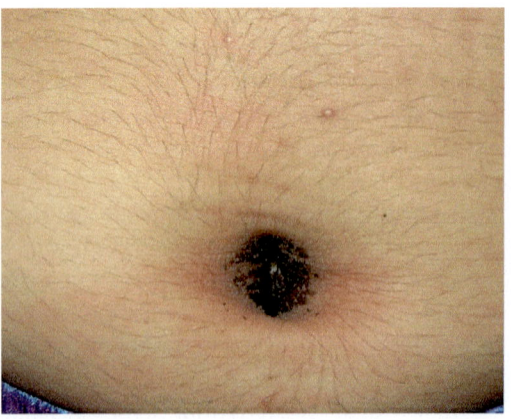

Fig. 31.12 A case of terra-firma forme dermatosis (TFFD) of the umbilicus

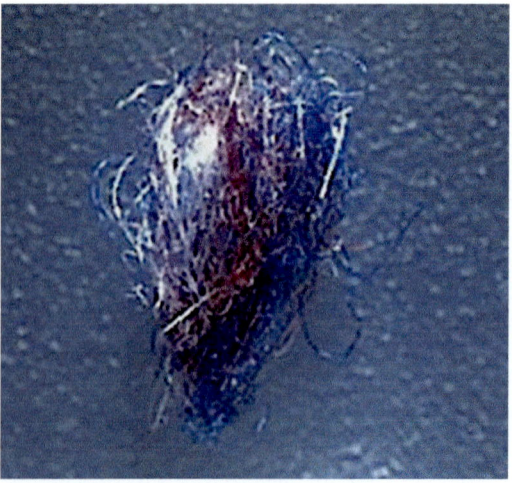

Fig. 31.13 A belly button lint

Predisposing factors:

- Obesity
- Deeply seated umbilicus.
- Poor hygiene

Hairball (navel trichobezoar) is also encountered as foreign body seen in hairy men.

31.4 Umbilical Dermoid and Epidermoid Cyst

Dermoid cyst is usually a congenital inclusion cyst, caused by the implantation of epithelial tissue into another structure, and most frequently occurs on the face and in midline structures.

It contains developmentally mature skin, with sweat glands, hair follicles, sometimes luxuriant clumps of long hair and often pockets of sebum, blood, fat, bone and cartilage, nails and teeth and thyroid tissue.

Because they contain mature tissue, these cysts are almost always benign, but it may turn to malignancy in rare occasions, usually solitary, and expand slowly over many years. These cysts are not tender unless they rupture.

Epidermoid cysts are similar in structure and origin to dermoid, and the two are often grouped together. Epidermoid cyst is usually acquired after surgery or skin trauma, and it is lined with stratified squamous epithelium (skin) as dermoids are, but does not contain the additional skin appendages; they are less likely to rupture [18].

Dermoid cyst of the umbilicus is a rare umbilical mass caused by inclusion of skin epithelium below or within the normal skin of the umbilicus, after cord separation.

Cullen's textbook of diseases of the umbilicus and urachus, published in 1916, described walnut-sized dermoid (or atheromatous) cysts of the umbilicus reported in only five patients; these cysts originate from the umbilicus; they contain sebaceous material that yields epithelial cells, fat droplets and cholesterin crystals; they are lined by squamous epithelium; and they do not contain hair [19].

Clinically: On examination, the umbilicus appears wider and darker in colour than normal, with a shiny small cyst occupying the whole umbilicus (Fig. 31.14).

Sometimes the cyst is small and dark in colour and appears beside the navel cicatrix (Fig. 31.15).

No inflammation is noted unless the cyst is infected. The diagnosis is made at surgery on finding the characteristic toothpaste-like

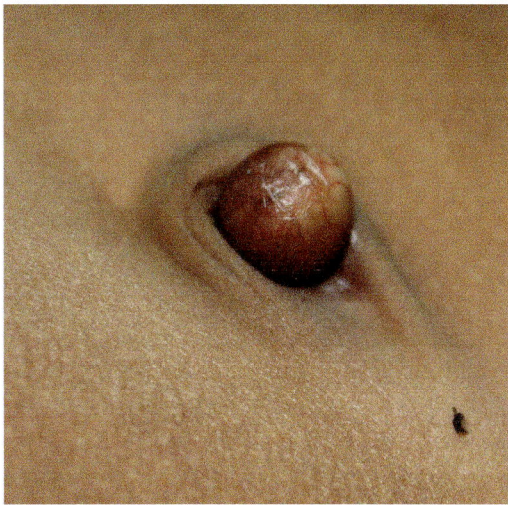

Fig. 31.14 A shiny dermoid cyst occupying the whole umbilicus

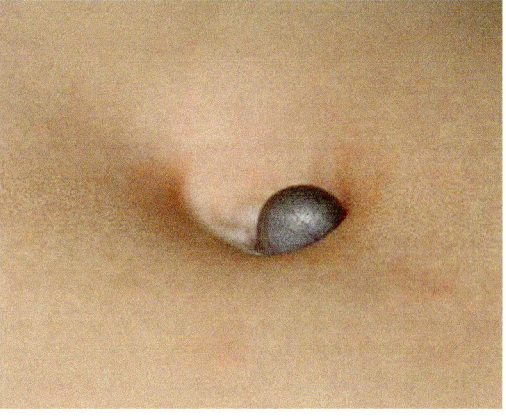

Fig. 31.15 Small *dark dermoid* cyst of the umbilicus

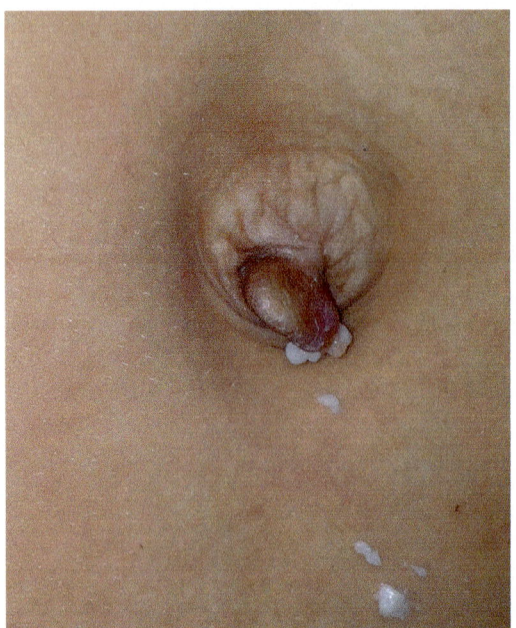

Fig. 31.16 A ruptured dermoid cyst with a sebaceous material coming out

sebaceous material within the umbilical mass (Fig. 31.16).

Ultrasound examination is helpful to rule out any other associated lesions and to detect the extent of the cyst, as dermoid cyst may be located in the retroperitoneal space [20].

Management: Complete excision of epidermoid cysts is recommended, without any reported recurrence. A large retained umbilical epidermal inclusion cyst may follow surgery at or around the umbilicus [21].

31.5 Umbilical Pilonidal Sinus (PNS)

Definition: Pilonidal sinus disease is a common chronic intermittent disorder characterized by a granulomatous reaction to a hair shaft penetrating epidermis from the external surface. Although it is a minor surgical condition, it is associated with considerable morbidity and has a significant social impact on the affected individuals. It is mainly seen in the sacrococcygeal region, but it may be encountered less frequently in other parts of the body such as web spaces of the hands,

axilla, perineum, suprapubic region, sole of the foot, amputation stump and umbilicus.

Historical Background: The first description of pilonidal sinus disease of the umbilicus was recorded 150 years ago [22].

Incidence: Although the umbilicus was first recognized as a site of pilonidal disease nearly 150 years ago, some reports indicate that it is more common in the general population than was generally thought. The most common atypical sites of pilonidal sinus was umbilicus (91%), followed by hand (4%). A total of 272 cases of umbilical PNS were reported till 2017 [23].

Etiology: Although the view is divided about the etiology of sacrococcygeal pilonidal sinus, there is little doubt about the origin of umbilical pilonidal sinus as an acquired disease.

Umbilical pilonidal sinus is characterized by penetration of hairs, foreign body reaction and formation of sinus with granulation tissue. It has been speculated that the hairs shed from the chest, and the abdomen is pulled down into the deep umbilical recess by the tugging action. Hairs caught in the umbilicus then possibly get hooked and puncture the umbilical recess, thereby inducing a foreign body inflammatory response. The resultant oedema may narrow the umbilical opening, converting it into a cyst, which may rupture with extrusion of its contents. If local infection is added, it will produce an acute abscess or omphalitis (Fig. 31.17).

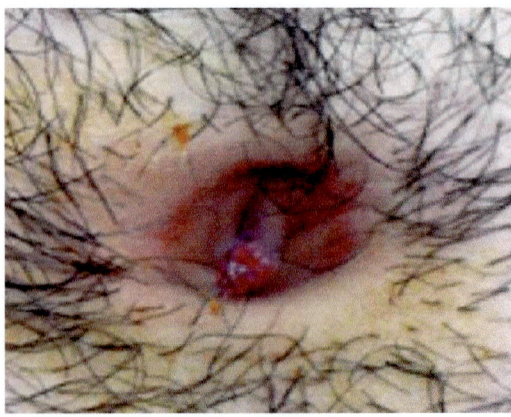

Fig. 31.17 An umbilical pilonidal sinus with granulation tissue around its punctum and inflammation in a hairy main

Predisposing Factors:

- About 90% of the patients were male. The male preponderance is perhaps due to hirsutism and the unique distribution of hairs around the umbilicus with the distal ends pointing towards the umbilicus, whereas in women the hairline is usually located well below the umbilicus.
- Obesity has been considered to be an important risk factor; this was observed in only 15% of patients [24].
- Hyperhidrosis is another risk factor; it was also found to be a factor for 23% of the patients [24].
- Deep navel, an important anatomic variation, was quite common in patients with umbilical pilonidal sinus.
- Inadequate personal hygiene was also noticed in the majority of patients.

Clinically: This is a disease of young, hirsute, adult males. Patients with umbilical pilonidal sinus usually present with pain and bloody or purulent discharge from the umbilicus. The pain was indolent, continuous and mild in nature. Local tenderness with redness was also noticed in nearly half of patients and may indicate abscess formation [25].

Sometimes an umbilical mass that makes the diagnosis difficult could be an associated symptom.

Differential Diagnosis of the umbilical pilonidal sinus with other umbilical disorders including umbilical hernia, endometriosis in women, metastatic tumors (Sister Mary Joseph nodule, etc.), remnant of omphalomesenteric ducts, congenital pathologies such as urachus anomalies, pyogenic granulomas and benign tumors like epidermoid cyst should not be neglected as the differential diagnosis.

Because umbilical pilonidal sinus disease is rarely reported, most doctors are unfamiliar with the disease, which may easily misdiagnosed and mistreated, so preoperative imaging with an ultrasound may help in this regard [26].

Treatment: The treatment of pilonidal sinus disease is not uniform. Most of the cases reported in the literature were treated with surgical excision. Authors who suggest the surgical excision assert that there is a risk of peritoneal extension of inflammation; however, no report in the literature indicates that peritonitis develops from untreated or conservatively treated umbilical pilonidal sinus disease [22]. Therefore, some other authors advocate conservative treatments, which include hair extraction, abscess drainage, antibiotic therapy and shaving of hairs around the umbilicus to prevent recurrence. Patients who failed the conservative treatment should undergo surgical excision and primary repair. Proponents of conservative treatment believe that because the disease is not congenital in origin, there is no need to excise the umbilicus. Besides, they believe that the disease would terminate naturally after the age of 30. There is no agreement concerning umbilical reconstruction among published series [27]. But I think if the umbilicus itself excised along the PNS, an attempt to reconstruct the umbilicus in another setting should be considered, specially for young patients (Fig. 31.18).

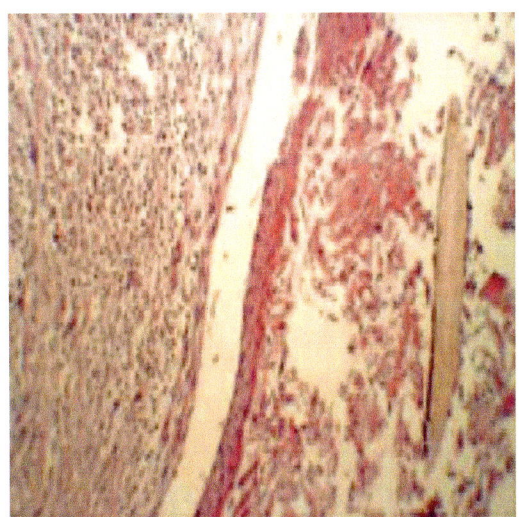

Fig. 31.18 The microscopic appearance of umbilical pilonidal sinus disease (H&E X40); hair shaft within the cavity is clear

31.6 Umbilical Keloid

Keloid is an abnormal pattern of dermal reaction to injury, resulting in excess collagen deposition, affecting 5–10% of general population [28].

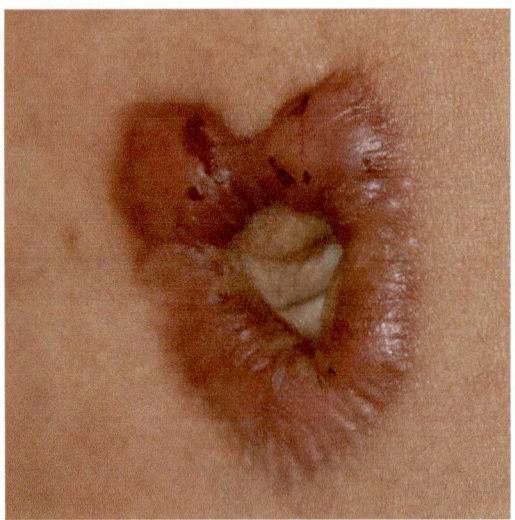

Fig. 31.19 Umbilical keloid complicating silver nitrate application for treatment of granuloma

but familial occurrences have also been described. There's no sex prevalence among affected individuals. They can be either solitary or numerous and may vary in size from small papules to large masses.

Umbilical keloid is a rare disease and could be seen in different forms and at different age group:

- Umbilical stump keloid in infancy [30].
- Keloid complicating granuloma or as a complication of umbilical burn after application of silver nitrate for granuloma management (Fig. 31.19)
- Keloid complicating umbilical piercing, in individuals who are prone to develop keloid (Fig. 31.20).
- Umbilical keloid after umbilical surgery, for hernia repair, or rarely after using umbilicus as a port for laparoscopy [31].

The lesion may be seen merging from the umbilical indentation, as a small pink solid or firm mass (Fig. 31.21) or as circular lesion around the umbilicus (Fig. 31.19); such small lesion should be differentiated from the excessive scaring of the umbilicus, where a normal skin may be seen over protruding from the navel 'protruded or prominent mamelon' (Chap. 20) (Fig. 31.22).

Very rarely, in the neglected or recurrent cases, the keloid mass may form a fungating swelling, which is difficult to differentiate from a neoplastic lesions (Fig. 31.23).

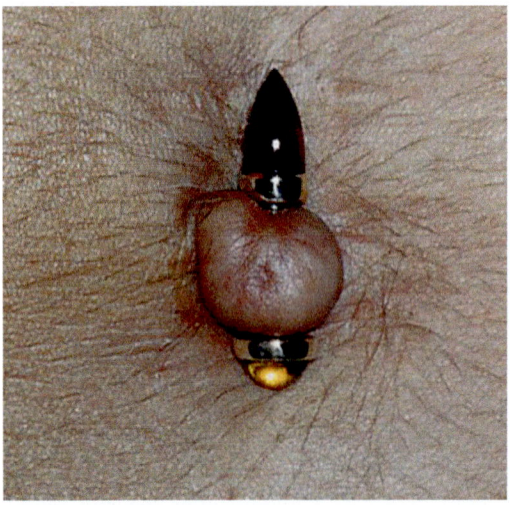

Fig. 31.20 Umbilical keloid around an umbilical ring, as a complication of piercing

Various types of injuries are on record, such as surgery, trauma, burns, inflammatory skin diseases (folliculitis, acne), viral dermatological diseases (chickenpox), vaccinations and foreign body injuries; occasionally the injury may be clinically inapparent. The pathogenesis is unknown, but genetic, hormonal or local factors may be involved [29]. Keloids may occur at any age, but they are more common in the young; black and coloured people. It is usually sporadic,

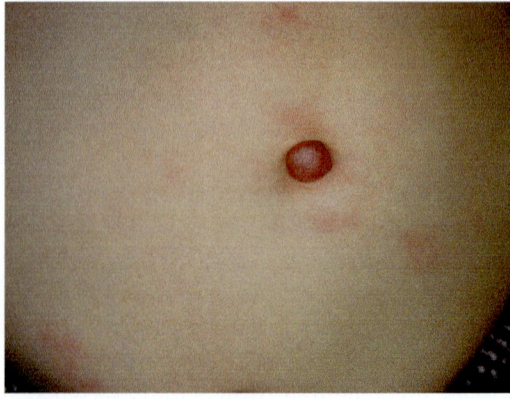

Fig. 31.21 Small firm umbilical mass, proved to be a keloid after excision

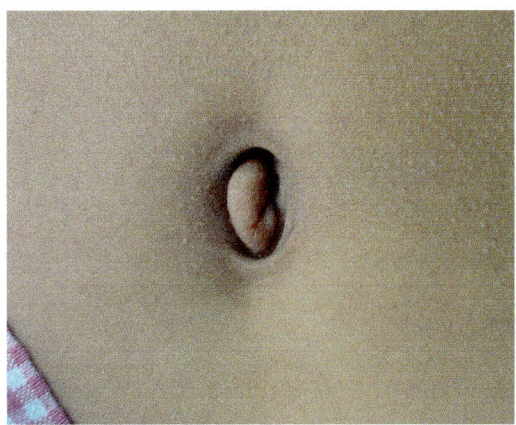

Fig. 31.22 A normal umbilicus with a normal skin protruded from the umbilical dimple 'prominent mamelon'

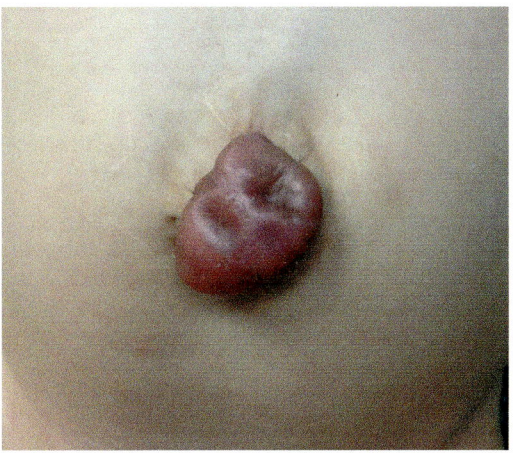

Fig. 31.23 Umbilical keloid presented as a large cauliflower mass merging from the umbilicus

Symptoms may vary from mild local distress (pain and/or pruritus) to cosmetic discomfort or anatomic disabilities, even to disfiguring deformities, associated with dramatic psychological and social side effects.

Keloids should be differentiated from hypertrophic scars, which remain confined to the site of injury and gradually involute over time. In contrast, keloids usually outgrow the boundaries of the original insult; they also are more often pedunculated. Sometimes it is impossible to differentiate keloid from metastatic lesions or endometriosis, except after excision and histopathological studies.

Investigations: Ultrasound, computed tomography and MRI of the abdomen may be indicated to reveal the tumor extension from the dermis to the rectus sheath and the peritoneum and also to rule out the possibility of neoplastic umbilical neoplasm in doubtful cases [32].

Treatment: There is no universally accepted treatment protocol standardized for treatment of keloid, but several choices are available according to several factors (site, size, clinical history, prior treatments); keloids are often resistant to treatment and have a high rate of recurrence. It may be effectively treated with intralesional corticosteroids, but large lesions may require surgical excision followed by intralesional corticosteroid, silicone gel sheeting or radiotherapy. Cryosurgery and cytotoxic drugs like bleomycin and 5-fluorouracil had been also tried with some success.

However, excision alone results in a high recurrence rate (45–100%) [33]. Usually the umbilicus is sacrificed along surgical excision of keloid, with the need for a subsequent umbilicoplasty. Few cases reported with deep extension of the keloid to the rectus sheath or the peritoneum, which needs wide excision [32].

References

1. Quijano FE, Rey MM, Echeverry M, Axt-Fliedner R. Body stalk anomaly in a 9-week pregnancy, case report. Case Rep Obstetr Gynecol. 2014;3:357285. doi:10.1155/2014/357285.
2. Rapini RP, Bolognia JL, Jorizzo JL. Dermatology: 2-volume set. St. Louis: Mosby; 2007.
3. Kanzler MH, Smoller B, Woodley DT. Congenital localized absence of the skin as a manifestation of epidermolysis bullosa. Arch Dermatol. 1992;128(8):1087–90.
4. Queizán A, Rivas S, Hernández F, Martínez L. Body wall dysplasia: a rare case of abdominal hernia. J Podiatry Surg. 2005;40(5):877–8.
5. Goltz RW, Peterson NC, Gorlin RJ, Ravits HG. Focal dermal hypoplasia. Arch Deruro. 1962;86:708.
6. Christison-Lagay ER, Kelleher CM, Langer JC. Neonatal abdominal wall defects. Semin Fetal Neonatal Med. 2011;16:164–72.
7. O'Marcaigh AS, Folz LB, Michels VV. Umbilical morphology: normal values for neonatal periumbilical skin length. Pediatrics. 1992;90(1 Pt 1):47–9.
8. Shinohara H, Matsuo K, Kikuchi N. Umbilical reconstruc-tion with an inverted C-V flap. Plast Reconstr Surg. 2000;105:703–5.

9. Lee YT, Kwon C, Rhee SC, Cho SH, Eo SR. Four flaps technique for neoumbilicoplasty. Archives of Plastic Surgery. 2015;42(3):351–5. doi:10.5999/aps.2015.42.3.351.

10. Hong YG, Cho JJ. Reconstruction of scarred umbilicus us-ing an inverted c-v flap: a case report. J Korean Soc Plast Re-constr Surg. 2007;34:653–5.

11. Friedman SJ, Liles WJ. Omphalokeratolith. Cutis. 1987;40(2):144–6.

12. Porter MF. Umbilical concretions. Report of case. J Am Med Assoc. 1920;75(9):599–600.

13. Sheehan D, Hussain S, Vijayaraghavan G. Umbilical concretion. J Radiol Case Rep. 2011;5(4):25–31. doi:10.3941/jrcr.v5i4.705.

14. Ichiki Y, Kitajima Y. Omphalith. Clin Exp Dermatol. 2009;34(3):420–1.

15. Mahdi HR, El Hennawy HM. Omphalolith presented with peritonitis: a case report. Cases J. 2009;2:8191. doi:10.4076/1757-1626-2-8191.

16. Ashique KT, Kaliyadan F, Goyal T. Terra firma-forme dermatosis: report of a series of 11 cases and a brief review of the literature. Int Jour Dermat. 2016;55(7):769–74.

17. Steinhauser G. The nature of navel fluff. Med Hypotheses. 2009;72:623–5. doi:10.1016/j.mehy.2009.01.015.

18. Andreadis AA, Samson MC, Szomstein S, Newman M. Epidermal inclusion cyst of the umbilicus following abdominoplasty. Plast Surg Nurs. 2007;27(4):202–5. doi:10.1097/01.PSN.0000306186.72942.ae.

19. Cullen TS. Embryology, anatomy, and diseases of the umbilicus: together with diseases of the urachus. Philadelphia, PA: WB Saunders; 1916. p. 253–7.

20. Agbreta N, Boutens A, Debodinance P. Dermoid cyst of the urachus: a case report and review of the literature. J Gynecol Obstet Biol Reprod (Paris). 2006;35(1):75–8.

21. McClenathan JH. Umbilical epidermoid cyst: an unusual cause of umbilical symptoms. Can J Surg. 2002;45(4):303–4.

22. Hull TL, Wu J. Pilonidal disease. Surg Clin North Am. 2002;82:1169–85.

23. Salih A, Kakamad F, Essa R, et al. Pilonidal sinus of atypical areas: presentation and management. PSJ. 2017;3(1):8–15.

24. Eryilmaz R, Sahin M, Okan I, Alimoglu O, Somay A. Umbilical pilonidal sinus disease: predisposing factors and treatment. World J Surg. 2005;29:1158–60.

25. Silva JH. Pilonidal cyst: cause and treatment. Dis Colon Rectum. 2000;43:1146–56.

26. Steck WD, Helwig EB. Umbilical granulomas, pilonidal disease, and the urachus. Surg Gynecol Obstet. 1965;120:1043–57.

27. Eryilmaz R, Sahin M, Okan I, Alimoglu O, Somay A. Umbilical pilonidal sinus disease: predisposing factors and treatment. World J Surg. 2005;29:1158–60. doi:10.1007/s00268-005-7895-9.

28. Marneros AG, Norris JE, Olsen BR, Reichenberger E. Clinical genetics of familial keloids. Arch Dermatol. 2001;137:1429–34.

29. Ford T, Widgerow AD. Umbilical keloid: an early start. Ann Plast Surg. 1990;25(3):214–5.

30. Ikard RW, Wahl RW. Umbilical stump keloid. South Med J. 1990;83:1494–5.

31. Matsushita K, et al. Umbilical keloid occurred after laparoscopically assisted vaginal hysterectomy. Hifu no kagaku. 2003;2(5):462–5. doi:10.11340/skinresearch.2.5_462.

32. Awad GA, Wilson P. Umbilical port site keloid extending through rectus sheath. Eur J Plast Surg. 2014;37:357–8. doi:10.1007/s00238-014-0935-7.

33. Alster TS, Tanzi EL. Hypertrophic scars and keloids: etiology and management. Am J Clin Dermatol. 2003;4:235–43.

Part V

Umbilical Disorders: Congenital Anomalies of Umbilicus

Congenital Hernia of Umbilical Cord (CHUC)

32

Pathophysiology: During early fetal life, there is physiological herniation of a greater portion of the intestines into the proximal part of the umbilical cord, which is called extracelomic cavity. At about 10–12 weeks gestation, intestines withdraw into the abdominal cavity after completion of the bowel rotation, the umbilical ring mostly closes, and the extracelomic cavity disappears leaving behind Wharton's jelly and umbilical vessels in the cord (Figs. 32.1 and 32.2).

In rare instances, the umbilical ring does not close, and variable portions of the intestines remain in the extracelomic cavity to present at birth as congenital hernia into the umbilical cord, which is a normal developmental herniation in early fatal life,

but it may persist and to be manifested at birth as a cystic swelling at the fetal end of the cord. The wall of the hernia formed of amnion and peritoneum; consequently, the intestinal loops within the sac are readily visible (Fig. 32.3).

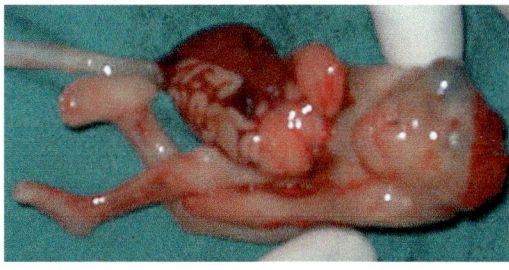

Fig. 32.2 An aborted human embryo at 5th week with physiological bowel herniation, bowel covered with amniotic membrane

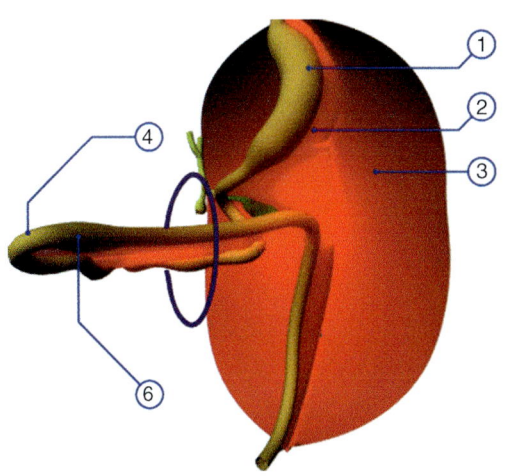

Fig. 32.1 Physiological bowel herniation in the early fetal life. 1. Stomach, 2. mesenterium, 3. parietal peritoneum, 4. intestinal loop, 5. cecum

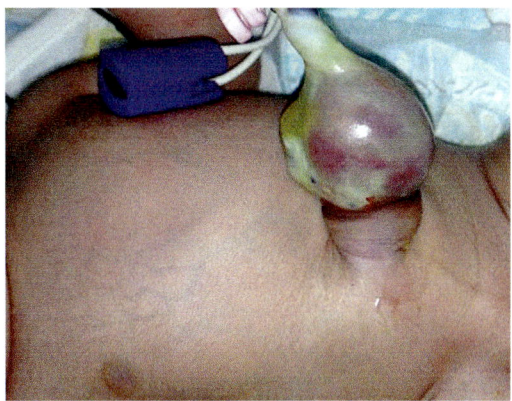

Fig. 32.3 A typical congenital umbilical cord hernia with normal umbilical ring width, strip of skin creeping over the cord and normal continuity of cord distal to hernia

© Springer International Publishing AG 2018
M. Fahmy, *Umbilicus and Umbilical Cord*, https://doi.org/10.1007/978-3-319-62383-2_32

Failure of the part of bowel to return to the abdominal cavity may be due to presence of adhesions between intestinal loops and the umbilical wall, which is usually seen during CHUC repair, or the failure of bowel return in the abdominal cavity may be due to constricting umbilical ring, but the former explanation is more acceptable.

Historically background: Power and D'Arcy [1] reported a case of CHUC at 1888 for the first time, and subsequently in 1929, Hempel-Jorgensen had reported two cases of this entity in a family and had coined the term 'familial congenital umbilical hernia' [2]. Tow in 1937 [3] described the characteristics and embryogenesis of this entity in couple of cases. Ever since only few case reports have been published clearly describing this rare anomaly, possibly poor understanding of CHUC has led to it's under reporting.

Significance: Hernia into the umbilical cord is a special entity, has been poorly understood, is easily missed and is often miscategorized as 'omphalocele minor'.

Few small and reducible congenital hernias of cord are left as such by the clinicians which finally get epithelialized and may be falsely diagnosed as 'cutis navel'. To the worst, inadvertent clamping of cord leads, with the presence of CHUC, leads to iatrogenic gut injury and faecal peritonitis. Also this anomaly usually associated with bowel atresia, adherent Meckel's diverticulum, malrotation and volvulus, which deserve investigations to rule out these associations.

Incidence: Incidence of CHUC is difficult to define, but in one review, it is estimated to be one in 5000, with a male preponderance (3:1), and association with prematurity in many series reports [4].

Clinically: CHUC characterized by a proximal cord swelling, covered by a strip of normal skin, which always enwraps the umbilical ring and a variable length of the proximal part of the cord, and the wall around the herniated bowel is variable: from a very thin membrane and intestinal loops within the sac which are readily visible to a thick wall similar to the rest of the cord wall (Figs. 32.4 and 32.5). Rarely the hernial wall is so thick to an extent that it looks like the skin, while the rest of the cord is usually normal (Fig. 32.6).

The umbilical vessels may be overstretched over the cord hernia, to be visibly congested and tortuous around the hernia sac (Fig. 32.7).

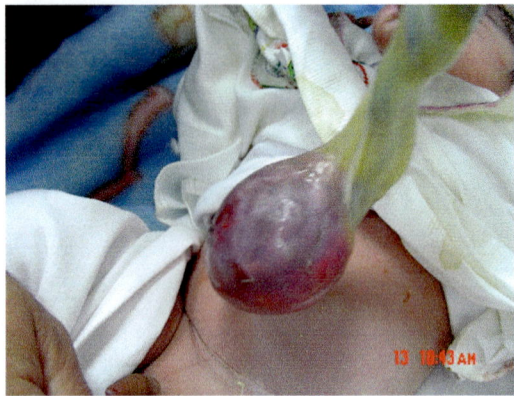

Fig. 32.4 CHUC with a thin wall sac, through which the herniated bowel seen easily

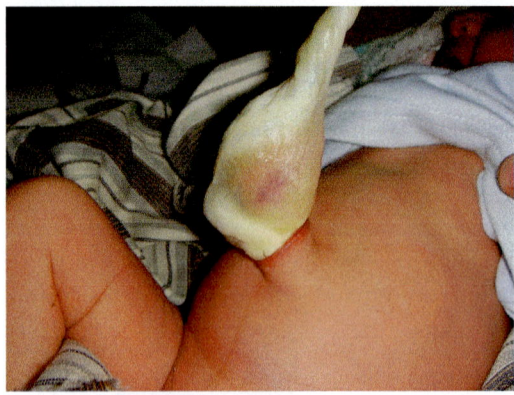

Fig. 32.5 CHUC with a thick wall

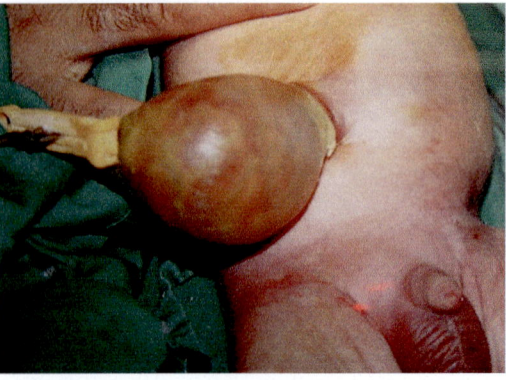

Fig. 32.6 The wall of CHUC looks like skin, but a demarcated abdominal wall skin could be seen proximally

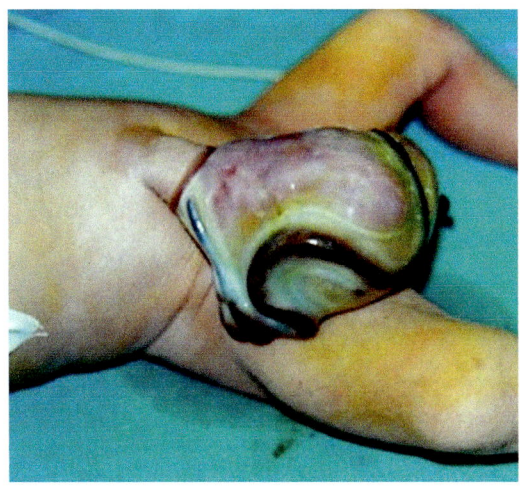

Fig. 32.7 A visible prominent umbilical vessels seen dilated and stretched over the hernia wall

32.1 Cardinal Signs for Diagnosis of CHUC

- In cases of CHUC, the body folds develop normally and form the umbilical ring, in which the bowel usually herniates into the base of a normally inserted umbilical cord.
- Presence of a well-formed complete umbilical ring, but it may be wider than normal (1.5–4 cm).
- A sac comprising of outer amnion and inner peritoneal lining.
- Complete union of the recti muscles in the midline and attachment to xiphoid process and costal margin [5].
- A cuff of skin is seen extending from the abdominal wall onto the neck of the sac (Fig. 32.7).

Herniated bowel into the umbilical cord may range from a small portion of the small bowel or part of the colon to the eviscerated bowel that floats freely into the amniotic fluid which may occasionally twist resulting in in utero volvulus, causing bowel obstruction and intestinal atresia. Mirza et al. [6] reported a case of congenital short gut and intestinal atresia associated with hernia of umbilical cord; similar in utero event would have led to poor outcome.

Associated anomalies: Unlike omphalocele, CHUC is believed to be a simple anomaly without any associated chromosomal or other organ involvements, except few cases reported with a persistent vitellointestinal duct (PVID) and cloacal anomaly. In contrast to omphalocele, which had an associated anomalies in 30–80% of cases, among which cardiac defects are more common, also chromosomal anomalies occur in 49% cases of omphalocele [7]. But Mirza and Waqas [6] found Tetralogy of Fallot, pulmonary stenosis, cleft lip and palate in a considerable number of cases.

Meckel's diverticula, colonic atresia and type IIIb ileal atresia are commonly associated with GI anomalies in the most reported series [8]. Some cases are associated with abnormal cord insertion in the abdominal wall, with either cephalic or caudal shift.

Antenatal Detection: Achiron et al. have demonstrated that CHUC occurs at early embryological stage and can be detectable at early second trimester on antenatal USG (Fig. 32.8).

Few of these might disappear before term and rest may persist as CHUC. No specific antenatal intervention has been advocated although a regular follow up is required as cord hematoma carries increased risk of fetal death [9].

Differential Diagnosis: Unlike omphalocele and gastroschisis, CHUC has an intact abdominal wall; omphalocele is a central defect of umbilical ring, resulting in persistent herniation of the abdominal contents. From an anatomical point of view, omphalocele is a defect involving both the umbilical and supraumbilical portion of the abdominal wall secondary to failure of progression of the lateral body wall folds, thus hindering the union of the recti muscles and causing the cranial circumference of the umbilical ring to remain open.

From an embryological point of view, the development of the two conditions occurs at different embryonic stages, being significantly earlier for omphalocele. In fact, hernia into the umbilical cord develops at around the 10th week, when the formation of the supraumbilical part of the abdomen has already taken place at the third week [10].

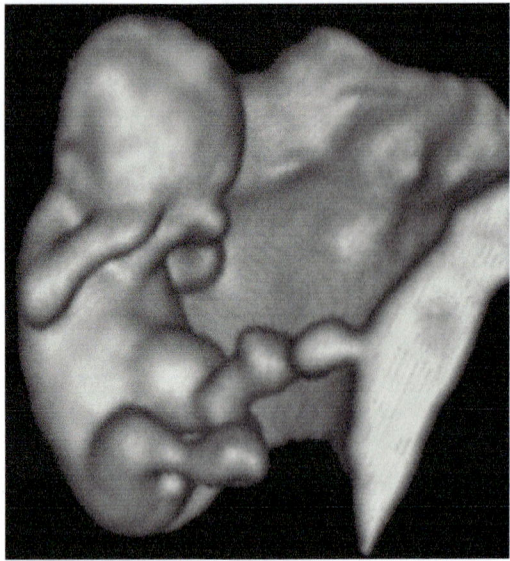

Fig. 32.8 Antenatal ultrasonography showing clearly CHUC and the fetal end of the cord

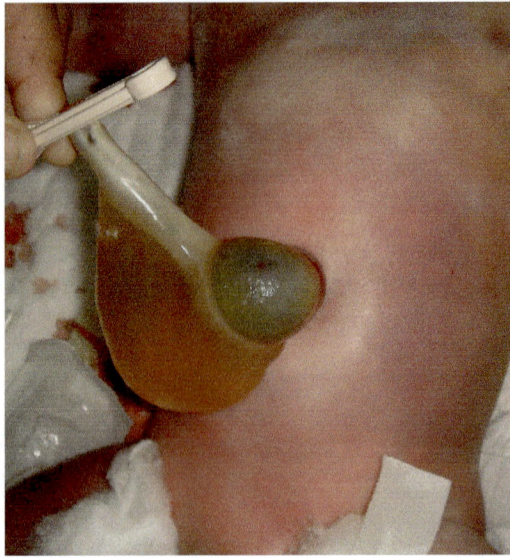

Fig. 32.9 A rare case of CHUC with an associated cord cyst

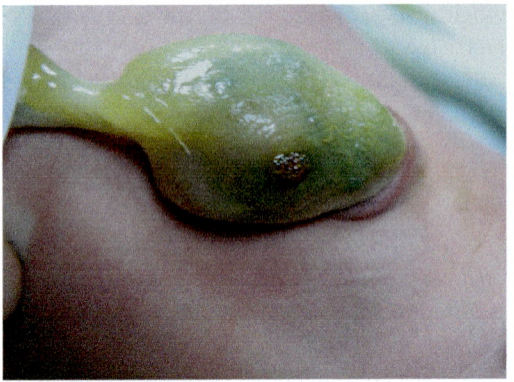

Fig. 32.10 Perforated bowel adherent to the wall of CHUC, with intestinal secretion coming out

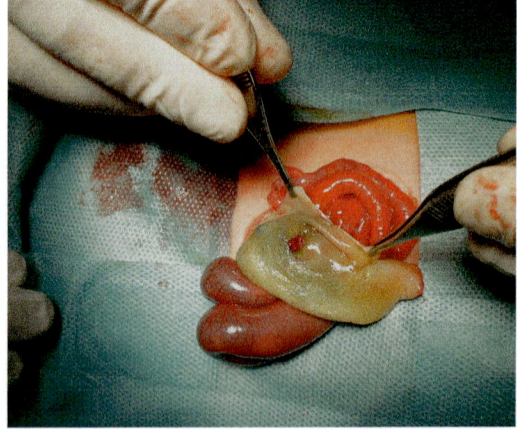

Fig. 32.11 Exploration of the case in Fig. 32.10, revealed a perforated Meckel's diverticulum, which was resected, and bowel anastomosed through the umbilical incision

Cord hematoma, cyst, giant cord, teratoma and other cord tumor should be differentiated during diagnoses for antenatally detected hernia of the cord, and, also postnatally, CHUC may confuse with other cord swellings, like true cord cysts (Fig. 32.9).

Complications: Bowel perforation, either antenatally or after delivery, is the most serious complication of CHUC, and adherent perforated Meckel's diverticulum is frequently encountered with this anomaly. So all cases should be investigated and explored to rule out any associated bowel anomalies (Figs. 32.10, 32.11, 32.12, and 32.13).

Another serious complication, which may happen due to unawareness of gynaecologists or midwives with CHUC, if they apply umbilical clamp proximal as usual, over a herniated bowel in an unrecognized CHUC, which will end with an iatrogenic bowel injury or perforation and a subsequent peritonitis (Fig. 32.14).

Management: All cases of CHUC require surgical exploration to rule out atresia or remnants of vitellointestinal duct. Outcome is excel-

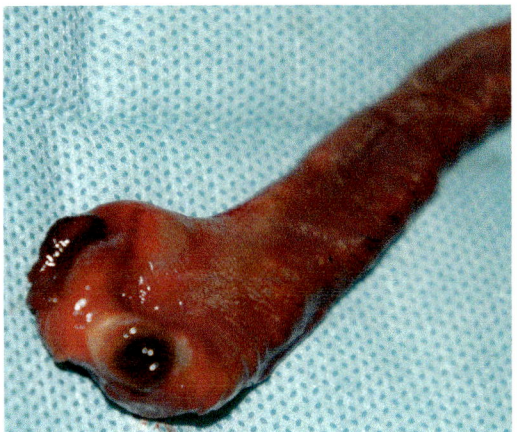

Fig. 32.12 Resected bowel with a perforated Meckel's diverticulum, same patient in Fig. 32.10

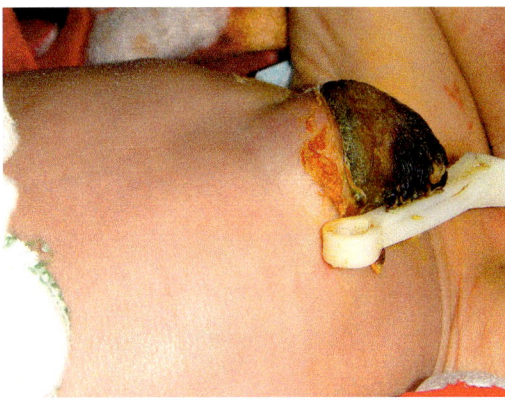

Fig. 32.14 Iatrogenic bowel gangrene due to proximal application of umbilical clamp over a herniated bowel in CHUC

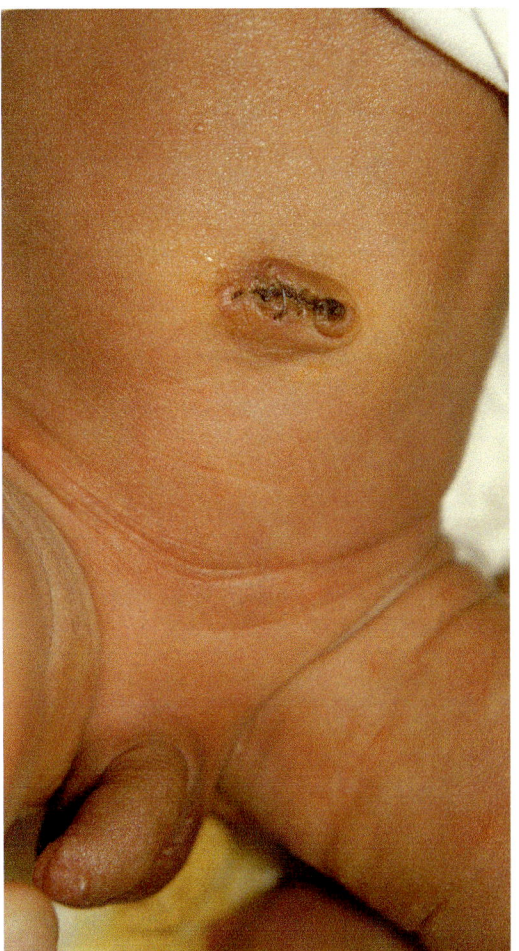

Fig. 32.13 A normally looked umbilicus after exploration, same patient in Fig. 32.10

lent in most cases, due to lack of association with other congenital or chromosomal anomalies.

The operation most commonly performed to repair either a hernia into the umbilical cord or a small omphalocele entails excision of the amniotic sac flush with the skin, individual ligation of the umbilical vessels at the level of the peritoneum, fascial closure and reconstruction of the skin with a circumferential subcuticular purse-string suture. However, this technique, despite being readily accepted, is often associated with a suboptimal cosmetic outcome owing to the lack of a normal looking umbilicus, which is instead characterized by the formation of a flat star-shaped umbilical scar [11] (Fig. 32.13).

Silvia Ceccanti et al. [10] described a simple method to repair a cord hernia with preservation of the umbilical cord elements and to leave it to dry as a stump; in an attempt to improve the cosmetic appearance of the umbilicus, this method is especially effective when the size of the fascial defect is less than 2.5 cm, [10] but the double purse-string technique is easy to apply and produces also a good cosmetic results for neonates with umbilical cord hernias [5] (Fig. 32.13).

32.2 Umbilicus Cutis

Nomenclature: Skin navel and cutaneous umbilicus.

It is another not uncommon anomaly that occurs when the abdominal skin is creeping

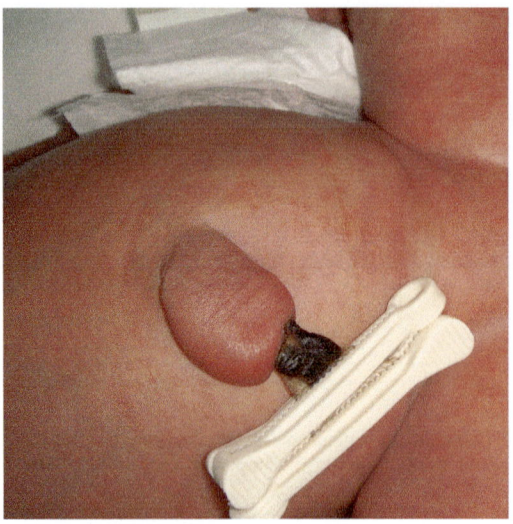

Fig. 32.15 Umbilicus cutis, with a long skin stump replacing the proximal part of the cord

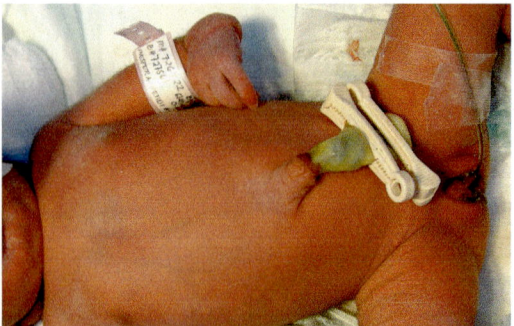

Fig. 32.16 A case of umbilicus cutis in a neonate with an absent radius

over the cord, without any umbilical or cord hernia; it appears in the umbilical region as a projecting cylinder of the skin, about 1–11 cm in length, at the apex of which the umbilical cord, or the wound after stump falling, is found (Fig. 32.15).

Umbilicus cutis is a harmless anomaly; with a subsequent prominent umbilical cicatrix and mamelon, which may be appreciated later on, if such cases followed up at adulthood. Umbilical cutis may be misdiagnosed as an umbilical hernia but is differentiated easily by the lack of fascial defect and by the fact that there is no further protrusion when the infant cries or strains; also umbilical hernia never happens early with the presence of cord stump. At the main time, this case should not interface with proboscoid umbilical hernia (Sect. 28.9).

This anomaly has been explained by assuming that the abdominal skin extends for an abnormally great distance over the cord. However, it is more probable that in a large number of instances, the cutis navel does not arise in this way but rather because of the failure of the physiologic infolding of the free margin of the skin of the cord, which should follow the separation of the cord [12].

Umbilicus cutis may be an isolated anomaly, but commonly it is associated with many syndromes and dysmorphology.

Rieger syndrome (an autosomal dominant disorder of morphogenesis) and Robinow syndrome commonly had such anomaly as an association [13] (Fig. 32.16).

References

1. Power D'A. A case of congenital umbilical hernia. Trans Path Soc London. 1888;xxxix:108.
2. Hempel-Jorgensen P. Familial congenital umbilical hernia. Ugesk f Laeger. 1929;91:273–4.
3. Tow. Diseases of the Newborn. NewYork: Oxford Medical Publication; 1937. p. 224–6.
4. Raju R, Satti M, Lee Q, Vettraino I. Congenital hernia of cord: an often misdiagnosed entity. BMJ Case Rep. 2015 Apr;21:2015. doi:10.1136/bcr-2015-209642.
5. İnce E, Temiz A, Ezer SS, et al. Poorly understood and often miscategorized congenital umbilical cord hernia: an alternative repair method. Hernia. 2016;21(3):449–54. doi:10.1007/s10029-016-1544-0.
6. Mirza B, Ali W. Distinct presentations of hernia of umbilical cord. J Neonatal Surg. 2016;5(4):53. doi:10.21699/jns.v5i4.400.
7. Brantberg A, Blaas HG, Haugen SE, Eik-Nes SH. Characteristics and outcome of 90 cases of fetal omphalocele. Ultrasound Obstet Gynecol. 2005;26:527–37.
8. Pal K, Ashri H, Al Wabari A. Congenital Hernia of the Cord. Indian J Pediatr. 2009;76:310–21.
9. Achiron R, Soriano D, Lipitz S, Mashiach S, Goldman B, Seidman DS. Fetal midgut herniation into the umbilical cord: improved definition of ventral abdominal anomaly with the use of transvaginal sonography. Ultrasound Obstet Gynecol. 1995;6:256–60. doi:10.1046/j.1469-0705.1995.06040256.x.

10. Ceccanti S, Falconi I, Frediani S, Boscarelli A, Musleh L, Cozzi DA. Umbilical cord sparing technique for repair of congenital hernia into the cord and small omphalocele. J Pediatr Surg. 2017;52:192–6.

11. Krummel TM, Sieber WK. Closure of congenital abdominal wall defects with umbilicoplasty. Surg Gynecol Obstet. 1987;165:168–9.

12. Friedman JM. Umbilical dysmorphology. The importance of contemplating the belly button. Clin Genet. 1985;28:343–7.

13. O'Marcaigh AS, Folz LB, Michels VV. Umbilical morphology: Normal values for neonatal periumbilical skin length. Pediatrics. 1992;90:47–9.

Gastroschisis

Definition: Gastroschisis (GS) means 'stomach cleft' which is a congenital defect of the abdominal wall, usually to the right of the umbilical cord insertion, and abdominal contents herniate into the amniotic space, without any covering sac (Fig. 33.1).

Nomenclature: Gastroschisis from Greek terms gastro (belly) and schism (rent or separation); other name is laparoschisis, which is not commonly used.

Historical Background: One such omen is recorded on Babylonian tablet YOS 1056: 'If (at birth) an anomaly's belly is already open and its intestines protrude, that land will experience famine…'. The tablet is one of a series that date to 2000–1600 BCE [1].

Ballantyne in 1904 used the term gastroschisis to refer to all somatic abdominal wall defects with the exception of physiologic hernia of the umbilical cord. "On the right side of the patient close to the insertion of the navel, a longitudinal appendage is visible which runs in a cranial direction. It gets smaller, ends abruptly and reminds of an intestinal segment".

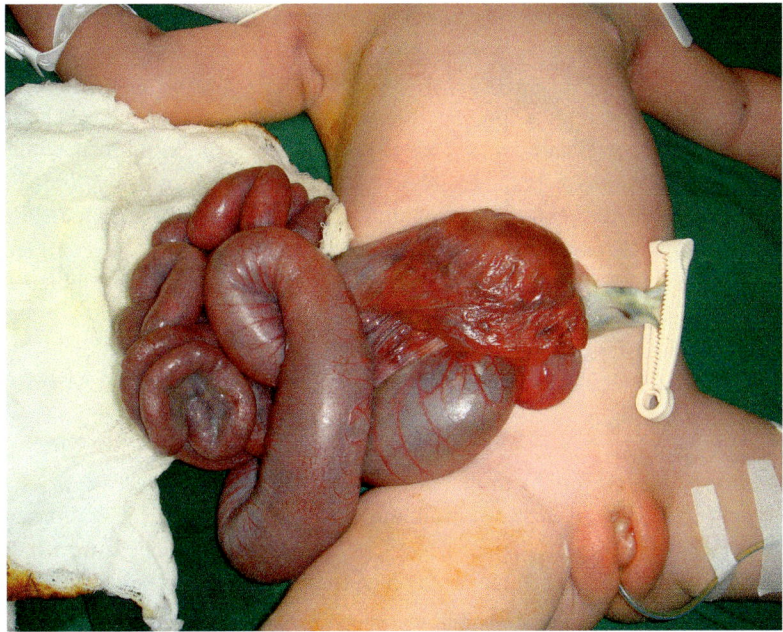

Fig. 33.1 Classical gastroschisis, with a normally looking gut herniated from a small defect at the left side of the cord

© Springer International Publishing AG 2018
M. Fahmy, *Umbilicus and Umbilical Cord*, https://doi.org/10.1007/978-3-319-62383-2_33

However, in 1953 Moore and Stokes [2] were able to find only five instances of gastroschisis evidence that the term had been redefined. They emphasized that gastroschisis was distinct from omphalocele in the absence of a membranous sac and in being an extraumbilical defect, usually to the right of the midline of the abdomen.

Incidence: The incidence of gastroschisis appears to be rising in developed nations; it becomes the most common abdominal wall defect along the last 30 years, epidemiological studies indicating association with young aged mothers, usually nulliparous and smoking. The reported incidence of gastroschisis is variable from 1 in 2.000 to 1 in 10.000 births [3].

There is general agreement that either gastroschisis or omphalocele has a geographic or racial predilection, but some data showed a greater risk for white women between 20 and 24 years of age, especially of Hispanic nationality (OR, 1.5), as well as recent data from some British records that indicate a higher incidence in England, with 2–3 cases for 10,000 births in total [4].

Etiology: The etiology of gastroschisis is not well known. The pathology appears to be a weakness in the body wall around the umbilicus, perhaps caused by defective ingrowth, cellular death or impaired cellular fusion, such that the intestines are extruded through the defective area into the amniotic cavity.

In summarizing the theories about causes of gastroschisis existing at the beginning of the twentieth century, Ballantyne at 1904 [5] included amniotic adhesions or rupture, short umbilical cord, injury to the fetal abdomen, smallness of the abdominal cavity, maternal impressions, twisting or retroversion of the vertebral column, defective development of the allantoic stalk and arrest of closure of the abdominal wall. Of these theories, only the last, arrest of closure of the abdominal wall, has survived. The other theories have largely lost favour and have been replaced in the past half century by those relating to mesodermal deficiency of the body wall and vascular disruptions.

Recent hypotheses have focused on a vascular aberration of umbilical and omphalomesenteric veins, interfering with the development of the somatopleure at the junction with the body stalk or a solution of continuity that is formed later than the development of the abdominal wall [6].

Risk Factors: Many risk factors had been incriminated as a predisposing factor for GS incidence:

- *Mother age*: Mothers under 20 years of age comprised 39% of the gastroschisis cases. There were very few mothers at 40 years or older who give a baby with gastroschisis. The reason for the younger maternal age, associated with GS, is still unknown [7].
- *Family history*: Most cases of GS are sporadic with recurrences and novelty; the risk of recurrence in the offspring is low (3–5%). Most cases (about 95%) are isolated except for related, presumably secondary anomalies of the gastrointestinal or genitourinary systems.
- *Genetics*: No genetic influence is known to play a significant causal role. Similarly, no environmental exposure has been clearly implicated [8].
  Some studies attribute a role to father's age, indicating an increased risk among fathers aged between 20 and 24 years compared to those aged 25–29 years [9].
- *Smoking*: Cocaine, smoking and ephedrine have long been suspects as teratogens for gastroschisis; these chemicals are vasoconstrictors, potentially causing occlusion of fetal abdominal wall arteries, with the defect resulting from inadequate blood supply [10].
- *Drugs*: Cyclooxygenase inhibitors (aspirin and ibuprofen), decongestants, acetaminophen, oral contraceptives and amphetamine had been implicated as a possible etiology [11].

Associated Anomalies: Additional malformations are encountered in patients with omphalocele (66% of the patients) as opposed to gastroschisis (23% of the patients). The overall incidence of malformations associated with gastroschisis was low; the vast majority of the additional malformations were jejunoileal or colonic atresias [12]. Cryptorchidism is reported in around 30% of cases, in some series [11].

Clinically: Classical cases of gastroschisis presented with a small defect at the right of a normal umbilical cord, with ileum, jejunum and part of the proximal colon herniated without any covering membrane (Fig. 33.1). Sometimes stomach and rarely liver may be also herniated; in some occasions the abdominal wall defect compromises the blood supply of the bowel resulting in ischaemia or even gangrene, specially in babies delivered at full term (Fig. 33.2). If surgical intervention, or baby transfer to a specialized delayed a fibrinous membrane start to cover the exposed bowel, which may be twisted and amalgamated in one mass (Fig. 33.3).

Fig. 33.2 Herniated bowel and stomach showing signs of ischaemia

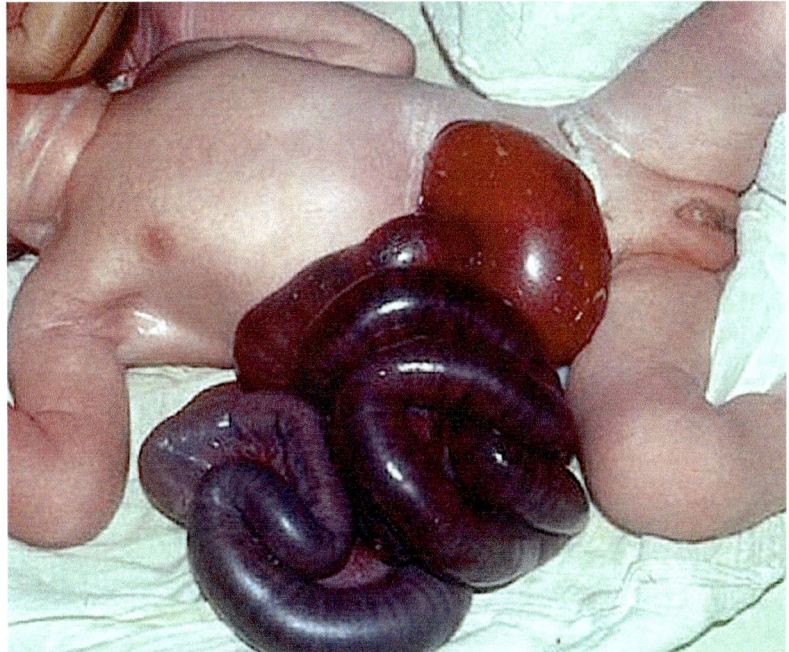

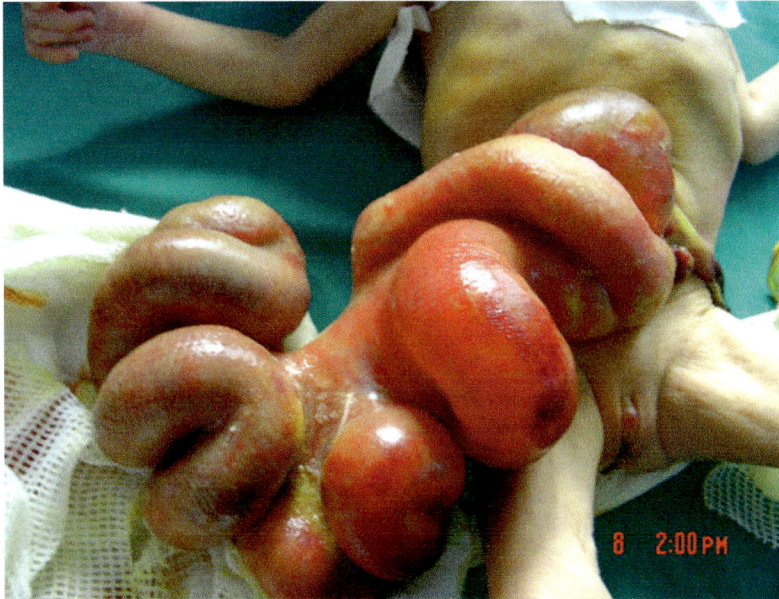

Fig. 33.3 Gastroschisis presented late, with fibrinous peel covering the bowel wall

33.1 Gastroschisis Variants

- Left-sided gastroschisis; few cases had been reported with a defect at the left side of the umbilical cord (Fig. 33.4).
- Vanishing GS, where the extruded bowel becomes ischaemic, gangrenous and subsequently atrophic and partially vanished with a different length of residual remnants (Fig. 33.5), such cases have to be differentiated from umbilical polyp and vitellointestinal duct anomalies (Chaps. 29 and 36).
- Closed GS: Very rarely the abdominal wall defect closes completely antenatally, and the herniated bowel became completely adherent to the skin defect around the umbilicus; in such cases it is extremely difficult to separate the intestine from the encircling skin ring (Figs. 33.6 and 33.7).
- Gastroschisis has been also classified into simple and complex forms. The latter correspond to the cases where there are intestinal atresia, perforation, ischaemia or necrosis and loss of bowel, which occurred in utero.

33.2 Prenatal Diagnosis

Prenatal detection is usually accomplished by the routine obstetrical procedures of midtrimester ultrasound and maternal serum screening. Less commonly, higher-resolution ultrasound performed for other anomalies, intrauterine growth retardation, polyhydramnios or oligohydramnios, may identify gastroschisis (Fig. 33.8).

Maternal serum screening conducted at 16–18 weeks gestation will show elevated alpha-fetoprotein levels; it is an albumin-related protein produced by the fetus, leaks from the exposed fetal bowel vasculature into the amniotic fluid and is transferred to maternal circulation in sufficient levels to be a reliable, but it is a nonspecific marker for gastroschisis. The

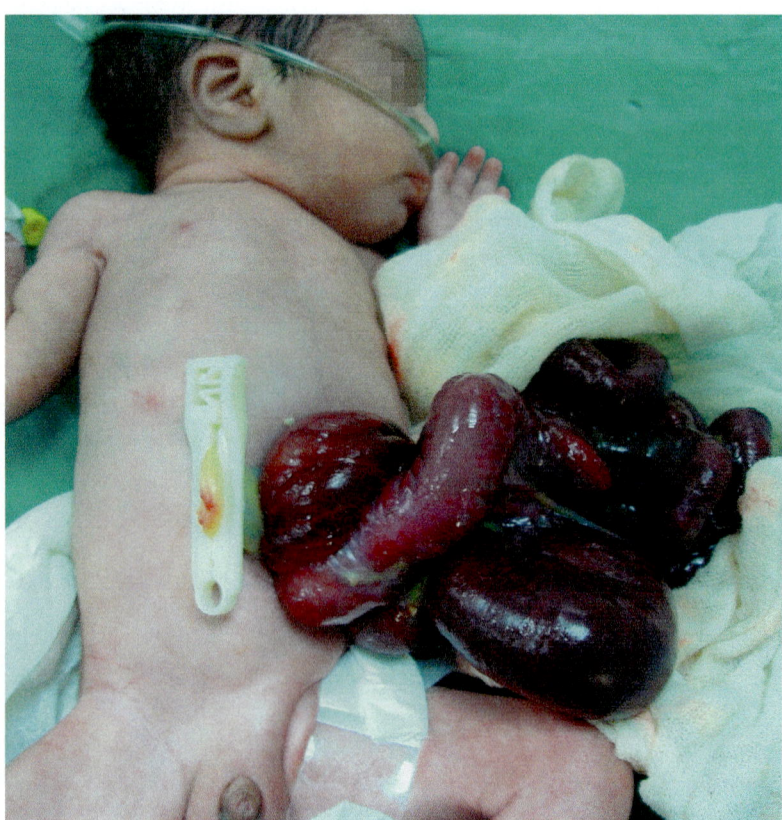

Fig. 33.4 Left-sided gastroschisis, with a defect to the left of the normal umbilical cord

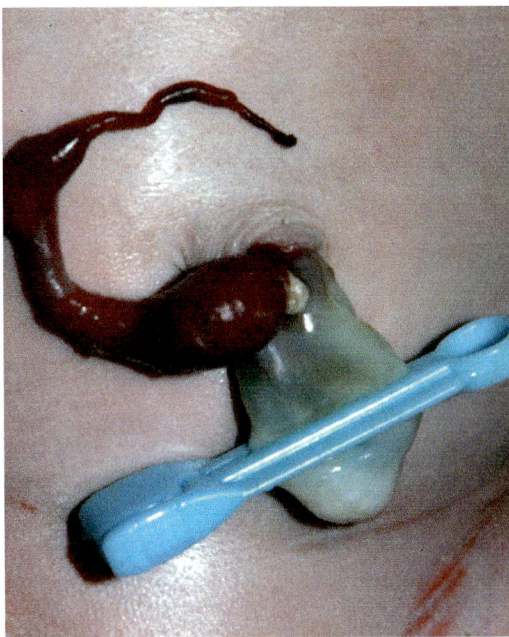

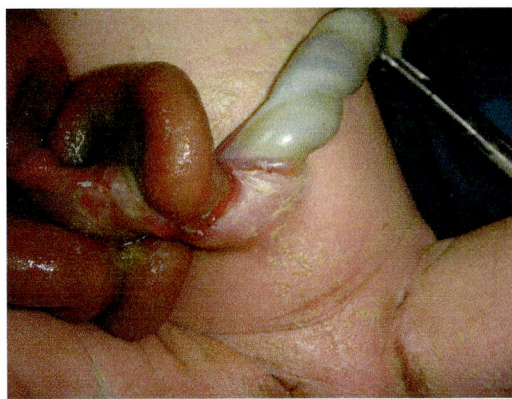

Fig. 33.7 Closed gastroschisis; the skin is completely adherent to the circumference of intestinal wall

Fig. 33.5 Vanishing gastroschisis; the herniated bowel becomes atrophic and represented as a small mucosal cord to the right of the umbilical cord

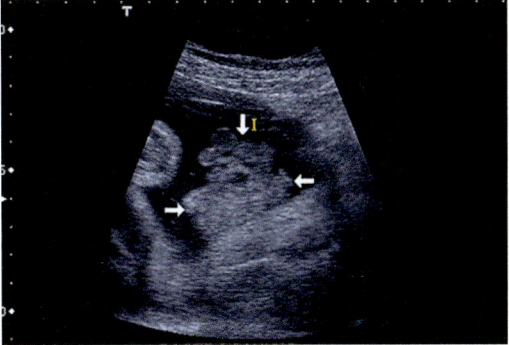

Fig. 33.8 Antenatally detected gastroschisis by US at 17th week; arrows indicate the boundaries of the defect, yellow one pointing to the umbilical cord

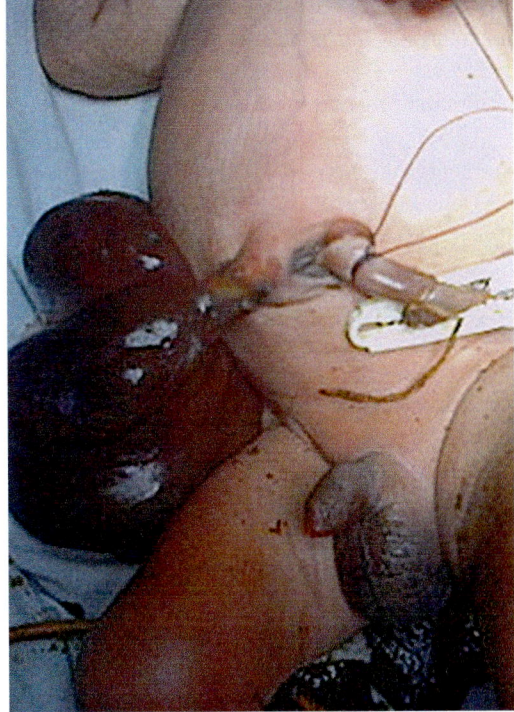

level at 16–18 weeks reaches 5–10 multiples of the usual maternal mean levels for that gestational age [13].

Prenatal detection has increased in recent decades so that the presence of gastroschisis is almost always known prior to delivery. In general, the frequency of prenatal ascertainment of gastroschisis increased from the 50–60% level in the 1980s, to 70–80% in the 1990s and 90–100% in the most recent decade. Early prenatal detection has meant that most affected pregnancies can be closely monitored during the second half of pregnancy and delivered at a tertiary medical centre' where paediatric surgery is available. The result has been a significantly improved survival with reduced morbidity [14].

Fig. 33.6 A case of closed GS with closed facial defect with normal skin and amalgamated bowel to the right of the cord

Among major series published in the past two decades, the average gestational age at delivery was 36.2 weeks, and the average birth weight was 2.4 kg. It is generally thought that intrauterine growth retardation results from nutrient loss through the exposed bowel. Lower levels of blood proteins in infants with gastroschisis support this notion. Salihu et al. [15] have pointed out that lower birth weight and prematurity may reflect low maternal age.

33.3 Complications

Prenatal complications: Bowel distension or perforation, polyhydramnios, oligohydramnios and intrauterine growth retardation are the common complications encountered in the antenatally diagnosed GS during follow-up, considered cases of closed gastroschisis as a parentally complicated case.

Gastrointestinal complications: A baby born with gastroschisis may have malabsorption, because of in utero exposure of the intestine to amniotic fluid, which may cause mucosal or muscularis dysfunction, or the anatomic defect may constrict the mesentery causing ischaemia and diminished intestinal length. In addition, there may be luminal obstruction from adhesions or bands associated with midgut malrotation, which accompanies all the anomalies in which the intestine remains outside the nascent abdominal cavity (Fig. 33.9).

Midgut volvulus, the complication most feared in babies with malrotation, is theoretically possible but unlikely, because of postsurgical adhesions. In addition, children with gastroschisis frequently have gastroesophageal reflux, which usually responds to medical therapy; fundoplication is rarely necessary.

33.4 Outcome

The mortality rate was 12.7% among gastroschisis patients; it is assumed that GS-related mortalities were preventable, or at least a lower mortality rates are feasible [11].

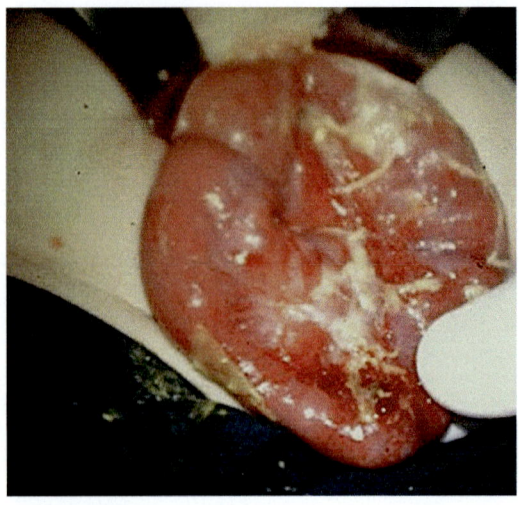

Fig. 33.9 Ileal perforation in an oedematous and matted bowel loop

The mortality of omphalocele relative to gastroschisis is 8:1. Irreversible pulmonary hypertension/right heart failure is the usual terminal condition [16].

Factors adversely influencing the management of babies with gastroschisis are as follows:

Prematurity and low birth weight

Hypothermia (exposure of the intestine to the ambient environment)

Dehydration (gastrointestinal losses, in addition to the above factors)

Sepsis (open wound)

Hypoglycaemia (stress with little metabolic reserve)

In utero growth restriction (protein loss from the extruded intestines)

Oligohydramnios

Fetal distress and birth asphyxia

Injury to the intestines during delivery (tearing or cutting the bowel or mesentery)

Improvements in respiratory care, pharmacology (antibiotics and total parenteral nutrition), anaesthesia and surgery have increased the survival rates for these babies from 60% during the 1960s to more than 90% in more recent years [17].

Certain patients with gastroschisis seem to be more at risk of a complicated course than others. In several outcome analyses, the presence of marked prematurity or intestinal pathology with malrotation, volvulus, infarction, atresia, perforation or stenosis has been recognized as factors associated with adverse outcome (Fig. 33.9).

33.5 Management

Early delivery is often prompted by fetal distress. Ultrasound monitoring after 28 weeks gestation and fetal heart rate monitoring after 32 weeks have been advocated to reduce the risk of intrauterine demise and determine the optimal time of delivery; there are some data to support this approach. A small series using home fetal monitoring was unsuccessful in reducing mortality [18]. Fetal signs that have been found to associate with increased morbidity and mortality include a dilated bowel with an echogenic wall and a dilated stomach. Bowel dilation of 17 mm provides reasonably good specificity, sensitivity and positive predictive value for gastroschisis-associated morbidity [18].

Mode of Delivery: The optimal method of delivery is controversial. Elective caesarean delivery is routinely performed at some medical centres, while a trial of labour is preferred at others. A trial of labour and the presence of ruptured membranes do not appear to increase morbidity or mortality, and there is no evidence that caesarean delivery has benefit. The majority of pregnancies given a trial of labour ultimately result in caesarean delivery because of fetal distress [19].

Bowel Status in Gastroschisis: In gastroschisis, bowel is usually covered with a thick fibrinous peel (Fig. 33.3). Some investigators have explained the appearance of peel on the basis of gestational age, abdominal wall defect and changes of amniotic fluid electrolyte composition with the onset of fetal kidney function. Although amniotic fluid exchange and amnion infusion are among therapeutic and prophylactic strategies to prevent or limit intestinal damage, the concept that amniotic fluid dilution prevents intestinal damage is not widely accepted. In some studies, effects of amnion infusion on intestinal damage of chick embryos were studied, but its feasibility in human is not established [20].

33.6 Surgical Management

Some data did show that neonates receiving immediate closure had a shorter time to reach full enteral feeding and lower incidence of wound infection [21].

Primary closure of the abdominal wall defect is possible only if inflammation of the intestine is minimal. Surgical repair has to be done as soon as possible to prevent the baby from abdominal sequelae. Gastroschisis is associated with a hypoplastic abdominal wall, with a reduced abdominal cavity which could not accommodate the herniated bowel, and closure of the defect may result in an elevation of the diaphragm with increasing ventilator pressure as a consequence, so we routinely put such babies postoperatively in mechanical ventilation for a couple of days (Fig. 33.10).

In some favourable cases, with a roomy abdominal cavity and normal bowel, primary closure is feasible through a small incision around the umbilical stump, which may be sacrificed at the end of surgery, or preserved, to fall off as usual; the baby will end with a near normal umbilicus without any extra scar (Figs. 33.11, 33.12, and 33.13).

If primary closure is not possible, many other options are available:

- Silastic sheets may be used temporarily, and secondary closure performed later.
- Closure of the abdominal wall defect may necessitate a use of silo to contain the eviscerated intestine; the silo should be removed within a week because of the risk of wound infection.
- Goretex patch may be used for staged repair.

Parenteral nutrition is used until the baby passes 'starvation stools.' If this has not occurred within 3–4 weeks, a mechanical

Fig. 33.10 Hypoplastic abdominal wall and reduced abdominal cavity which cannot accommodate the herniated bowel

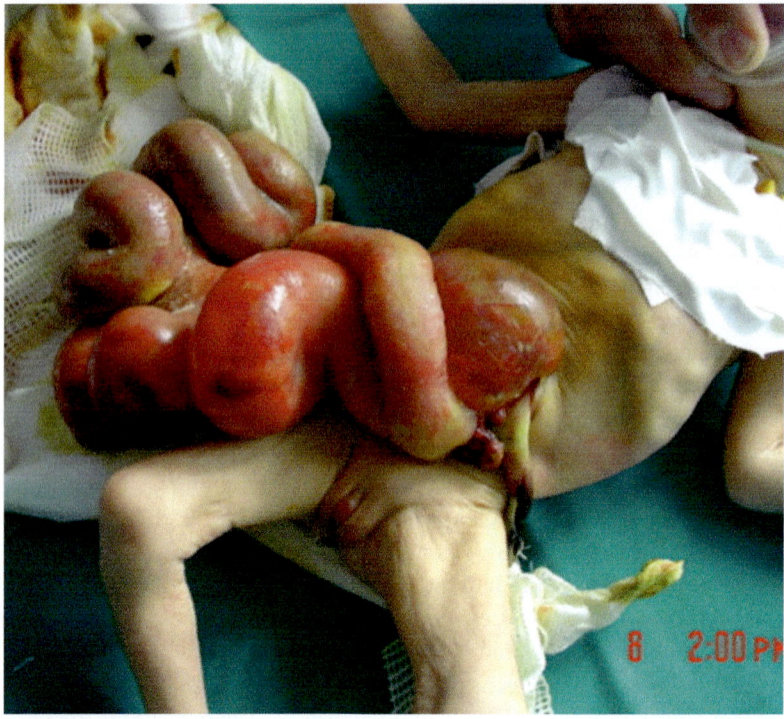

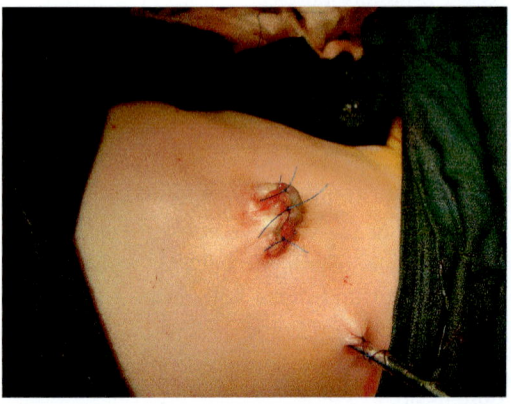

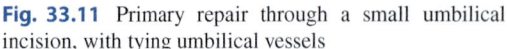

Fig. 33.11 Primary repair through a small umbilical incision, with tying umbilical vessels

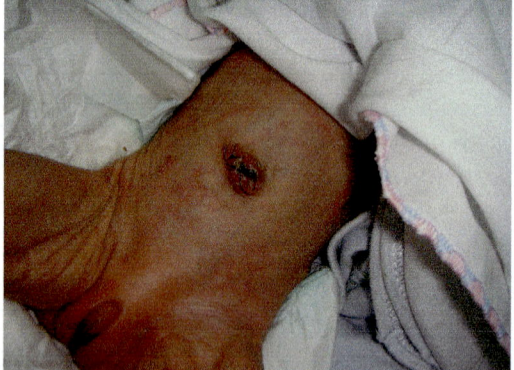

Fig. 33.12 Baby ends with a normal umbilicus without any extra scar

obstruction, rather than an ileus, should be suspected; upper GI/small bowel radiography should be performed to assess the transit of contrast through the intestinal tract. If this study demonstrates an intestinal obstruction, laparotomy is indicated.

Recently, with recognition of the benefit of early surgical intervention, gastroschisis became among surgical anomalies which is amenable for ex utero intrapartum treatment (EXIT); it is a modified caesarean delivery, where the baby is operated immediately, while he is still connected to the mother via the umbilical cord and uninterrupted utero-placental circulation. Such procedure creates a challenge for the obstetric anaesthesiologist who has to manage two anaesthetised patients concurrently. Surgical intervention is performed under general or even local anaesthesia, but general anaesthesia is preferable. The prenatal repair of abdominal wall defect is safe for the mother and the fetus, which could potentially improve the neonatal outcomes [22].

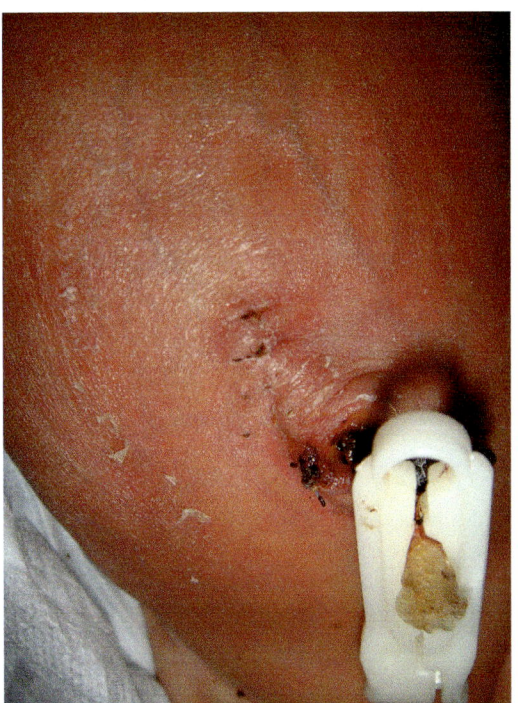

Fig. 33.13 Gastroschisis repair with preserving the umbilical cord

References

1. Leichty E. Texts from cuneiform sources. In: Oppenheim AL, editor. The omen series summa Izbu, vol. IV. Locust Valley: JJ Augustin Publisher; 1970. p. 201.
2. Moore TC, Stokes GE. Gastroschisis: report of two cases treated by a modification of the gross operation for omphalocele. Surgery. 1953;33:142.
3. Eggink BH, Richardson CJ, Malloy MH, Angel CA. Outcome of gastroschisis: a 20-year case review of infants with gastroschisis born in Galveston, Texas. J Pediatr Surg. 2006;41(6):1103–8. [Medline]
4. Insinga V, Lo Verso C, Antona V, Cimador M, Ortolano R, Carta M, La Placa S, Giuffrè M, Corsello G. Perinatal management of gastroschisis. J Pediatr Neonat Individ Med. 2014;3(1):e030113. doi:10.7363/030113
5. Ballantyne JW. Manual of antenatal pathology and hygiene. Edinburgh: The Embryo; 1904.
6. Feldkamp ML, Carey JC, Sadler TW. Development of gastroschisis: review of hypothesis, a novel hypothesis, and implications for research. Am J Med Genet Part A. 2007;143A:639–52.
7. Hwang P-J, Koussef BG. Omphalocele and gastroschisis: an 18-year review study. Genet Med. 2004;6: 232–6. doi:10.1097/01.GIM.0000133919.68912.A3.
8. Mastroiacovo P, Lisi A, et al. Gastroschisis and associated defects: an international study. Am J Med Genet Part A. 2007;143A:660–71.
9. Werler M, Sheehan JE, Mitchell AA. Association of vasoconstrictive exposure with risks of gastroschisis and small intestinal atresia. Epidemiology. 2003;14:349–54.
10. Zamakhshary M, Yanchar NL. Complicated gastroschisis and maternal smoking: a causal association? Pediatr Surg Int. 2007;23(9):841–4. doi:10.1007/s00383-007-1926-6.
11. Jayapal K, et al. Gastroschisis – 10 years study. J Evolution Med Dent Sci. 2016;5(44):2736–41.
12. Mayer T, et al. Gastroschisis and Omphalocele, an eight-year review. Ann Surg. 1980;192(6):783–7.
13. Burc L, Volumenic JL, de Lagasie P, et al. Amniotic fluid inflammatory proteins and digestive compounds profile in fetuses with gastroschisis undergoing amnioexchange. BJOG. 2004;111:292–7.
14. Tibboel D, Vermey-Keers C, Kluck P, et al. The natural history of gastroschisis during fetal life: development of the fibrous coating on the bowel loops. Teratology. 1983;33:267–72.
15. Salihu HM, Emusu D, Aliyu Z, et al. Mode of delivery and neonatal survival of infants with isolated gastroschisis. Obstet Gynecol. 2004;104:678–83.
16. Puligandla PS, Janvier A, Flageole H, et al. Routine cesarean delivery does not improve the outcome of infants with gastroschisis. J Pediatr Surg. 2004;39(5):742–5.
17. Jager LC, Heij HA. Factors determining outcome in gastroschisis: clinical experience over 18 years. Pediatr Surg Int. 2007;23:731–6. doi:10.1007/s00383-007-1960-4.
18. Wilson RD, Johnson MP. Congenital abdominal wall defects: an update. Fetal Diagn Ther. 2004;19: 385–98.
19. Chr V-K, Hartwig NG, van der Werff JFA. Embryonic development of the ventral body wall and its congenital malformations. Semin Pediatr Surg. 1996;5:82–9.
20. Langer J, Longaker MT, Crombleholme TM, et al. Etiology of intestinal damage in gastroschisis. I: effects of amniotic fluid exposure and bowel constriction in a fetal lamb model. J Pediatr Surg. 1989;24:992–7.
21. Baird R, Puliganda P, Skarsgard E, Laberge JM, Canadian Pediatric Surgical Network. Infectious complications in the management of gastroschisis. Pediatr Surg Int. 2012;28:399–404.
22. Dong L, et al. Anesthetic management of a neonate receiving prenatal repair of gastroschisis. Int J Clin Exp Med. 2015;8(5):8234–7.

Examophalos (Omphalocoele)

34

Nomenclature: Exomphalos, omphalocele, also spelled omphalocoele, exomphalos commonly used in British language, but an omphalocele is an American usage.

The word omphalocoele is derived from the Greek words 'omphalos' (Ομφαλός) meaning naval and 'cele', meaning pouch.

Definition: Omphalocoele is a rare congenital, central abdominal wall defect due to failure of normal return of intestines and other contents back to the abdominal cavity during the ninth week of intrauterine development that results in the herniation of the abdominal contents through an umbilical defect with an overlying membrane covering the contents. Characteristically, the origin of the umbilical cord is abnormally large. In the majority of cases, omphalocele is associated with other congenital anomalies of the gastrointestinal tract or cardiovascular system, syndromes or chromosomal aberrations (Fig. 34.1).

Historical background: Lycosthenes Chronicon at 1557 and Ambroise Pare's [1] classic text at 1634 both give a testimony that gastroschisis and omphalocele were known in the sixteenth century. The first reports of successful surgical treatment, which are those of Hey [2] and Hamilton [3]. Scarpa [4] drew attention to the association of exomphalos with other malformations and concluded that the condition was almost always fatal because of them or because the hernia was too large to be reduced. Ahlfeld [5] used alcohol dressings on the sac in a patient successfully treated without operation. Uncertainty and confusion concerning the embryology, clinical presentation and surgical treatment of these anomalies were continued until the past two decades.

34.1 Etiology

Embryological background: The midgut, positioned in umbilical cord, rotates 90° counterclockwise around the superior mesenteric artery. At tenth weeks of gestation, intestines return to the abdomen. The small intestines return first, followed by large intestines, which complete an additional 180° counterclockwise rotation. After the intestines return to the abdomen, they enlarge, lengthen and fuse to the abdominal cavity. The abdominal wall then closes and the body stalk constricts to become umbilical cord. Omphalocele results due to either the developmental arrest of the abdominal wall or failure of the abdominal viscera to return to the abdominal cavity [6].

Incidence: The reported incidence is approximately 1 in 3000 to 1 in 10,000 live births. Omphalocoeles occur more frequently in males than in females, at a ratio of 1.5–3:1 [7].

Predisposing factors:

- Several cases of omphalocele had been reported with advanced maternal age; maternal age > 35 years is a risk factor for some of the trisomies associated with omphalocoele [7].
- Some cases of omphalocele are believed to be due to an underlying genetic disorder, such as Edward's syndrome (trisomy 18) or Patau

© Springer International Publishing AG 2018
M. Fahmy, *Umbilicus and Umbilical Cord*, https://doi.org/10.1007/978-3-319-62383-2_34

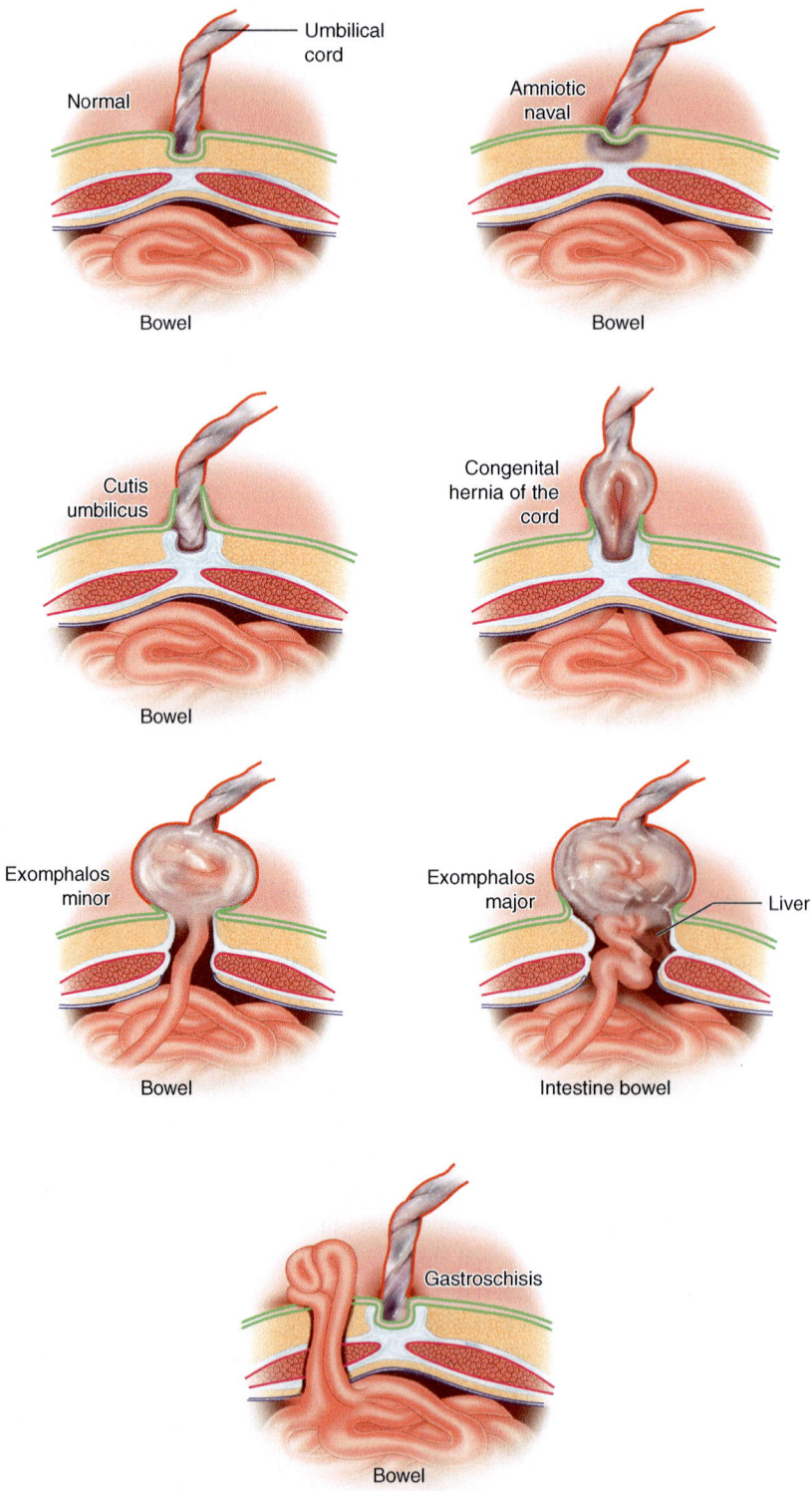

Fig. 34.1 A diagram showing the different forms of all addominal wall defects

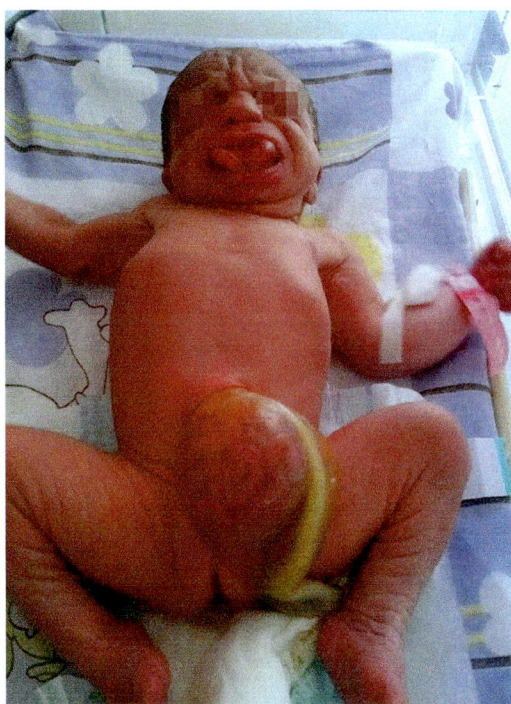

Fig. 34.2 A case of Beckwith–Wiedemann syndrome with exampholas; macroglossia is evident

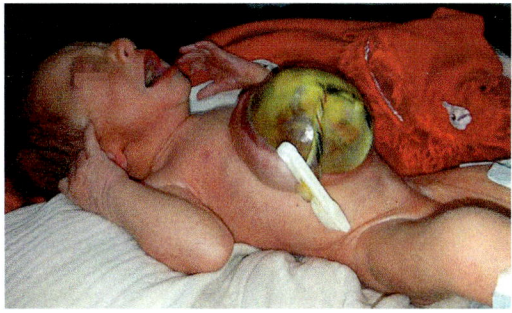

Fig. 34.3 Typical case of exampholas major; abdominal wall defect of 7 cm, covered with a thin membrane, umbilical cord inserted centrally at the dome of the sac and a rim of skin seen at the base

syndrome (trisomy 13). Beckwith–Wiedemann syndrome is also associated with omphalocele (1–114%) (Figs. 34.2 and 34.3).

- Folic acid deficiency, hypoxia and salicylates are implicated in the etiology of exampholas, as proved in experimental animals, but the clinical significance of these experiments is conjectural.
- Intraperitoneal injection of retinols induces omphalocele in 15% of the pregnant Swiss mice [8] (Fig. 34.4).

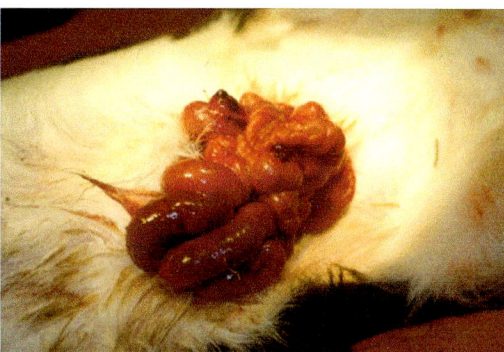

Fig. 34.4 Ruptured exampholas of the Swiss mice after injection of retinols

- The short- and long-term implications of HIV association with omphalocoeles are yet to be determined [9].
- Black infants had a higher incidence of omphalocele than gastroschisis, with gastroschisis, have worse survival outcomes, while those with omphalocele have better chances of survival than their White or Hispanic counterparts [10].

Associated anomalies: Associated anomalies are reported in 30–80% of cases of omphalocele among which cardiac defects are more common. Chromosomal anomalies occur in 49% of cases of omphalocele. Interestingly, multiple associated anomalies appear to be more common in omphalocele minor than omphalocele major (55 vs. 36%). Fifty percent of babies born with omphalocele have genitourinary, brain, lung, spine, heart and gastrointestinal defects [11].

GIT anomalies: The association of the intestinal atresia and omphalocele is not rare; some studies showed that G1T atresia was found in 30%. In a series of 45 infants that had omphalocele of 5 cm, seven had malrotation and volvulus, eight patients had Meckel's diverticulum and one had ileal atresia [10]. Intestinal anomalies are distinctly associated with omphalocele minor. The etiopathogenesis of atresia associated with omphalocele remains elusive. It is hypothesized that the intestinal atresia occurs because of mechanical compression of the intestines at the neck of omphalocele defect or because of the internal volvulus of the prolapsed segment during antenatal period. The small abdominal defect could divide the part of prolapsed gut, thereby causing the atresia. Atresia

Fig. 34.5 Ileal atresia
with exampholas major

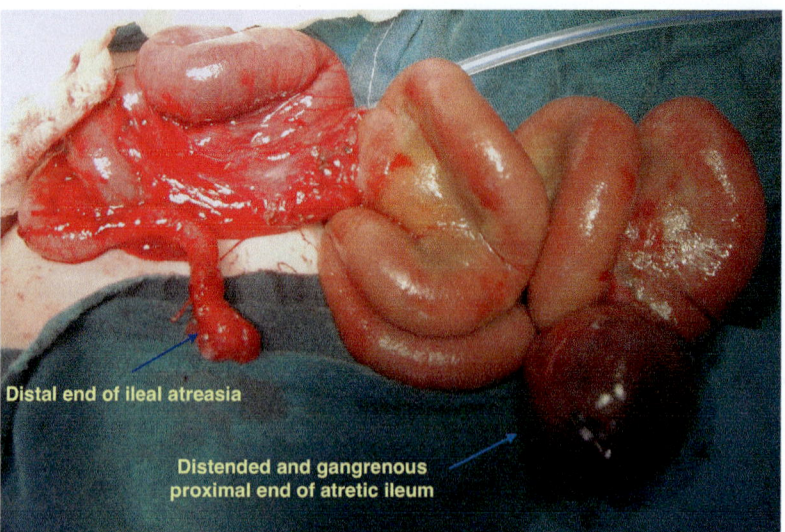

Distal end of ileal atreasia

Distended and gangrenous
proximal end of atretic ileum

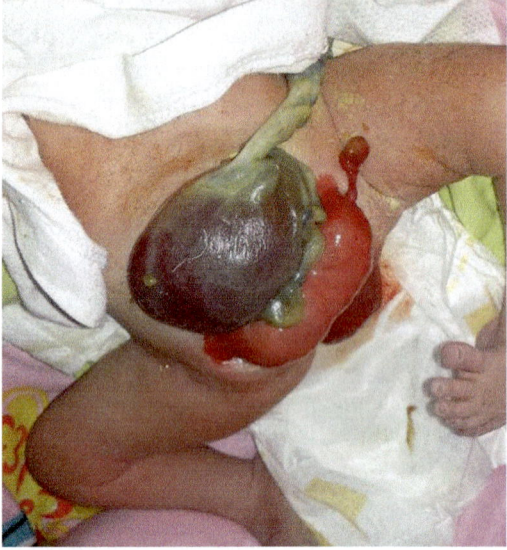

Fig. 34.6 Exampholas at the top of bladder exstrophy

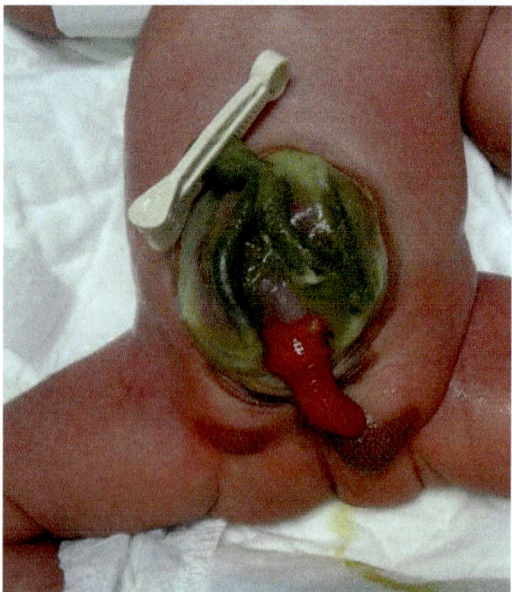

Fig. 34.7 Exampholas with cloacal exstrophy

could also result in such cases because of ischemia
subsequent to the interruption of blood supply at
the reentry point of intestines to the abdominal
cavity. In some patients, the intestinal obstruction was acquired either by the compression of the
neck of the defect or by the adhesions around the
omphalocele [12] (Fig. 34.5).

Bladder and cloacal exstrophy: Seventeen
percent of omphalocele patients had cloacal/
bladder exstrophy. The greatest therapeutic challenge in these children is not the omphalocele per
se but the additional midline, cloacal or bladder
anomalies [13] (Figs. 34.6 and 34.7).

Vesico-intestinal fissure: The term 'vesico-
intestinal fissure' was suggested by Schwalbe [14];
it is a very rare challenging anomaly due to the
lack of separation of the urogenital sinus and the
alimentary canal. In this complex anomaly, there
is an exomphalos which is of little capacity, and
the outer surface of exampholas does not bulge but
retains the contour of the abdomen. A classical case
of the malformation is shown in Fig. 34.8; beneath
the exomphalos, there is an ectopia vesicae with a
central area of ectopic intestinal mucosa; through
these passes, the terminal ileum which is frequently

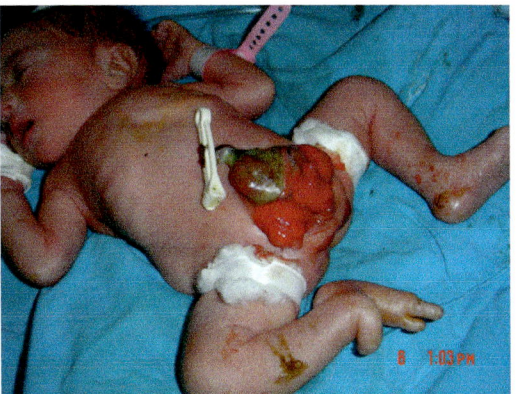

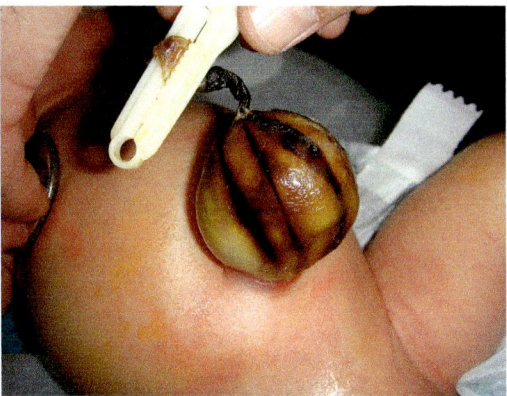

Fig. 34.8 A case of vesico-intestinal fissure; central non-capacious omphalocele, prolapsed terminal ileum, two halves of bladder plates at both sides, a bifid scrotum and imperforate anus

Fig. 34.9 Exampholas minor

prolapsed. Beneath this again, there opens a segment of colon which ends blindly in the pelvis; the anus is imperforate. Bladder mucosa is present on each side of the intestinal area, and the penis (or clitoris) is split and duplicated. Elective abortion is permissible for such cases in many countries, as the survivors are challenging for the paediatric surgeon with a poor outcome (Fig. 34.8).

Syndromes: Omphalocele forms the main pillar of many well-known syndromes:

- Beckwith–Wiedemann syndrome (Fig. 34.2)
- Omphalocoele, exstrophy, imperforate anus, spinal (OEIS) complex
- The pentalogy of Cantrell (full spectrum syndrome consists of a deficiency of the anterior diaphragm, a midline abdominal wall defect, a defect in the pericardium, various congenital intracardiac abnormalities and a defect of the lower sternum.) [15]
- Edward's syndrome (trisomy 18)
- Patau syndrome (trisomy 13)

34.2 Diagnosis

Omphalocoele size (minor vs major): The literature arbitrarily defines a major omphalocoele as >5 cm and containing liver or small bowel and minor as <5 cm. This definition is flawed as it does not consider the size of the baby or the visceroabdominal disproportion. It is, however, the only working definition that helps stratify

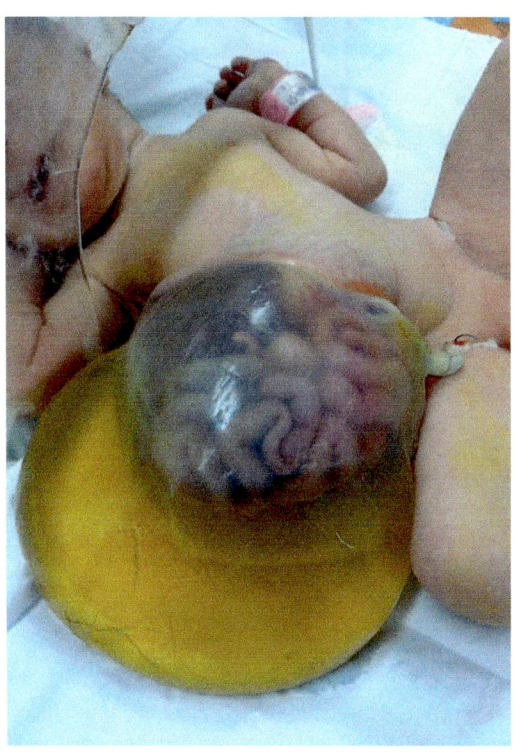

Fig. 34.10 A case of exampholas major with unusual extensive Wharton's jelly at the dome of the sac

omphalocoeles. Groves et al. [16] found that congenital abnormalities were commonly associated with a minor omphalocoele (Fig. 34.9).

Clinically: Omphalocele varies in size from 4 to 12 cm. At birth the sac is a shiny with pellucid membrane formed by a layer of amnion with peritoneum beneath it. Between these is stratum of pale yellow embryonic tissue (Wharton's jelly) of varying thickness and with occasional bulbous excrescences (Fig. 34.10).

Fig. 34.11 Cloudy, yellow exampholas sac, with opaque sticky area due to longer exposure to air without coverage

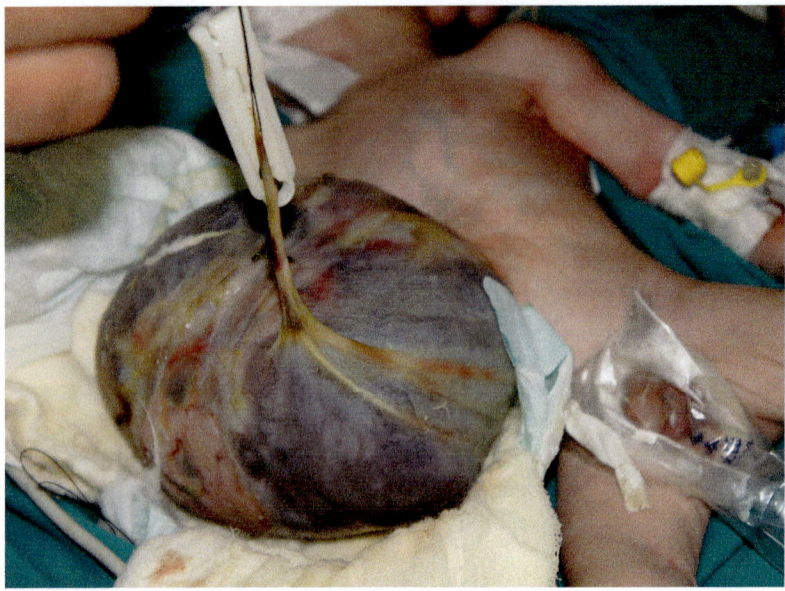

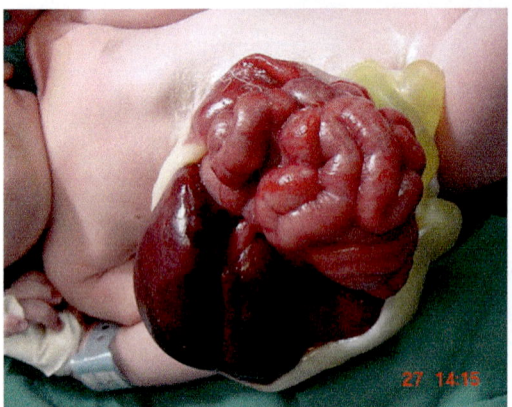

Fig. 34.12 Ruptured exampholas major during vaginal delivery; sac remnants could be appreciated at the periphery

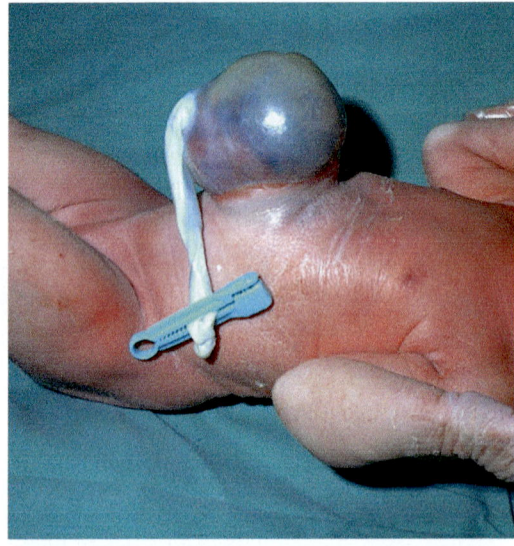

Fig. 34.13 Caudal insertion of the umbilical cord, with a considerable rim of skin at the base of the sac

At the periphery of the sac, there are some blood vessels beneath the peritoneum, but they are apparently inadequate, for death of the sac commences at the moment of birth. Other factors such as the drying effect of contact with the air and perhaps increase in intra-abdominal pressure may contribute to necrosis of the sac, which within 6–12 h, becomes cloudy, yellow and opaque, and the surface becomes granular, sticky and malodorous. With longer exposure, it becomes an inelastic eschar liable to rupture with evisceration (Fig. 34.11).

When rupture occurs before birth, the gut spills into the amniotic cavity, and such cases could be differentiated from gastroschisis by the presence of a smaller defect and an intact cord in the latter. Ruptured sac may occur after birth, specially in cases with a wide defect and major contents, which is not diagnosed antenatally and delivered vaginally (Fig. 34.12).

In contrast to the gastroschisis, not only the intestine but the liver and other organs are herniated and may be eventrated inside the exampholas defect.

The insertion of the umbilical cord is usually located at the centre of the omphalocele sac (Fig. 34.1); in few cases the cord may be located caudal and cephalic or at one side of the sac (usually the right side) (Figs. 34.13 and 34.14), and the connection between the sac and the abdominal may be either narrow or large, but at least it is wider than the defect seen in cases of CHUC. Cases of exampholas minor usually have a thick oedematous cord with an ectopic insertion in the sac (Fig. 34.15). An irregular rim of the skin may be appreciated at the base of omphalocele sac (Fig. 34.16).

Differential diagnosis: If the clinical picture of both malformations (exampholas and gastroschisis) is well known, and a precise and careful clinical evaluation is performed in the individual case, there is no differential diagnosis. Superficially, exampholas cases may be confused with a sternal cleft, a bladder or a cloacal exstrophy (vesicointestinal fissure); in case of a tiny omphalocele,

with a variant of the normal umbilical cord insertion, it should be differentiated from congenital hernia of umbilical cord (CHUC), which would be disastrous for the newborn in case of erroneous cord ligation.

It may be extremely difficult to differentiate some cases of CHUC from exampholas minor, unless the criteria, which we will discuss later on, are applied (Fig. 34.17). In Fig. 34.18 a rare case of ectopia cordis, with sternal and diaphragmatic defect as well as a small umbilical defect, without thorough investigations, such case may be wrongly diagnosed as a simple exampholas minor.

Investigations: Immediately after birth photographs of the clinical findings and additional examinations for evaluation of associated

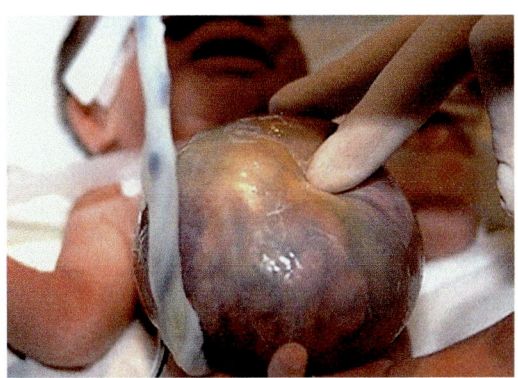

Fig. 34.14 Abnormal cord insertion at the *right side* of the sac, in a case of large exampholas

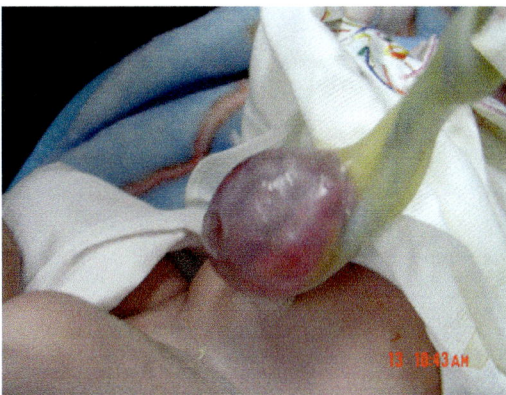

Fig. 34.15 A case of exampholas minor with oedematous thick cord

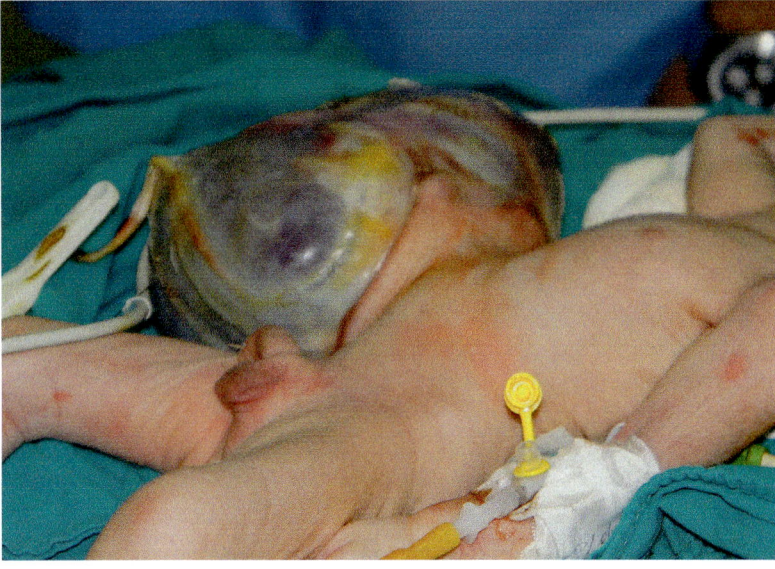

Fig. 34.16 Variable length of skin creeping to the base of the sac

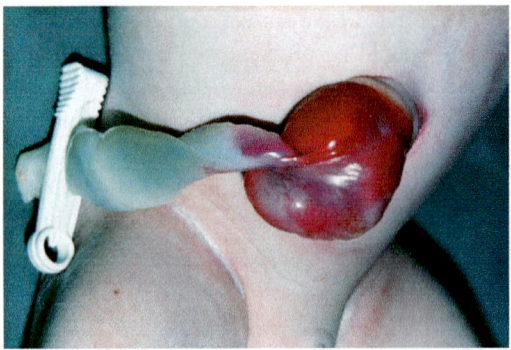

Fig. 34.17 A case of exampholas minor mimic a congenital hernia of the umbilical cord

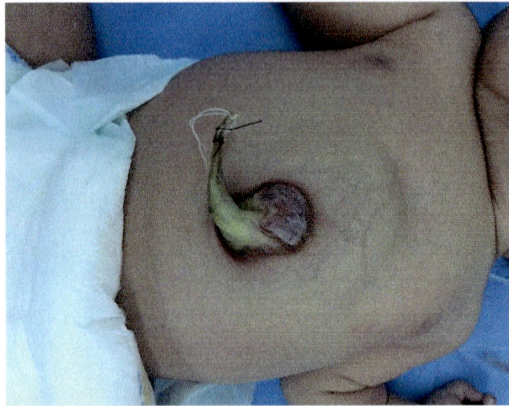

Fig. 34.18 A variant of ectopia cordis; superficial look may give an impression of exampholas minor

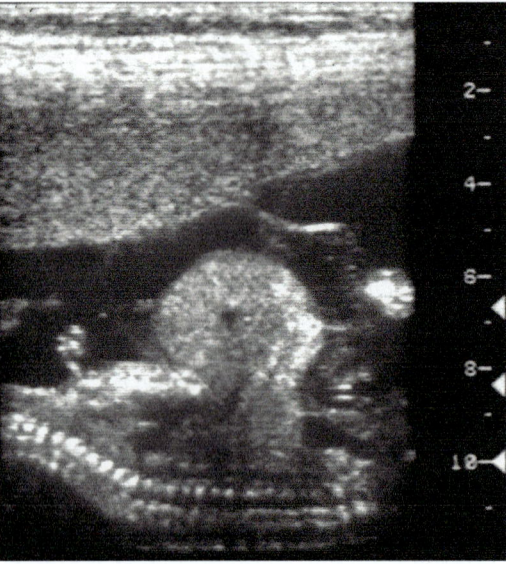

Fig. 34.19 Ultrasound at 14 weeks showing an exampholas with a herniated liver

malformations, cardiovascular and intestinal anomalies should be done. Special care should be paid for suspected cases of Beckwith–Wiedemann syndrome with the inherent danger of hypoglycaemia due to pancreatic islet cell hyperplasia. It is advisable to admit all cases to neonatal intensive care unit for evaluation, specially the premature or small-for-date newborns and cases suspected to have combined intestinal malformations.

Antenatal ultrasound: Prenatal diagnosis may influence timing, mode and location of delivery. Prenatal ultrasound in the second trimester of pregnancy (>12 weeks) and level II fetal ultrasound determine the type of omphalocele with the abdominal organs in the umbilical sac and even whether the sac is ruptured (free-floating bowel or the liver outside of the abdomen) (Fig. 34.19).

Ultrasound findings:

- Multiple bowel loops (and on occasion liver) herniate into a membrane-covered defect (i.e. not free flowing).
- The umbilical cord insertion is directly into the omphalocoele.
- US may also show evidence of polyhydramnios.
- The abdominal circumference may be smaller as a result of bowel herniation.
- An allantoic cyst is often present.

Plain radiograph may be helpful in cases with a suspicion of bowel obstruction or perforation.

CT scan allows direct visualization of herniation content +/− evidence of any malrotation or associated anomalies.

MRI, as with CT, allows better direct visualization; the herniated liver is often of low T2 signal and the bowel of high T2 signal (Fig. 34.20).

Other investigations which may be done for some cases are amniocentic analysis to confirm chromosomal abnormalities, ultrafast fetal MRI for central nervous system anomalies and fetal echocardiogram to confirm heart defects. Elevation of maternal serum alpha-fetoprotein (MSAFP) is associated with omphalocele and gastroschisis. An elevated MSAFP warrants

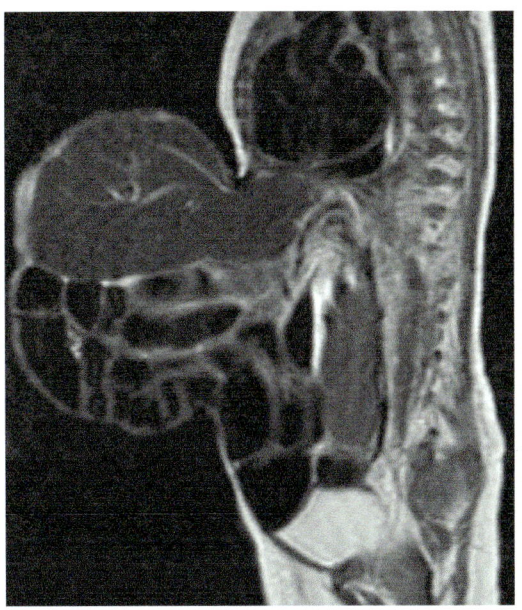

Fig. 34.20 MRI, sagittal T2 of a case of giant omphalocele. 'Case courtesy of A. Prof Frank Gaillard, Radiopaedia.org, rID: 35853'

ultrasonography to determine if structural abnormalities are present in the fetus. If the study is suspicious for an omphalocele, amniocentesis is indicated to determine any associated genetic abnormality.

34.3 Management

Mode of delivery: Delivery of foetuses with antenatally diagnosed abdominal wall defects varies; How et al. [17] report that such cases can be safely delivered by the vaginal route and elective caesarean delivery be opted for obstetric indications. The outcome depends upon the size of the herniation and the presence of defects. In small omphalocoeles primary repair is done by putting the herniated organs back into the abdominal cavity and closing the defect in layers. The survival rate of isolated omphalocoele is as high as 96%, but this drops significantly in the presence of associated abnormalities.

Surgical closure: The size of the omphalocele and abdominal cavity influences the approach to the surgical management. Closure of a small or moderate-sized omphalocele, with

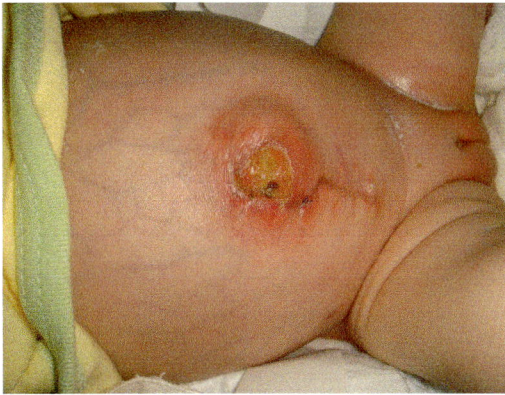

Fig. 34.21 Repair of exampholas with umbilical cord preservation

bowel anomalies, is accomplished without difficulty through a small semicircular incision, with or without cord preservation; this will end with a near-normal umbilical scar (Fig. 34.21).

In giant omphalocele with the liver and other organs, a staged repair (Schuster procedure) is done where a mesh is sewn to the fascia, and the muscle on each side of the omphalocele defect and the two pieces of mesh or silastic sheet are then sewn together over the defect creating a silo and the omphalocele sac remains intact; the mesh/silo is tightened over days or weeks to return the organs into the cavity and mesh is removed and closure done. This process provides time for the abdominal wall to stretch so as to enclose the viscera and promotes lung growth and expansion [18] (Fig. 34.22).

Sometimes the protruding organs may prevent closure when a technique called 'paint and wait' is employed, where the sac covering the omphalocele is painted with an antibiotic cream or other antiseptic solutions and covered with elastic gauze. This promotes epithelialization. This provides extra length and mobility by separating the fascia and muscles, but there is a possibility of a hernia or defect that may develop at the site of repair (Fig. 34.23).

Conservative: If primary reduction is not possible because of high intragastric pressure (>16 mmHg) or inability to reduce the bowel, a spring-loaded silo is indicated. The cord is wrapped in Vaseline gauze and kept moist, while the silo is in place in preparation for use after the

Fig. 34.22 Schuster procedure; silo sutured in the abdominal wall defect

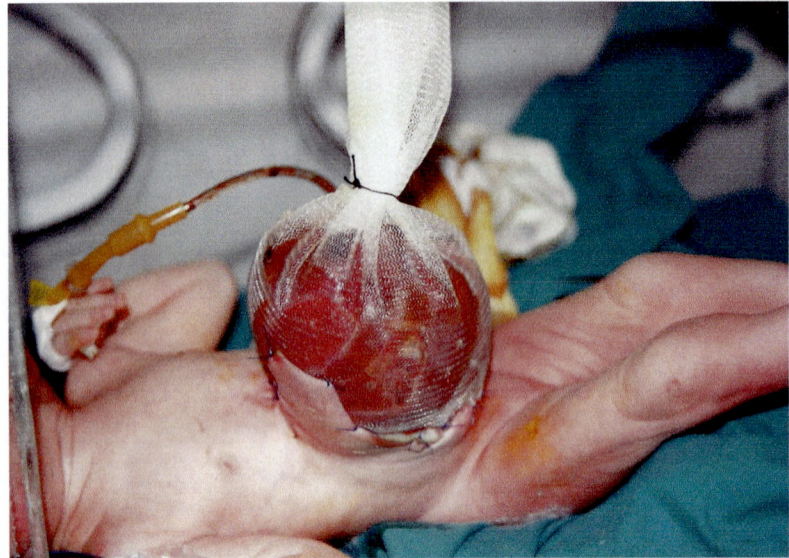

Fig. 34.23 'Paint and wait'; the exampholas wrapped with a sterile towel and painted daily with bovoiodine

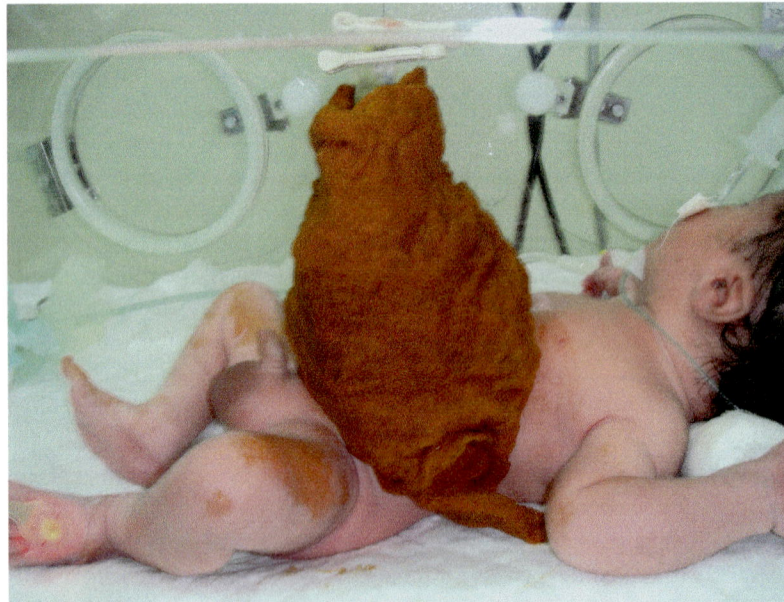

silo is removed. Cord traction is helpful to reduce some herniated contents, while the baby is waiting for surgery (Fig. 34.24).

After daily progressive reduction of the bowel, the silo is removed when it no longer maintains its intra-abdominal position or when the intestine is completely reduced. The remaining defect is then allowed to close spontaneously. The opening is initially reinforced with Tegaderm, and if the umbilical cord remains viable, it also is included as the biologic dressing, held in position by the Tegaderm dressing. Dry dressings are substituted for the plastic dressing once the bowel is fixed in the abdominal cavity, and granulation tissue starts to cover the open defect. Percutaneous intravenous catheters are placed for parental nutrition [19].

Conservative management or even surgical repair of large exampholas usually ended with a ventral hernia [20], which could be repaired later on, with an acceptable outcome, either with or without using a mesh (Figs. 34.25 and 34.26).

Fig. 34.24 Cord traction in incubator

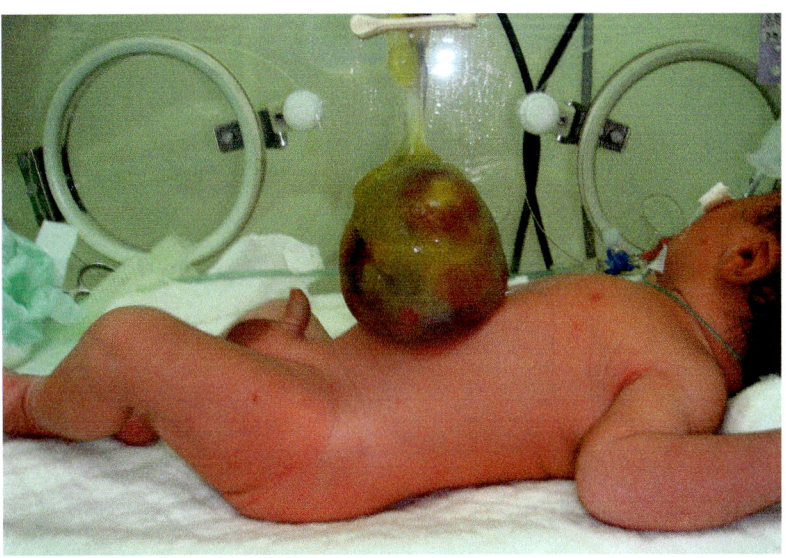

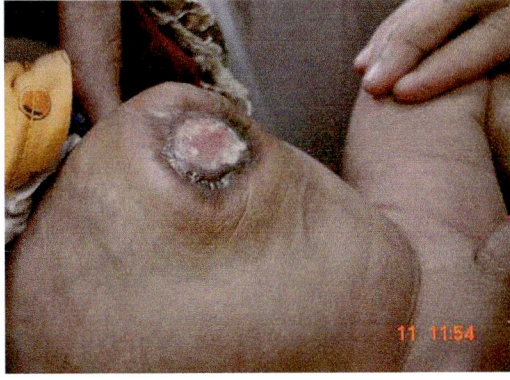

Fig. 34.25 Residual ventral hernia with granulation tissue after conservative management of a large exampholas

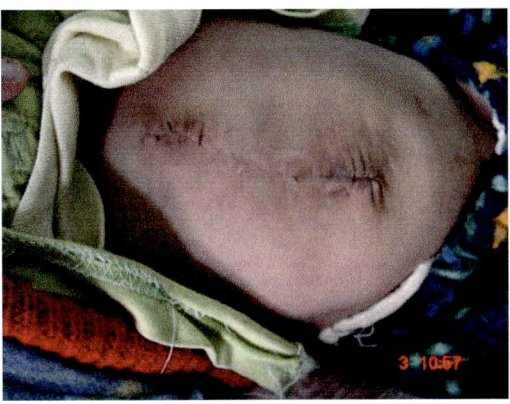

Fig. 34.26 Late repair of the residual ventral hernia, with an acceptable outcome

References

1. Pare A. The works of that famous Chirurgeon. London: Th. Cotes and R. Young; 1634. p. 59. Book 24.
2. Hey W. Practical observations in surgery. London: Cadell and Davies; 1803. p. 226.
3. Hamilton J. In Cooper, A. (1807). The anatomy and surgical treatment of Crural and umbilical hernia, part 2. London: Longman; 1806. p. 56.
4. Scarpa A. Traite pratique des Hernies. Paris: Gabon; 1812.
5. Ahifeld F. Der Alkohol bei der Behandlung inoperabeler Bauchbriiche. Mschr Geburtsh Gynak. 1899;10:124.
6. Dillon PW, Cilley RE. Newborn surgical emergencies. Gastrointestinal anomalies, abdominal wall defects. Pediatr Clin N Am. 1993;40:1289–314.
7. McNair C, Hawes J, Urquhart H. Caring for the newborn with an omphalocoele. Neonatal Netw. 2006;25(5):319–32. doi:10.1891/0730-0832.25.5.319.
8. Quemelo PRV, et al. Teratogenic effect of retinoic acid in swiss mice. Acta Cir Bras. 2007;22(6):451.
9. Singh S, Madaree A. Omphalocoeles: A decade in review. S Afr J Child Health. 2016;10(4):211–4. doi:10.7196/SAJCH.2016.v10i4.1149.
10. Salihu HM, et al. Omphalocele and Gastroschisis: black-white disparity in infant survival. Birth Defects Res A. 2004;70:586–91.
11. Van Eijck FC, Hoogeveen YL, van Weel C, Rieu PN, Wijnen RM. Minor and giant omphalocele: long-term outcomes and quality of life. J Pediatr Surg. 2009;44:1355–9.
12. Hamid R, Mufti G, Wani SA, Ali I, Bhat NA, et al. Importance of the early management of omphalocele minor. J Neonatal Biol. 2015;4:169. doi:10.4172/2167-0897.1000169.

13. Mayer T, et al. Gastroschisis and omphalocele, an eight-year review. Ann Surg. 1980;192(6):783–7.
14. Schwalbe E. Die Morphologie der Missbildungen des Menschen und der Tiere. Jena: Fischer; 1909.
15. Cantrell JR, Haller JA, Ravitch MM. A syndrome of congenital defects involving the abdominal wall, sternum, diaphragm, pericardium, and heart. Surg Gynecol Obstet. 1958;107(5):602–14.
16. Groves R, Sunderajan L, Khan AR, et al. Congenital anomalies are commonly associated with exomphalos minor. J Pediatr Surg. 41(2):358–61. doi:10.1016/j.jpedsurg.2005.11.013.
17. How HY, Harris BJ, Pietrantoni M, Evans JC, Dutton S, Khoury J, et al. Is vaginal delivery preferable to elective cesarean delivery in fetuses with a known ventral wall defect? Am J Obstet Gynecol. 2000;182(6):1527–34. doi:10.1067/mob.2000.106852.
18. Hamid R, Mufti G, Wani SA, Ali I, Bhat NA, et al. Importance of the early Management of Omphalocele Minor. J Neonatal Biol. 2015;4:169. doi:10.4172/2167-0897.1000169.
19. Cohen-Overbeek TE, Tong WH, Hatzmann TR, et al. Omphalocele: comparison of outcome following prenatal or postnatal diagnosis. Ultrasound Obstet Gynecol. 2010;36(6):687–92. doi:10.1002/uog.7698.
20. Wakhlu A, Wakhlu AK. The management of exomphalos. J Pediatr Surg. 2000;35:73–6.

Urachal Anomalies

35

Nomenclature: Detailed definition of vesicourachal abnormalities helps surgeons to determine the extent of surgery and makes important contribution to the success of surgical outcome.

There are a lot of confusion between allantois and urachus in literatures and textbooks, and there is no landmark between both; many descriptions are given for allantois, and it actually means urachus. This could be related to the fact that in literature, observations have been extrapolated to the human from many different species including mice, rats and other animals, so many questions rise in this regard, which will be answered at the conclusion:

Is allantois another name given to urachus?

Is allantois developed into urachus?

Does allantois persist as the urachus does and form pathological features?

Allantois (noun): 'a-lan'tō-is' [Gr. allas, a sausage] n. It is a membranous sac-like appendage for effecting oxygenation in the embryos of mammals, birds and reptiles.—adjs. Allantō'ic, Allan'toid.

It is a vascular fetal membrane that lies below the chorion and develops from the hindgut in many embryonic higher vertebrates (reptiles, birds and mammals) (Fig. 35.1).

So allantois is an extraembryonic membrane of reptiles, birds and mammals arising as a pouch, or sac, from the hindgut. In reptiles and birds, it expands greatly between two other membranes, the amnion and chorion, to serve as a temporary respiratory organ, while its cavity stores fetal excretions. In mammals other than marsupials, the allantois is intimately associated with the chorion, contributing blood vessels to that structure as it forms in conjunction with the endometrium, or mucosal lining, of the uterus (Fig. 35.2).

In human the allantois forms at postconceptional day 16, as a small diverticulum from the lower wall of fetal yolk sac that eventually becomes the primitive hindgut (the cloaca), so allantois becomes contiguous to the cloaca. The cloaca then divides into the hindgut posteriorly and the urogenital sinus anteriorly. The allantois remains connected to the urogenital sinus and extends into the base of the umbilical cord. The umbilical cord is formed from the fusion of the body stalk (containing the allantois) and the umbilical vessels and yolk stalk (containing the omphalomesenteric duct) [1] (Fig. 35.3).

So allantois disappears after formation of the proper umbilical cord at the sixth week and replaced by urachus, most of the recorded anomalies related to the urachus and not the allantois, and should be defined as urachal and not allantoic anomalies; few cases of allantoic cyst were reported early in pregnancy before urachal formation.

© Springer International Publishing AG 2018
M. Fahmy, *Umbilicus and Umbilical Cord*, https://doi.org/10.1007/978-3-319-62383-2_35

Fig. 35.1 Allantois in continuity to the hindgut; it is embedded in body stalk before formation of umbilical cord

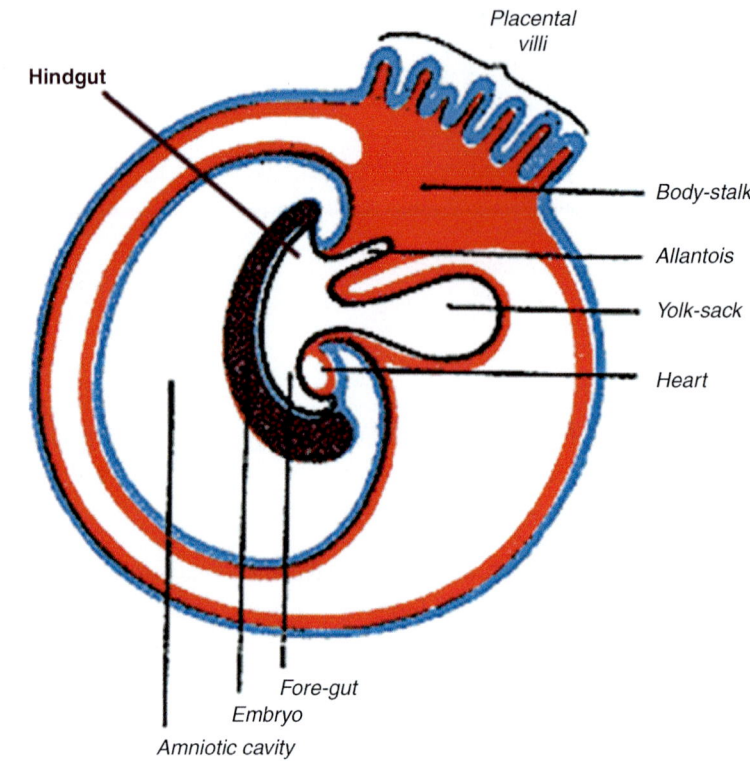

Fig. 35.2 Allantois in continuity with hindgut at the cloaca stage. *al* allantois, *fg* foregut

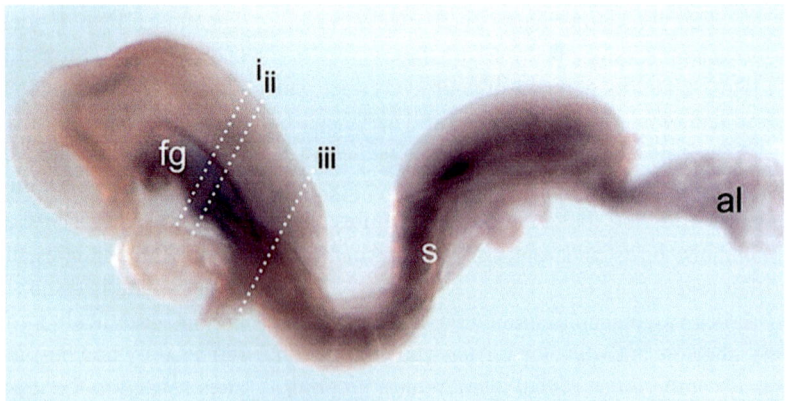

Urachus: 'ū′ra-kus' [Gr. ourachos—ouron, urine]

The urachus is a fibrous remnant of the allantois, a canal that drains the urinary bladder of the fetus that joins and runs within the umbilical cord. This fibrous remnant lies in the space of Retzius, between the transversalis fascia anteriorly and the peritoneum posteriorly. The urachus is an embryonic remnant of the allantois [2].

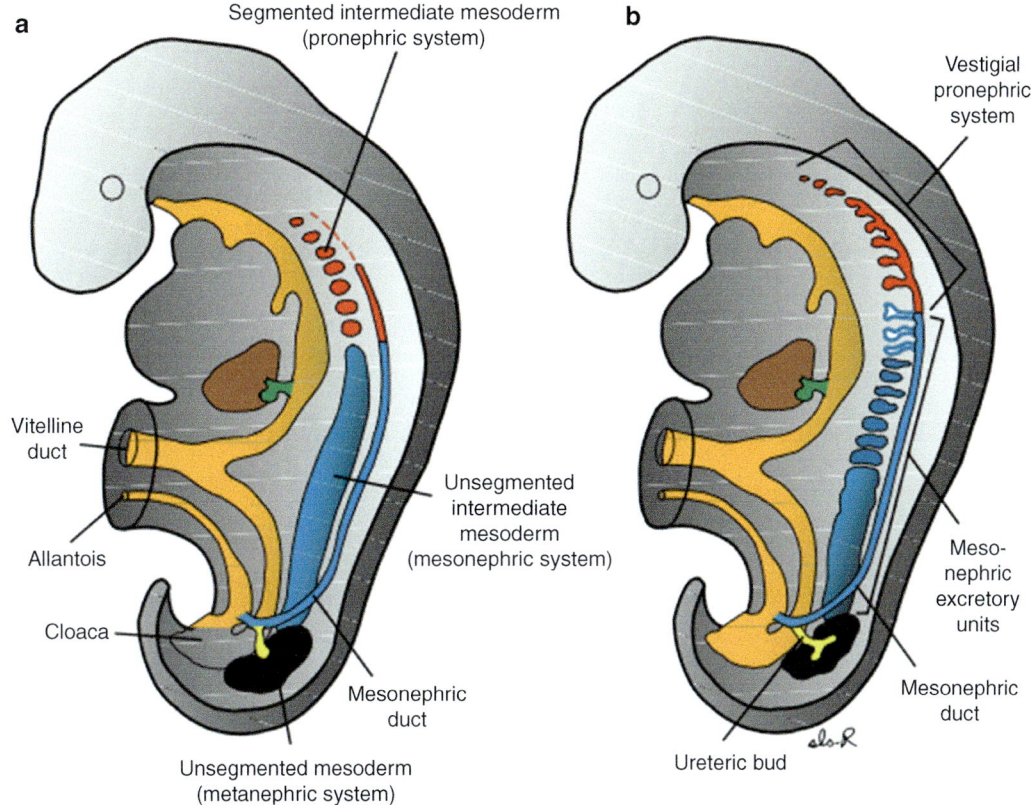

Fig. 35.3 (**a**) Relationship of the intermediate mesoderm of the pronephric, mesonephric and metanephric systems. (**b**) Excretory tubules of the pronephric and mesonephric systems in a 5-week-old embryo

35.1 Embryology of Urachus

A basic knowledge of urachal development is necessary to suspect and diagnose urachal disease; also understanding of the embryonic development of the urachus is mandatory for the radiologist to diagnose the wide variety of urachal anomalies.

Embryologically the allantois develops on about the 16th day of life as a diverticulum of the yolk sac, and it is invaginated later on into the umbilical cord to become a urachus in humans. With the division of the cloaca, the allantois loses its hindgut connection but remains connected to the urogenital sinus through a narrow and elongated tube called urachus which extends from the apex of the bladder to the umbilical ring (Fig. 35.4).

Therefore, anatomically allantois is the extra-abdominal, and urachus is the intra-abdominal component of common allantoic–urachus–vesical communication. Allantoic–urachal lumen undergoes obliteration by around 6 weeks of gestation, and umbilical cord differentiation is completed at approximately 10 weeks.

Failure of this obliteration may result in different types of urachal remnants, e.g. complete patency or vesicoumbilical fistula, vesicourachal diverticulum, urachal sinus and urachal cyst (Fig. 35.5a–d).

However, persistence of allantoic structures has been rarely encountered. There have been reports of antenatally detected cysts of umbilical cord in the first and second trimester presenting postnatally as patent urachus only without the evidence of any cystic structures.

Fig. 35.4 (1) Urachus,
(2) posterior wall,
(3) ureteral orifice,
(4) bladder neck,
(5) prostate, (6) trigone,
(7) anterior wall,
(8) lateral wall and
(9) dome

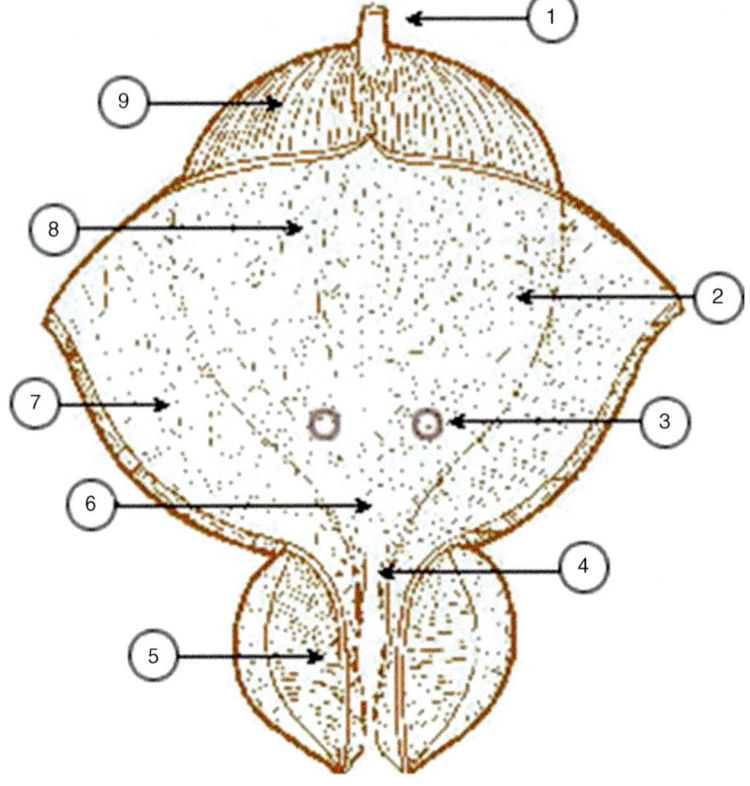

These disappearing vesico-allantoic cysts observed on prenatal ultrasound have been poorly understood. Subvesical pseudo-obstruction and rupture of allantoic wall have been postulated as the etiology [3].

When the fetal bladder descends from the umbilicus into the pelvis around the fourth or fifth month of gestation, the urachus stretches and progressively narrows to an epithelialized fibromuscular tubular structure, the urachus, which progressively obliterates by fibrous proliferation and remains as a fibrous band lying in the pyramidal, retropubic, preperitoneal perivesical space between the transverse fascia and the parietal peritoneum. Its length varies from 3 to 10 cm and from 8 to 10 mm in diameter.

In adulthood, the urachus is formed by a fibrous band that measures from 5 cm to 10 cm in length and from 8 to 10 mm in diameter, also known as the median umbilical ligament, which extends upward the anterior dome of the bladder towards the umbilicus.

35.2 Ontogenetic and Structural Study of the Urachus

At higher gestational ages, the urachal lumen area was smaller. In 13th WPC (weeks postconception) fetuses, the urachal lumen area was 16,301 μm^2, and in 17th WPC fetuses, the urachal lumen area was 1676 μm^2. The urachal lumen was closed from the 17th WPC in all fetuses [4].

Histologically, it is composed of three layers: an innermost layer of modified transitional epithelium similar to urothelium, surrounded by a submucosal connective tissue layer, a middle fibroconnective tissue layer and an outer layer of smooth muscle continuous with the detrusor. Lumen lined by a transitional epithelium is seen commonly in the fully developed infant. Occasionally, the urachus may merge with one or both of the obliterated umbilical arteries, and there may be a slight deviation to the right or left of the midline.

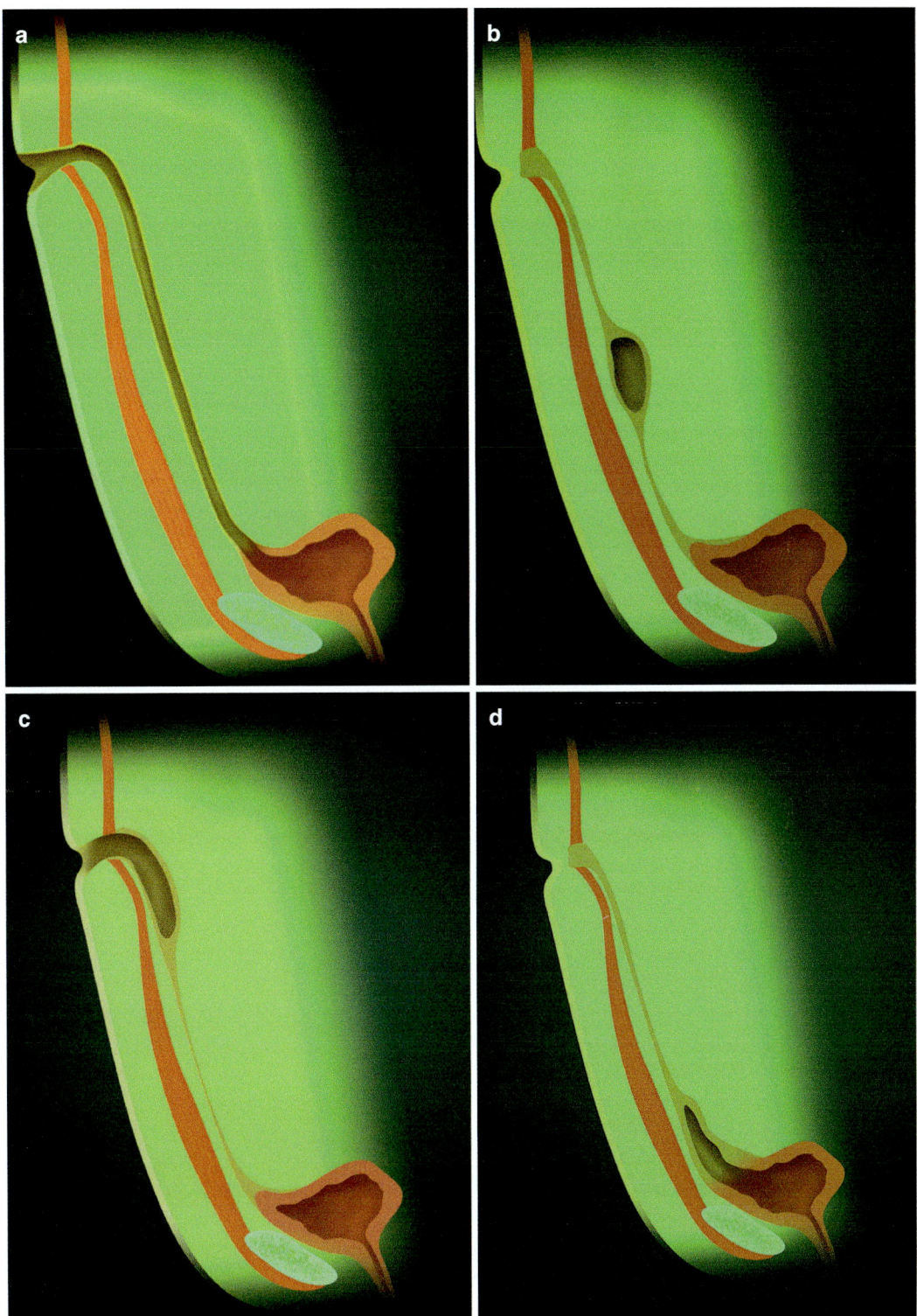

Fig. 35.5 Common urachal anomalies; (**a**) Patent urachus. (**b**) Urachal cyst. (**c**) Urachal sinus. (**d**) Urachal diverticulum

Three portions of the urogenital sinus can be distinguished: The upper and largest part is the urinary bladder (Fig. 35.3). Initially the bladder is continuous with the allantois, but when the lumen of the allantois isobliterated, a thick fibrous cord, the urachus, remains and connects the apex of the bladder with the umbilicus. In the adult, it is known as the median umbilical ligament. The next part is a rather narrow canal, the pelvic part of the urogenital sinus, which in the male gives rise to the prostatic and membranous parts of the urethra. The last part is the phallic part of the urogenital sinus. It is flattened from side to side, and as the genital tubercle grows, this part of the sinus will be pulled ventrally.

When the lumen of the intraembryonic portion of the urachus persists, a urachal fistula may cause urine to drain from the umbilicus (Fig. 35.5a). If only a local area of the urachus persists, secretory activity of its lining results in a cystic dilation, a urachal cyst (Fig. 35.5b). When the lumen in the upper part persists, it forms a urachal sinus; this sinus is usually not connected to the urinary bladder (Fig. 35.5c). It lies in the space of Retzius, extending between behind the transversalis fascia and anterior to the parietal peritoneum, and is bordered laterally by the obliterated umbilical arteries (medial umbilical ligaments); persistence of the most distal part of the urachus, with complete obliteration of the proximal part, will result in different sizes of bladder diverticulum which may be manifested in cases of obstructive uropathy (Fig. 35.5d).

35.3   Patent Urachus (PU)

During the late second and early third trimester, when the bladder has descended into the pelvis, the urachus progressively narrows and obliterates, even though, a microscopic lumen may continue to communicate with the bladder in up to a third of adults. A pathological patent urachus occurs because of failure of the entire tubular urachus to close, leaving an open epithelialized channel between the bladder and the umbilicus. It accounts for approximately 50% of congenital

urachal anomalies [5]. Patent urachus usually presents in the neonate with urine leaking from the umbilicus.

35.3.1 Historical Background

The first report of patent urachus was attributed to Bartholomaeus Cabrolius in 1550; Begg [6] was able to collect 58 cases from the literature in a review at 1927, and Bilchert and Nielsen [7] found another 92 reports from 1927 to 1971. PU is sometimes seen in animals like horses and cattle as an extra-urine stream from the umbilicus (Fig. 35.6).

35.3.2 Incidence

Patent urachus is the commonest type of urachal remnant anomaly; it accounts for approximately 50% of congenital urachal anomalies, but there are some reports of 15% clinically important urachal anomalies that have an incidence of 2 in 300,000 births [8].

In a paediatric autopsy studies, incidences of 1 in 7610 cases for patent urachus have been documented [5]. Urachal anomalies are found in 1.6% of children less than 15 years of age and in 0.063% of adults. There may be a slight male gender, with a ratio of 1.2:1–2:1 in paediatric and adult patients, respectively, but rates vary among series given the low numbers reported [9].

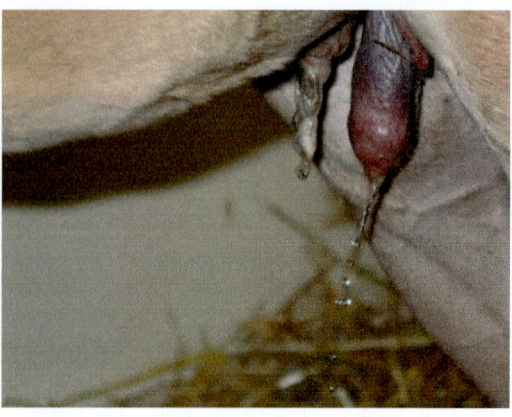

Fig. 35.6 A horse with a PU leaking urine

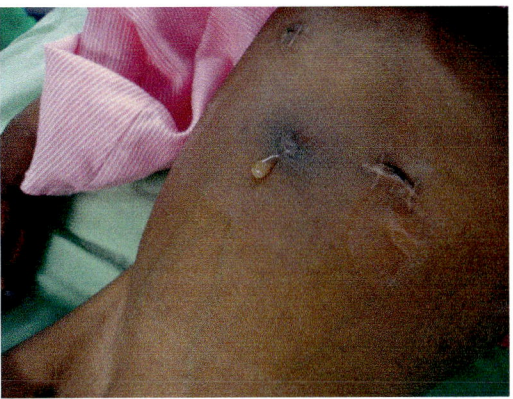

Fig. 35.7 PU leaking urine in a 12 years girl with a progressive obstructive uropathy

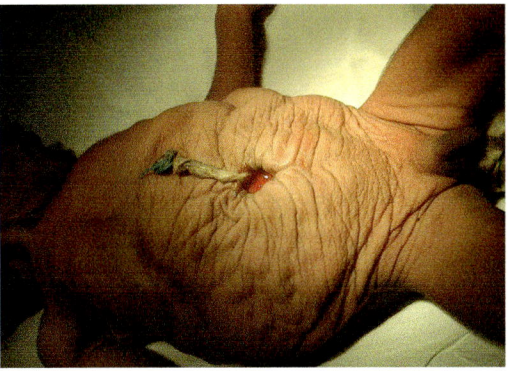

Fig. 35.8 PU with prune belly syndrome, mucosal lining of the urachus seen distal to umbilical cord

35.3.3 Pathogenesis

PU may be presented obviously in a newborn due to failure of its natural closure, but a dormant open urachus may be presented late in adulthood and will be only manifested in cases of bladder outlet obstruction (Fig. 35.7). Obstructing lesions at the bladder neck, urethra or prostate can lead to a reopening of the once-closed urachal canal, causing what is considered as an acquired patent urachus; also this has been noted in infants with the 'prune belly syndrome' as well as adult patients with bladder outlet obstruction; such cases are usually not infected and not usually associated with malignancy, and therefore, whether a given urachal abnormality is congenital or acquired depends on the existence and timing of contributing factors.

35.3.4 Patent Urachus and Fetal Obstructive Uropathy

Most urachal anomalies (e.g. patent urachus, urachal cyst, urachal sinus and urachal diverticula) seem to result from delayed closure of the urachus, which may also arise from lower urinary tract obstruction at less than 12 weeks of gestation.

General mesodermal failure as in cases of prune belly syndrome (PBS) may be associated with PU or urachal diverticulum in 25–50% of the cases; mesodermal defect theory implies that a noxious event to the mesoderm prevents normal development of the abdominal muscles and urinary tract muscles [10]; however, the exact mechanism of PBS is still not known; some researchers considering an early obstructive uropathy is merely responsible for both the characteristic defective abdominal musculature and PU which is associating this syndrome [11] (Fig. 35.8).

Bladder outlet obstruction caused by the urethral obstruction of posterior urethral valves or urethral hypoplasia may be detected from 4 weeks of gestation concurrent with the absorption of the mesonephric duct and the resorption of the urogenital membrane. Congenital urethral developmental anomalies may present early with features of congenital obstructive uropathy or later with voiding dysfunction; these include urethral hypoplasia, urethral agenesis, urethral valves, syringocele and urethral duplications [12]. It is hypothesized that the increased pressure within the urinary tract kept the urachus patent, this allowing the fetus to empty his bladder and protect him from the usual complications of PUV. This emphasizes the importance of detection and characterization of umbilical cord cysts on antenatal ultrasound examination and suggests that obstructive uropathies should be included in the differential diagnosis of umbilical cord cyst communicating with the fetal bladder. [13]

Normal ovine fetal urinary tract function and drainage depend on urachal function and the timing of urachal closure. Therefore, fetal hydronephrosis is associated with this alteration in bladder function, but it may also be associated with other factors, such as bladder sphincter maturation or prostate development. Experiment done to show that premature urachal closure and its role in induction of hydronephrosis in ovine proves that hydroureteronephrosis develops in ovine fetuses when all bladder drainage occurs only via the urethra, without the sharing of urachus. This condition may be an amplification of the differences in bladder outlet resistance in human fetuses, which may explain the male predominance in the various forms of hydroureteronephrosis [14].

Patent urachus frequently coexists with PUVs in about one-third of cases; the increased incidence of vesicoureteric reflux (VUR) in cases of urachal anomalies (UA) had also been reported, but the combination of these three entities has been reported occasionally; VUR was demonstrated in 14 of the 22 children (64%) with UA [15] (Fig. 35.9).

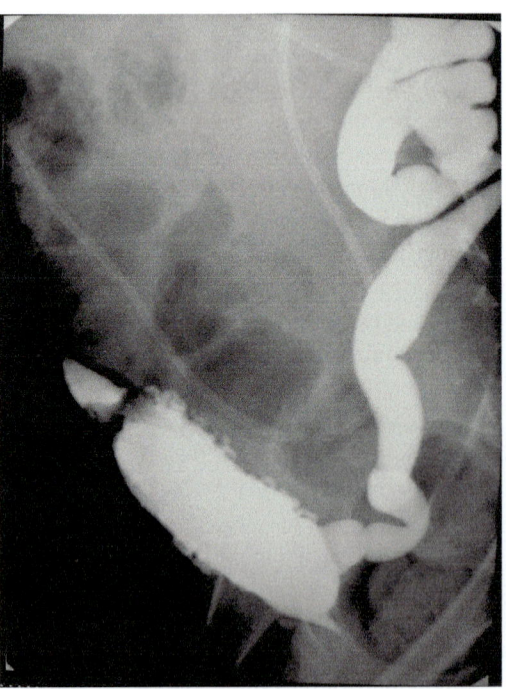

Fig. 35.9 A case of combined PU, PUV and significant VUR

Urethral tubularization occurs after the urachal lumen obliterates during fetal development. Subsequently, it suggests that infravesical obstruction has little influence on urachal development [16]. This could explain why urachus is not patent in all cases of PUV and other cases of obstructive uropathy.

It seems that for the urachus to be patent, several factors are required:

- Defective obliteration of the wall, as a part of general mesodermal failure, as in cases of prune belly syndrome.
- Early lower urinary obstruction before urachal closure at 12th week of gestation, which will result in PU in a neonate.
- Late obstructive uropathy with an incompletely closed urachus will result in late or adulthood PU.

Associated Anomalies: Associated anomalies were reported in 46% of children presenting with urachal anomalies, including omphalocele, omphalomesenteric remnant, meningomyelocele, unilateral kidney, hydronephrosis and vaginal atresia. Careful fetal evaluation to rule out associated anomalies is indicated when patent urachus is diagnosed in utero. Different rare cases of ureteral and bladder neck obstruction may be linked with PU; it can also be associated wisth omphalocele and umbilical cord anomalies, mainly cysts (Chap. 14). Prune belly syndrome is associated with different spectrum of urachal anomalies (Fig. 35.8). Few cases of PU had been reported with different variants of bladder and cloacal exstrophy.

I had an interesting case of PU associated with one moiety of bladder duplication (anterior small one) (Fig. 35.10).

Symptoms: Patent urachus may be diagnosed antenatally, in neonates, at childhood or late at older age; it may remain asymptomatic but usually presents with urine leaking from the umbilicus during the neonatal period, and other variable presentations could be a diagnostic challenge. When cord separation is delayed in healthy infants with no local or systemic infections, an important diagnostic consideration is a urachal anomaly [17].

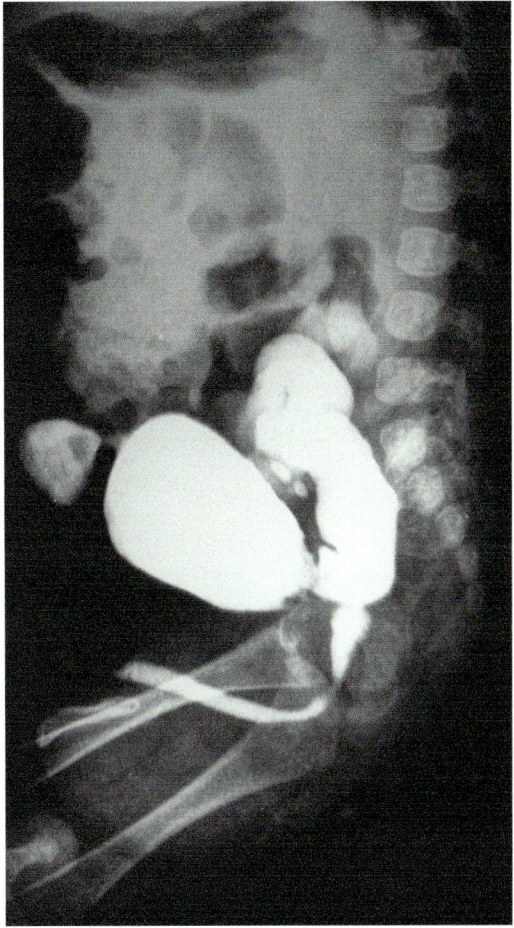

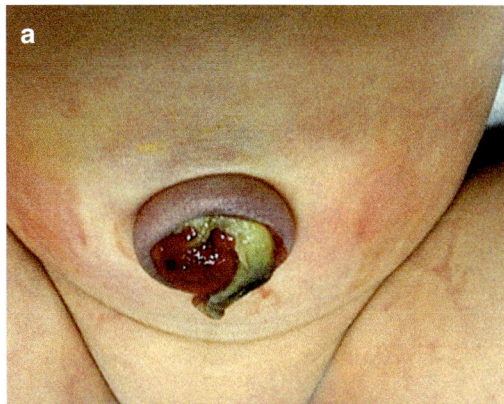

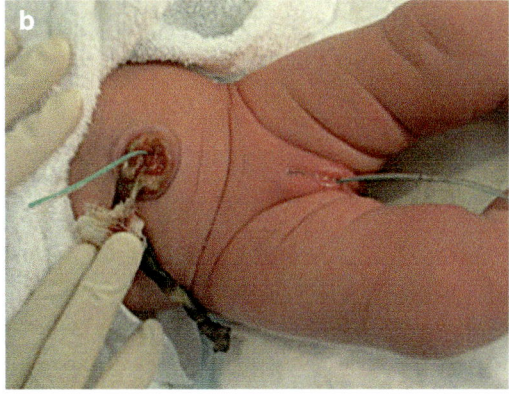

Fig. 35.11 Abnormal umbilical swelling in a neonate girl, mimic granuloma or polyp (**a**), with urine leaking, and when a fine catheter passed, it passed directly to the urethra (**b**)

Fig. 35.10 PU with bladder duplication (the anterior moiety)

Symptoms of a patent urachal anomaly include umbilical discharge, abnormal umbilical swelling, local infection, lower abdominal pain and urinary tract infection [17].

The abnormal or atypical appearance of the umbilicus may be a sign of urachal anomalies; presence of any opening or minute tract at the summit of umbilical stump is highly suspicious for the presence of PU, especially if there is some clear discharge appreciated at the umbilical stump (Figs. 35.11 and 35.12). Such presentation may be similar to cases of vitellointestinal anomalies (Chap. 36). Very rarely the bladder wall may be prolapsed through a widely patent urachus, with its characteristic mucosa, giving a false impression of an omphalocele (Fig. 35.13).

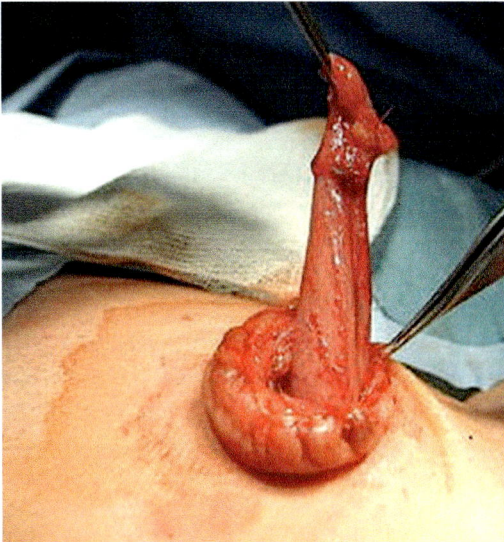

Fig. 35.12 The same patient in Fig. 35.11 during surgery, with a wide patent urachus

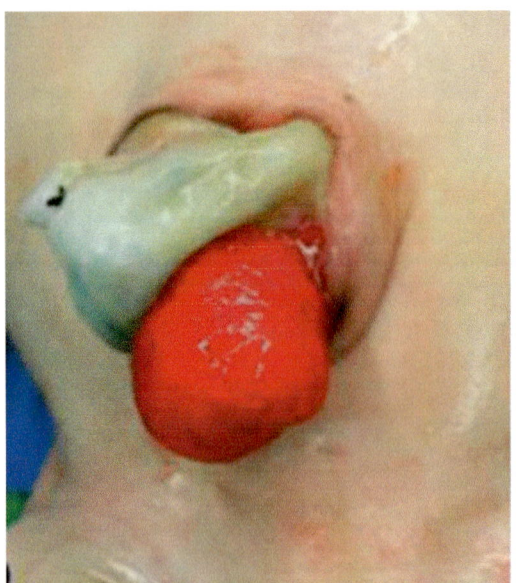

Fig. 35.13 Urinary bladder prolapsed through a patent urachus

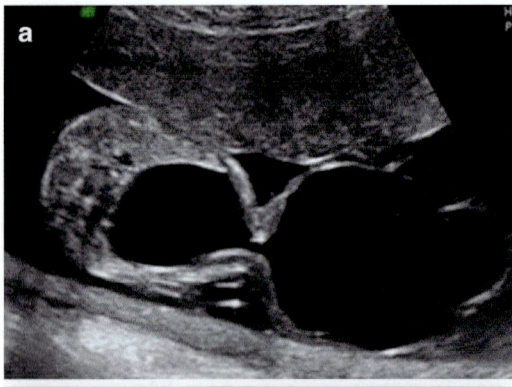

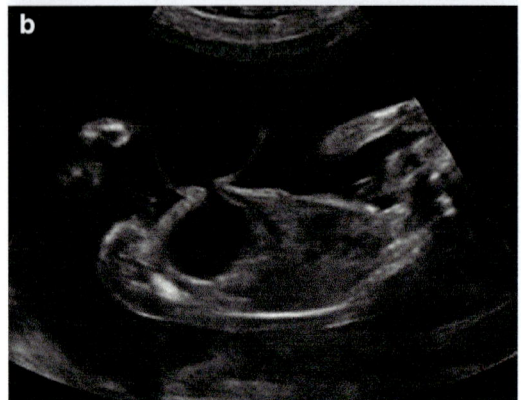

Fig. 35.14 Ultrasonography at 14 gestational weeks demonstrates a cystic formation, corresponding with the bladder in transverse (**a**) and sagittal plane (**b**)

Antenatal Diagnosis: The most common sonographic finding is the presence of a cystic mass located in the base of the umbilical cord, communicating with the bladder and flanked by the umbilical arteries. Moreover, a reduction in size (or even disappearance) of the mass over the course of pregnancy is also a feature of this pathology [18]. Differential diagnoses include omphalocele, bladder exstrophy, persistent omphalomesenteric duct and umbilical oedema.

It was considered that the overflow of urine from urachal remnants to omphalomesenteric remnants caused the extraordinary oedema of the umbilical matrix, and finding of progressive umbilical cord oedema may indicate a patent urachus with a coexisting allantoic and omphalomesenteric remnants. Enlargement of the umbilical cord observed initially at 28 weeks' gestation is an indication of presence of PU. The efficiency in prenatal diagnosis of 3D and 4D ultrasound examinations could help paediatrician surgeons to explain to a couple about neonatal surgical repair and plastic reconstruction in the prenatal period (Fig. 35.14). SonoAVC (sonography-based automated volume count) is a new software tool, which can help in early diagnosis of patent urachus (Fig. 35.15).

Investigations: Ultrasonography has been described as an excellent modality for evaluation of the urachus and has been recommended as the initial imaging tool in urachal diagnostics, either antenatally or postnatally. Furthermore, US results depend on the examiner who needs expertise in US technique and knowledge of the anatomy of the urachal remnant.

The diagnosis can be confirmed with a contrast study, usually an MCUG, or by the introduction of contrast into the umbilical end of the tract, or cannulation of any visible tract at the vicinity of the suspected umbilical swelling (Fig. 35.16); however many authors may not recommend

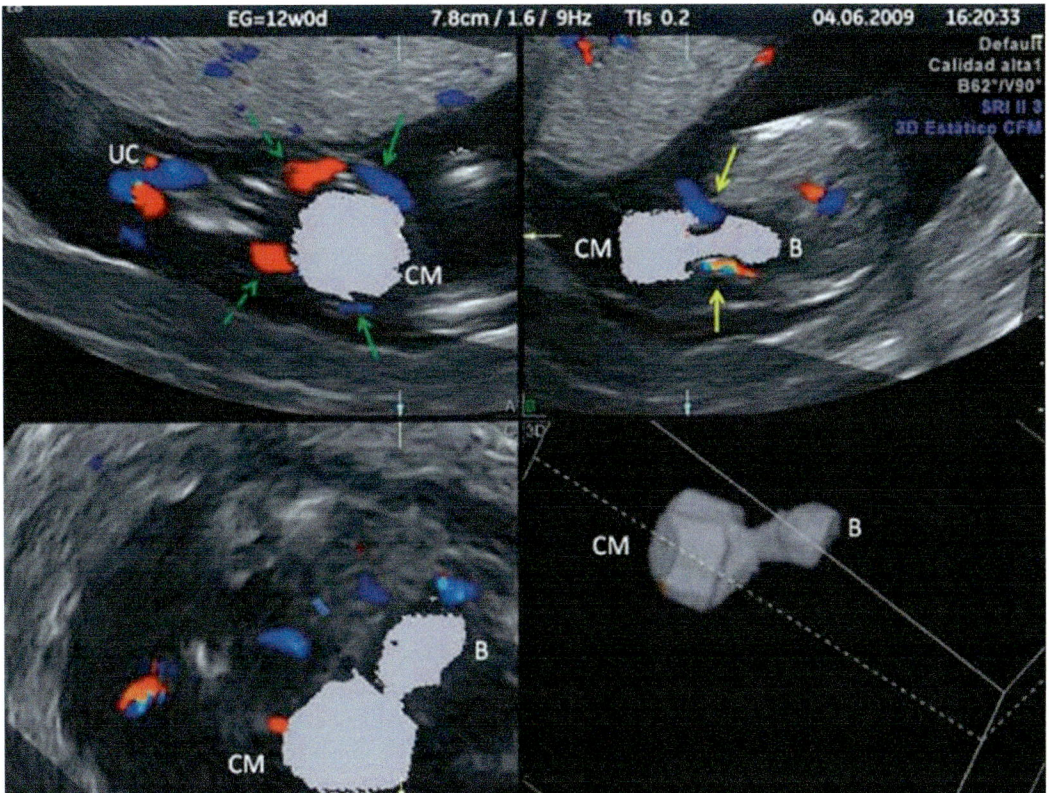

Fig. 35.15 SonoAVC with 3D Doppler ultrasound showing umbilical arteries running around the bladder (B), passing through the abdominal wall defect (*yellow arrows*) and surrounding laterally the cystic mass (CM) (*solid green arrows*) to end in the umbilical cord (*dashed green arrows*). *UC* umbilical cord vessels

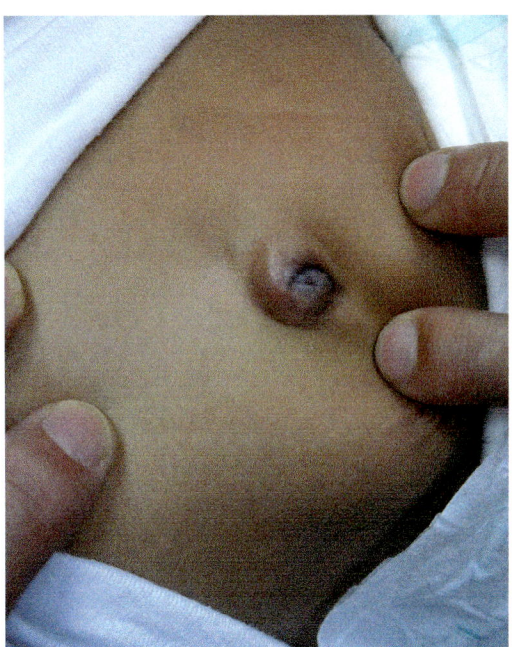

Fig. 35.16 Abnormal umbilicus with a minute opening as an indication of PU

using contrast studies in such cases as they consider it invasive and inconvenient to the child [19], but in my opinion, contrast study is helpful for detection of any associated obstructive uropathy as well as other rare urinary anomalies which may associate PU (Figs. 35.9 and 35.10).

Computed tomography (CT) and magnetic resonance urography (MRU) are ideally suited for demonstrating urachal remnant diseases in details. A patent urachus is demonstrated at longitudinal US and occasionally at CT as a tubular connection between the anterosuperior aspect of the bladder and the umbilicus (Fig. 35.17). CT may help in detection of any

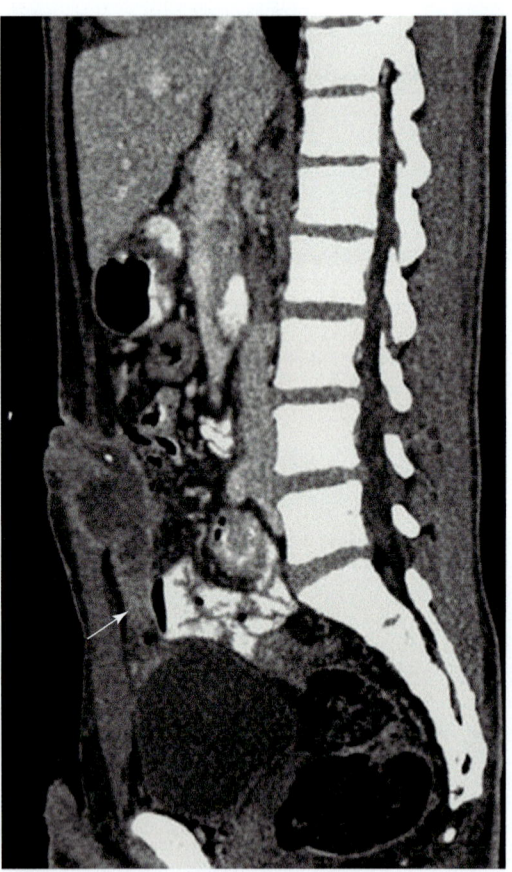

Fig. 35.17 Enhanced CT examination demonstrates a tubular, fluid-filled structure in the midline, consistent with patent urachus, with an inflammation that leads to an increase in wall thickness (*arrow*)

possible complication in a PU: like infection or neoplastic changes (Fig. 35.17). Analysis of the umbilical fluids may provide another means of diagnosing a urachal anomaly; fluid analysis would include measuring the umbilical fluid for content of urea and creatinine. Fetal MRI is a modality with multiplanar capabilities that yields high soft-tissue contrast without ionizing radiation. This technique has proved helpful in detecting and elucidating abnormalities of urachus, which are not clearly visible on sonography. Recently MRI using TWI sequences represents a safer and more useful second-line cross-sectional imaging modality than CT to arrive at this diagnosis.

Complications: PU may get infection, and to be presented late with an abscess at or below the umbilicus, and few cases reported after rupture of infected urachus, of course patent urachus as an open channel between urinary bladder and outside environment, that may result in repeated attacks of UTI and chronic urinary infections. PU may present in a neonate with severe umbilical bleeding. Few cases of stone formation in a PU had been reported. Neglected and undiagnosed cases may be complicated with necrotizing fasciitis as a rare complication of an infected urachal remnant in adults. Very rarely a specific granulomatous infection, like xanthogranulomatous infection, actinomycosis or tuberculosis, may affect a PU. A case of urachal–colonic fistula had been reported [20]. Bladder prolapse through a patent urachus may be a fetal or neonatal feature of PU; this prolapse can be predicted by prenatal ultrasound and has a distinct neonatal appearance (Fig. 35.13) [21].

Neoplastic transformation: The risk of urachal malignancy in adults is high, and the prognosis is poor; this will be discussed under a separate heading.

Management: PU found in neonates <6 months old usually resolve spontaneously without the need for any surgery; those found in older patients require management and should uniformly be resected, as chronic exposure to urinary stasis increases the risk for infection and inflammation, and are of utmost importance in adults, due to an increased risk of neoplastic changes. Galati et al. retrospectively reviewed 23 patients treated for a PU and found that in an overall 50 and 80% in children less than 6 months, the PUs resolved nonoperatively [22].

The traditional surgical approach for the excision of persistent urachal remnants is a lower midline laparotomy or semicircular infraumbilical incision. The excised urachal tissue should be examined carefully for any neoplastic changes.

Laparoscopy is a useful alternative for the management of persistent or infected urachus, especially when its presence is clinically suspected despite the lack of sonographic evidence. The procedure is associated with low morbidity, although a small risk of bladder injury exists, particularly in cases of severe active inflammation. Recurrence is uncommon and was caused by inadequate excision of inflammatory tissue [23]. Robotic-assisted laparoscopic surgery may be an attractive alternative to the open approach, which has only been studied in few case reports. Urachal pathology is well suited to robotic-assisted laparoscopic surgery, the urachus is immediately visualized upon entry into the abdomen, and the procedure can be performed safely, with short hospitalization and minimal narcotic requirement for pain control (Fig. 35.18) [24].

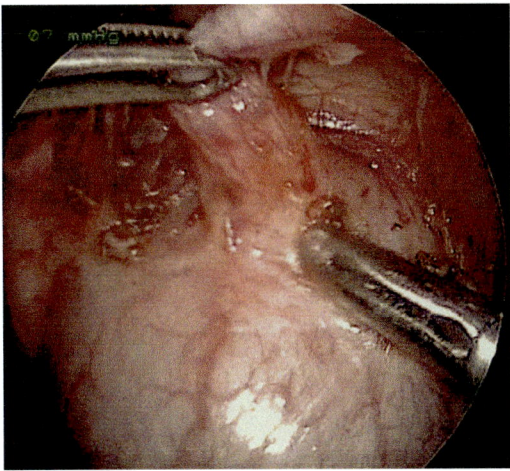

Fig. 35.18 Laparoscopic dissection of a patent urachus

35.4 Urachal Cyst

Urachal cysts are noncommunicating urachal duct remnants that occur anywhere along a line between the bladder and the umbilicus but are most commonly found near the dome of the bladder. In a completely walled off urachal cyst, and usually, there is no discharge at the umbilicus (Fig. 35.5b).

These cysts are small and remain undetected, being discovered in infancy in only one-third of cases. If left untreated, a urachal abscess can develop, which may rupture either through the umbilicus or into the peritoneal cavity causing peritonitis.

Incidence: Urachal cyst represents 30% of urachal anomaly; in paediatric autopsy studies, the incidence of 1 in 5000 cases for urachal cysts have been documented [25].

It is postulated that the patent urachus and the cyst formation were secondary to the increased pressure in the urinary tract. Intrauterine cystic perforation, which may complicate many cases, allowed the fetus to empty his bladder thus preventing renal damage and oligohydramnios. It is possible that the urachus was initially patent, but the presence of the stenotic meatus kept it open and probably caused formation of the cyst [13].

Diagnosis: Ultrasounds in the second and third trimesters can easily diagnose almost all urachal cyst, but confusion may arise if the cyst arises from the distal part of umbilical cord, in such case the cyst could be a true or false umbilical cyst or a vitellointestinal remnant (Chap. 36) (Fig. 35.19). Very rarely the uncomplicated urachal cyst may be detected in a child as a small abdominal wall swelling, and in such cases ultrasound could confirm the diagnosis (Fig. 35.20).

Clinical presentation is usually associated with superadded infection of the urachal cyst. Infected urachal cysts present with various symptoms: low abdominal mass, umbilical discharge, tenderness with erythema, fever, urinary tract infection, haematuria and peritonitis. Infected urachal cyst can occasionally lead to urachal abscess and can develop to systemic septic condition. With a severe urachal cyst infection, pyourachus can form a fistula with bladder, bowel or umbilicus. Abscess rupture due to expansion of

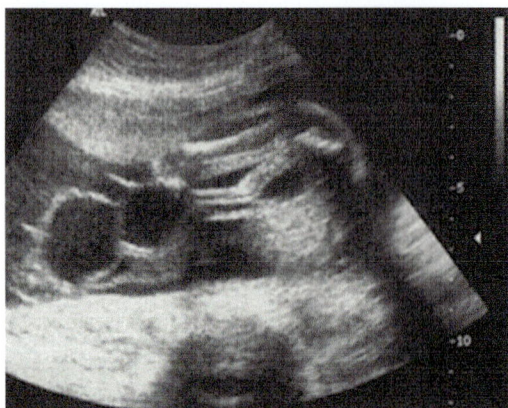

Fig. 35.19 Ultrasound for an antenatally detected urachal cyst

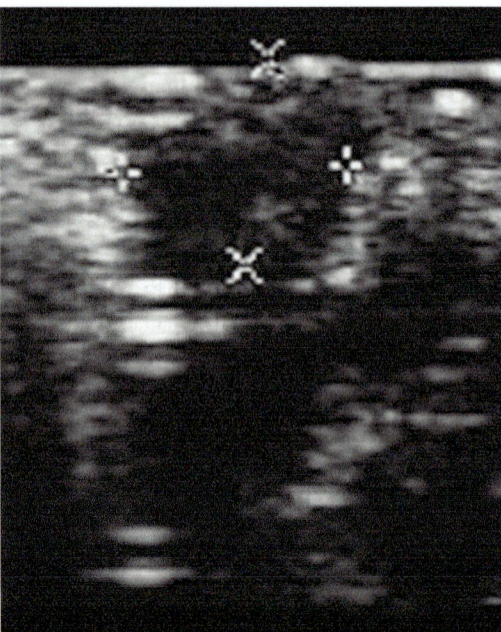

Fig. 35.20 Small urachal cyst between the peritoneum and abdominal muscles, seen by US

infected urachal cyst can cause acute abdomen requiring emergency surgery.

As cyst infection being the usual mode of presentation, the route of infection may be haematogenous, lymphatic, direct or ascending from the bladder, and the commonly cultured microorganisms from the cystic fluid include *Escherichia coli*, *Enterococcus faecium*, *Klebsiella pneumonia*, *Proteus*, *Streptococcus*

viridans and *Fusobacterium*. Infected may be presented with a vague abdominal pain, erythema of abdominal wall and fever, and unrecognized cases may be presented with septicaemia. Intracystic haemorrhage is rare, but it is possible specially in large one; herein I'm presenting a case of 8 cm urachal cyst in a 2-month-old girl presented with a lower abdominal swelling, and exploration revealed an intracystic haemorrhage; the cyst is connected with the ileum by a fibrous band (Figs. 35.21 and 35.22).

Fetal MRI may also be an additional tool to help characterize the cyst [26]; also CT scan and

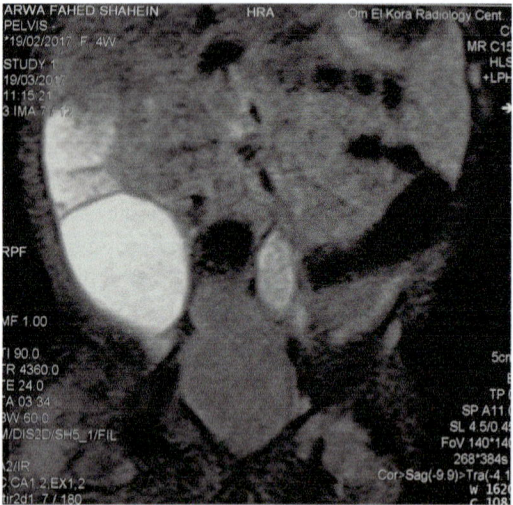

Fig. 35.21 MRI of a large urachal cyst in 2-month-old girl

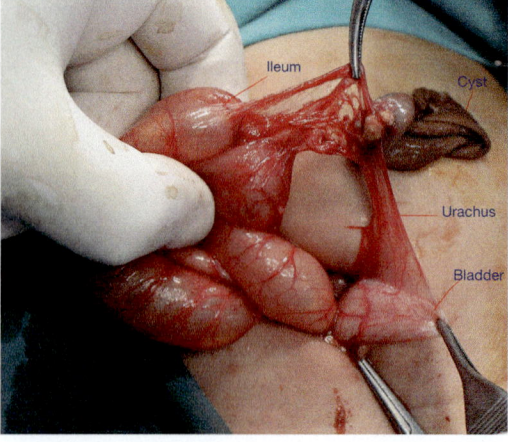

Fig. 35.22 Urachal cyst with fibrous connection to the terminal ileum

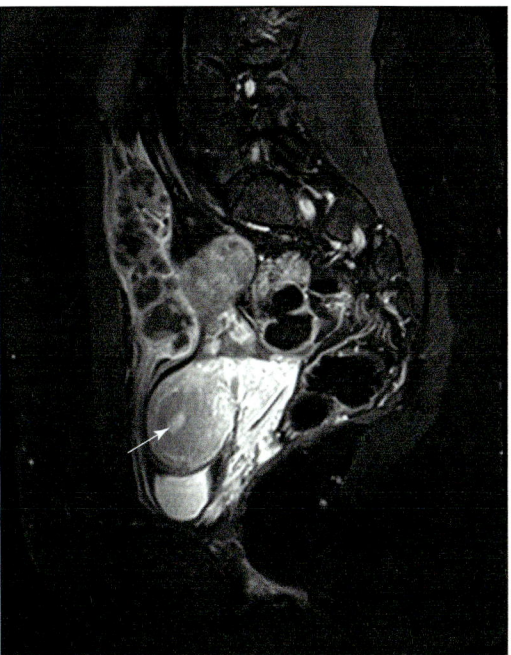

Fig. 35.23   MRI of a large urachal cyst in the sagittal plane (*arrow*)

MRI may be helpful for detection of the complicated cases (Fig. 35.23).

Theoretically the urachal cyst had no luminal connection with either the urinary bladder or the umbilicus, but we encountered few cases of cystic urachal dilation with a microscopic connection to the bladder, which allow contrast inject in the bladder during an ascending cystography to delineate a small dormant urachal cyst as in Fig. 35.24, where in Fig. 35.25, a small urachal cyst detected accidentally during contrast study for av case of isolated epispadias, those cases where a minute connection established between bladder and the cyst is considered as a combined patent urachus and urachal cyst.

Complications of urachal cyst:

Rupture into the peritoneal cavity leading to peritonitis [27].

Internal haemorrhage

Rare fistulous connection with a bowel loop (uracho-colonic fistula).

Stone formation.

Neoplastic transformation: the risk of malignant degeneration towards an adenocarcinoma of

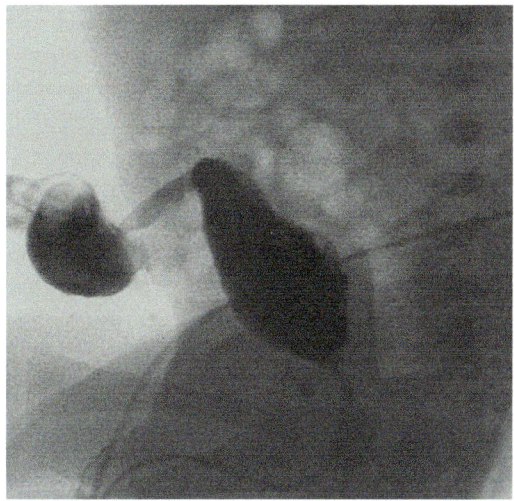

Fig. 35.24   Urachal cyst with a minute patent urachus, detected accidentally during cystography

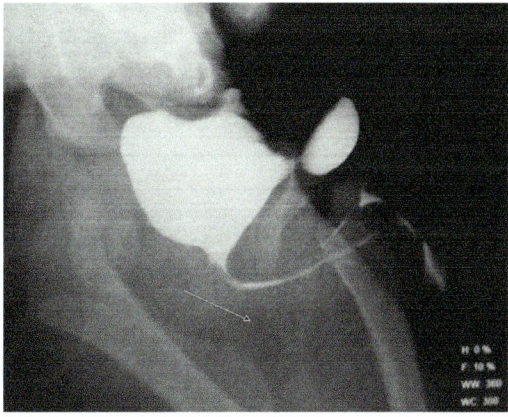

Fig. 35.25   A small urachal cyst discovered accidentally investigation of a case of isolated epispadias

the urachus representing 0.35% of bladder adenocarcinomas, and this risk in adults is high with a poor prognosis [28].

Management: Blichert–Toft and Nielson [29] reported that up to 31% of infected cysts recurred when not excised in the absence of infection; urachal cyst excision provides the most benign postoperative course. It is generally recommended that all urachal remnants should be excised to avoid recurrent disease. Classical treatment of urachal cysts involves complete excision. If a urachal cyst is not completely removed, the reinfection rate is 30% [30]. A complicated urachal cyst requires surgical excision to prevent symptom recurrence and complications, most notably malignant degeneration. However, a traditional open excision is associated with significant morbidity and prolonged convalescence, especially in children. Laparoscopic excision of the urachal remnant is feasible through a transpirational approach, by using three ports, so the urachus could be excised and separated from the bladder dome, the efficacy and outcome of this approach as a minimally invasive alternative deserve a comparative study for evaluation [31] (Fig. 35.26).

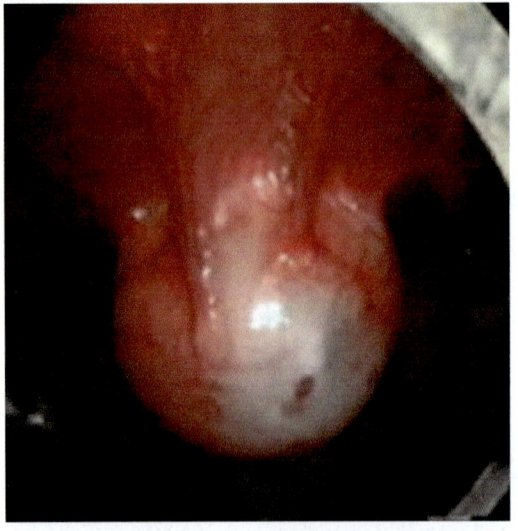

Fig. 35.26 Urachal cyst as seen via laparoscopy

When infection is present, management by perioperative drainage and antibiotics followed by subsequent elective excision may represent the most effective surgical option. Excision of the urachal cyst may be done openly or may be performed laparoscopically. Simple drainage of the cyst is not recommended due to high recurrence rates (approximately 30%) [31]. If the patient has a huge size of abscess with poor general condition, it is better to perform percutaneous drainage of the urachal abscess before surgical excision. Because of the high recurrence rate and possibility of developing carcinoma in the urachal remnant, it is a key point to complete resection of the cyst wall throughout its length during operation [32]. Operation may include removal of cuff of the bladder if there is communication between the urachal cyst and the bladder. Open excision has been performed as the treatment of choice, traditionally. However, recently, the laparoscopic method has been accepted as an alternative option because of faster recovery, less postoperative pain and better cosmetic results. At older age a meticulous search with ordinary and specific staining should be carried out to detect any neoplastic changes in the excised urachal cyst, which normally appear histologically with a complex architecture; the lining epithelium is predominantly flat cuboidal epithelium, interspersed with glandular-type epithelium (Fig. 35.27).

Fig. 35.27 Histology of urachal cyst with a complex architecture, predominantly flat cuboidal epithelium, interspersed with glandular epithelium

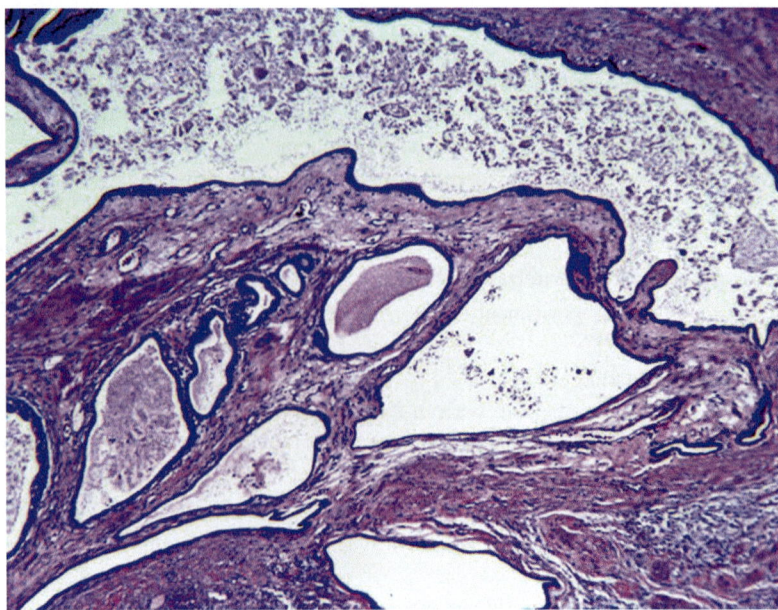

35.5   Urachal Sinus

A urachal sinus most likely represents a proximal patent urachus with obliteration of the distal part at the bladder connection or a urachal cyst that becomes infected and dissects the abdominal wall to have an access to the umbilicus (Fig. 35.5c). Additionally, a urachal sinus may drain into the bladder, or it may drain into either the umbilicus or the bladder and is termed an alternating sinus [33].

Urachal sinus represents about 15% of the detectable urachal anomalies. Yiee et al. reported that there were approximately two cases of urachal abnormality per 100,000 hospital admissions in adults [34].

Symptoms: Patients with urachal sinus typically present in childhood with periumbilical pain and tenderness and may have umbilical erythema, excoriation or reactive granulation tissue (Fig. 35.28). Persistent clear fluid leakage (likely urine) in an infant is highly suggestive of a patent urachus, while cloudy serous or bloody fluid is more indicative of an urachal sinus or cyst.

Common age presentation is of 3 years. The clinical signs and symptoms are nonspecific and variable. In most cases urachal sinus are asymptomatic unless they become infected. Clinical trial of symptoms including a tender midline infraumbilical mass, umbilical discharge and sepsis should arouse suspicion of urachal sinus [35]. A fistulogram is usually diagnostic and will help to delineate the extent of the sinus tract, but this should be done cautiously in patients with suspected or proved infection.

Differential diagnosis of this condition includes anomalies of the vitelline ducts (such as Meckel's diverticulum), patent omphalomesenteric duct, infected umbilical cyst, appendicitis or omphalitis.

Ultrasonography could help in establishing the diagnosis in 77% of patients. An umbilical–urachal sinus manifests at US as a thickened tubular structure along the midline below the umbilicus. Enhanced CT scan may be indicated to diagnose precisely complicated or doubtful cases (Fig. 35.29).

Urachal sinus can be complicated by stone and abscess formation; other reported complications include rupture into the peritoneal cavity leading to peritonitis, uracho-colonic fistula and neoplastic transformation. The risk of urachal malignancy in adults is high and the prognosis is poor [36].

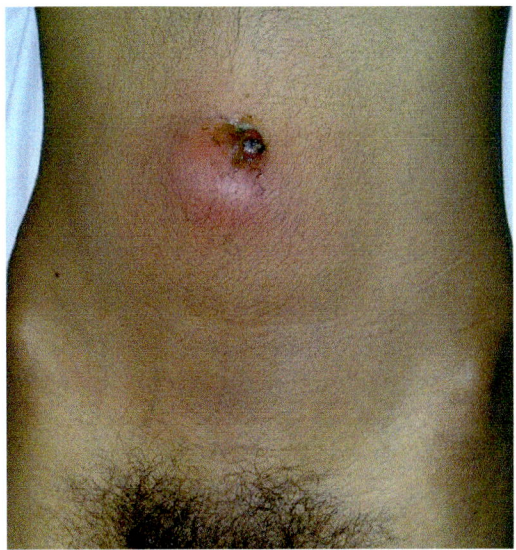

Fig. 35.28 Erythema and excoriation around the umbilicus due to urachal sinus

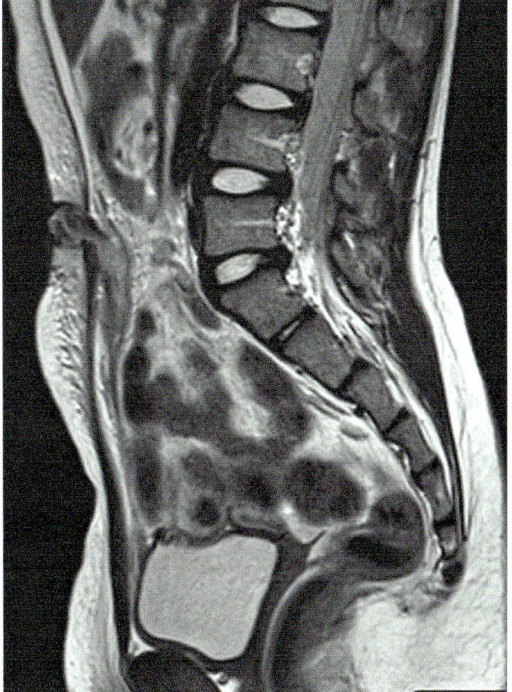

Fig. 35.29 CT scan showing a urachal sinus in a sagittal plane

After treatment of the acute infection, surgical excision of the sinus tract is recommended.

35.6   Urachal Abscess

Acquired urachal remnant disorders are mainly due to infection or neoplasm. Infection within an urachal cyst is uncommon with a peak incidence in infancy and then again in early adulthood [37]. The adult presentation may be a consequence of partial opening of the urachus which may have closed at birth. Umbilical urachal sinuses and infected cysts close to the abdominal wall will result in umbilical discharge. Infected cysts close to the bladder and vesicourachal diverticuli may present with urinary symptoms; a large infected cyst may rupture into the peritoneal cavity and cause peritonitis. Urachal abscess is rare in adulthood but should be considered as differential diagnosis of abdominal pain, because it may require emergency surgical management.

Urachal anomalies may get secondarily infected via lymphatic, haematogenous or vesical route by a wide spectrum of microorganisms and may form a urachal abscess. Fever, severe abdominal pain and pus discharge may ensue. In rare cases infected urachal abscess may burst into the peritoneum causing severe peritonitis. Ultrasound may show collection with complex echogenicity or septations. Ultrasound and CT are both reliable modalities for diagnosis of urachal abscess (Fig. 35.30). Demonstration of a

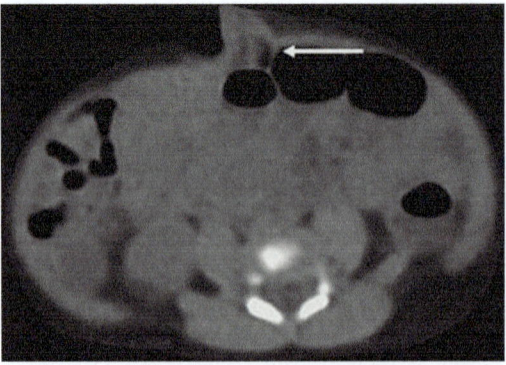

Fig. 35.30 Non-contrast CT scan of the abdomen demonstrates a urachal abscess (*arrow*) separated from the bladder

midline fluid containing structure within the anterior abdominal wall and extension into the umbilicus with or without umbilical discharge is virtually diagnostic of a urachal abscess. In some complex abscesses, the mixed echoes on US, heterogeneous enhancement on CT may mimic a urachal carcinoma, and an image-guided FNAC or biopsy is then indicated for definitive diagnosis and therapeutic planning.

Treatment includes complete excision of the urachal remnant. In case of infection/abscess, initial control of infection/pus drainage should be followed by surgery. A complete excision of the wall is important as there is a high probability of reinfection and chances of development of malignancy in residual remnants. Direction of drainage of infected urachal fluid depends on the type of urachal patency.

35.7   Urachal Diverticulum (UD) 'Vesicourachal Diverticulum'

Vesicourachal diverticula are the most rare of all symptomatic urachal anomalies, accounting for only 3–5% of all urachal anomalies in the Blichert–Toft [38] study of 315 documented cases of urachal anomalies. The diverticulum mouth seems to be the critical factor in determining presenting symptoms; if the mouth is small, debris can collect, urinary calculi can from, intermittent occlusion of the diverticular lumen, and presenting complaints can relate to infection, mass or rupture. If the mouth is large and allows free movement of urine, the diverticulum can remain asymptomatic or manifest as an umbilical mass that disappears with urination. Common symptoms associated with UD are repeated attacks of UTI, dysuria, haematuria and urgency.

Diverticulum usually looks saccular with rounded wall as in Fig. 35.31, but it could be tubular, and in such case, it looks like a distally patent urachus communicated with the bladder lumen as in Fig. 35.32. US usually diagnoses most cases, but sometimes CT scan or MRI is indicated to diagnose unusual large cyst or the associated anomalies [39].

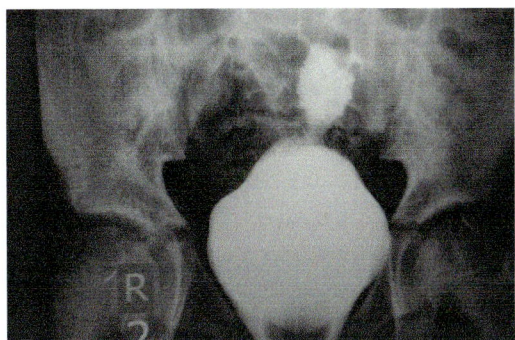

Fig. 35.31 Saccular urachal diverticulum seen at the bladder dome during VCUG

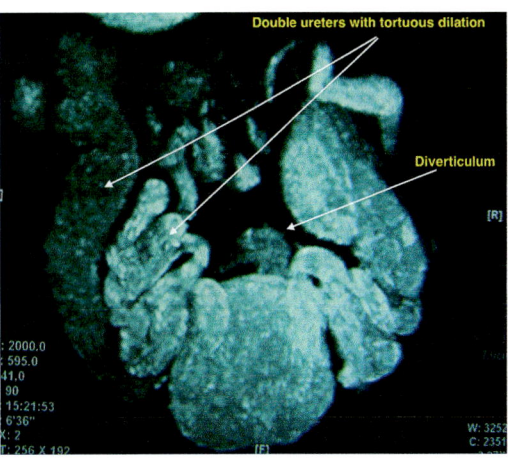

Fig. 35.33 MRI in a case of prune belly syndrome with hugely dilated ureters, double left ureter and urachal diverticulum

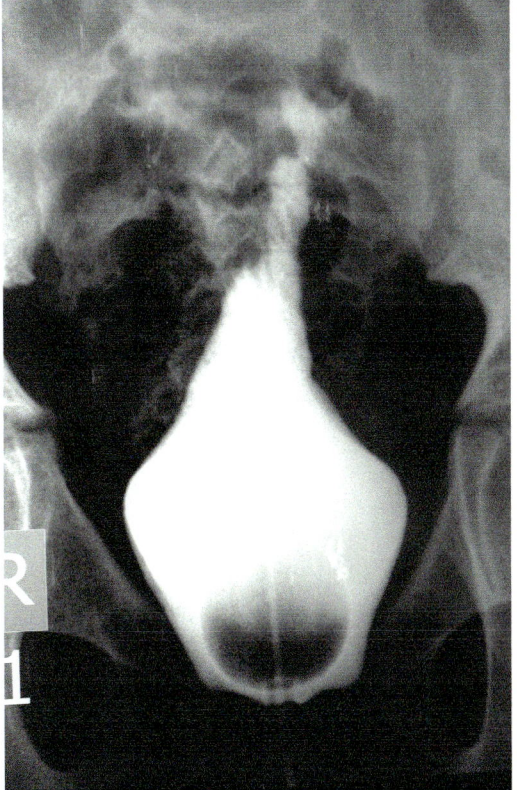

Fig. 35.32 Tubular urachal diverticulum looks like a partial patent urachus

Usually UD, specially the manifested one, is associated with a high intravesical pressure as in cases of bladder neck obstruction or defective musculature of the urinary system as in cases of prune belly syndrome. In Fig. 35.33 a magnetic resonance urography (MRU) shows a urachal diverticu-

lum, which was detected in a case of prune belly syndrome with double tortuous dilated ureters in the left side and a marked hydroureter in the other side, due to high intravesical pressure; UD may be also associated with vesicoureteric reflux or a multiple distal bladder diverticula as in Fig. 35.34.

Complications of UD include stone formation [40] and a possibility of neoplastic changes on the long term; presence of a radiopaque stone in a DU may raise a confusion with urachal carcinoma, which usually presented with calcifications (Fig. 35.35).

Accidentally discovered vesicourachal diverticulum rarely requires treatment except in these conditions:

- Large cyst with poor emptying due to a narrow neck or paradoxical contraction: this could be proved by the presence of contrast in the UD in the post voiding film, during MCUG.
- Cases complicated with stone formation also deserve excision.
- UD with suspicious thickened wall.

Simple excision of UD through a small infraumbilical incision, either transverse or longitudinal, may be enough if there are no any other associated anomalies, with two layers closure of the bladder wall (Fig. 35.36).

Fig. 35.34 Urachal
diverticulum with
another three distal
smaller diverticula,
bilaterally dilated ureters
are obvious

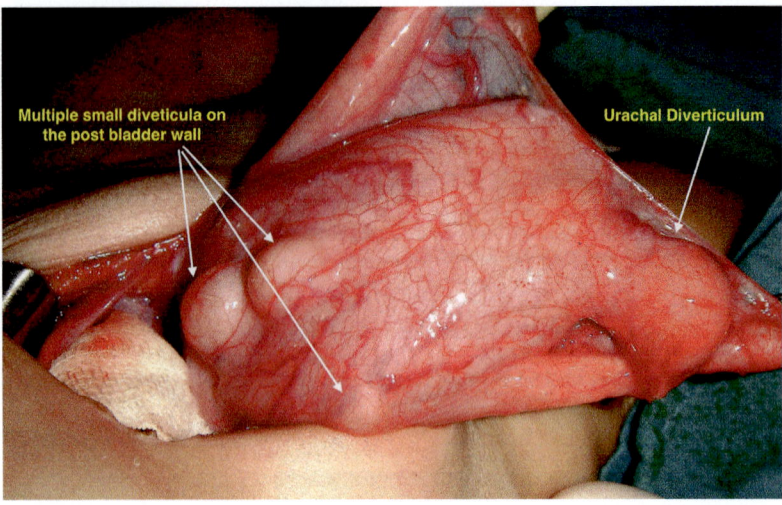

**Multiple small diveticula on
the post bladder wall**

Urachal Diverticulum

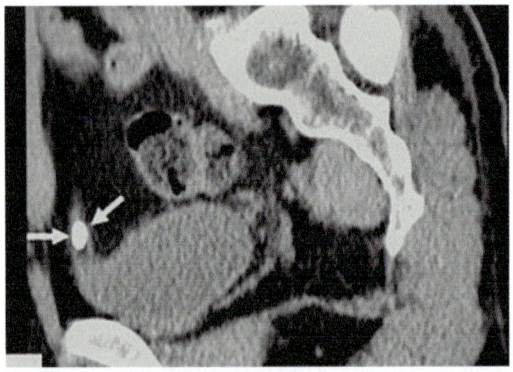

Fig. 35.35 A well-formed stone in a small urachal
diverticulum

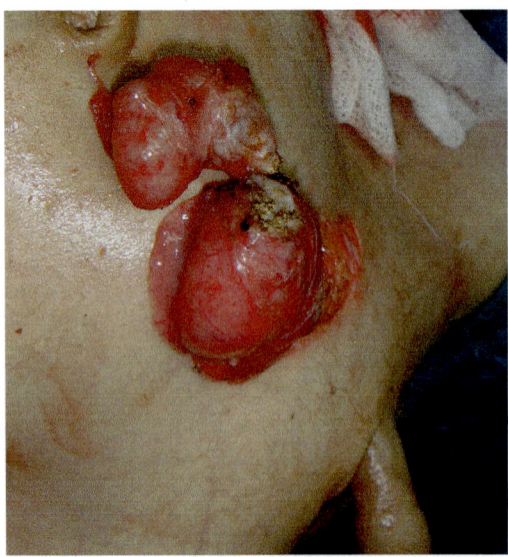

Fig. 35.36 An excised large UD with its pedicle

35.8   Urachal Neoplasm

Urachal carcinoma (UraC) is a rare and poorly
investigated complication of the urachal remnant.

Historical Background
Urachal cancer was mentioned for the first time
by Hue and Jacquin in 1863 followed by an elaborate work by T. Cullen in 1916, detailed diagnostic and staging schemes were proposed by
Sheldon et al. in 1984, which are widely used
today [41].

Incidence: The incidence of urachal carcinoma was 0.2% of all bladder cancers and
about 20% of all bladder adenocarcinomas.
The incidence ranges from 0.55 to 1.2% of
bladder tumors, but in Japan it is 0.07%–0.7%.
The vast majority (91%) of UraCs are diagnosed at later stages, when the tumor invades
the urinary bladder. About 21% of patients
have distant metastasis at first presentation
[42]. Ninety-four percent of UraCs were adenocarcinoma; conversely 34% of bladder adenocarcinomas are of urachal origin. Other
histologic subtypes like sarcomatoid, squamous or transitional cell elements have been
reported; the male-to-female ratio is 1.4:1, and
median patient age was 58 years (range 20–90)
(Fig. 35.37) [43].

Other primary epithelial tumors of the urachus
include villous adenoma, transitional cell carcinoma and, rarely, squamous cell carcinoma.

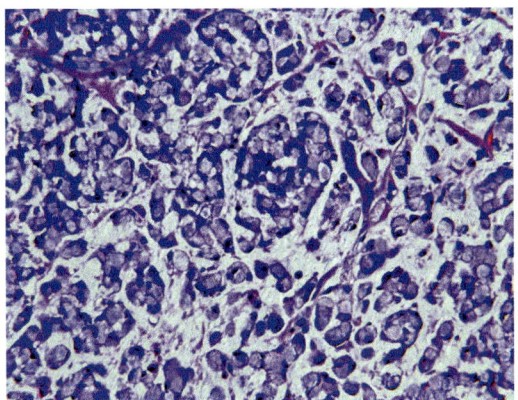

Fig. 35.37 Histopathology of UraC with a typical picture of adenocarcinoma

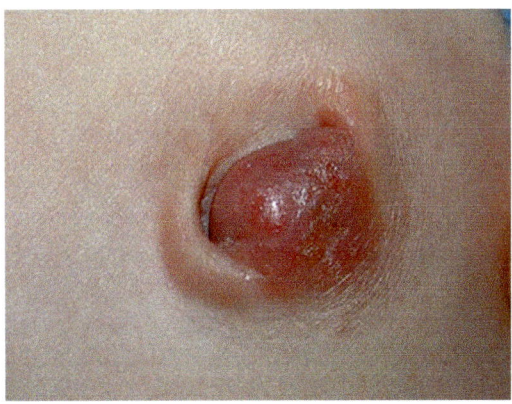

Fig. 35.38 Urachal carcinoma, with redness and signs of infection

Primary extragonadal germ cell tumors of the urachus are exceedingly rare [44].

Diagnosis: Most acceptable criteria for diagnosis of UraC are the one proposed by Sheldon et al. [41]:

1. Tumor is located in the dome/anterior wall of the bladder.
2. Epicentre in the bladder wall.
3. Absence of cystitis cystica and cystitis glandularis.
4. Lack of known primary adenocarcinoma (ADC) elsewhere.

Carcinoembryonic antigen (CEA) marker was elevated in 40–60% of patients.

Symptoms: The most frequent symptom of UraC is macroscopic or microscopic haematuria, which was reported in 73% of patients followed by abdominal pain in 14%, dysuria in 13% and mucosuria in 10%. Other less frequent clinical presentations included pollakisuria, pyuria, urinary tract infection, umbilical discharge (e.g. blood, urine or mucus), vaginal discharge and nonspecific symptoms (nausea, vomiting, diarrhoea, weight loss or fever) [45].

UraC may be presented as an umbilical swelling; the presence of signs and symptoms of infected umbilical swelling doesn't rule out presence of malignancy, which may look like an infected urachal cyst (Fig. 35.38).

A typical work-up includes cystoscopy with biopsy of any suspicious bladder lesion, and radiographic evaluation by US, CT and MR imaging which have the ability to display a cross-sectional images and therefore are ideally suited for demonstrating urachal anomalies. US may demonstrate a midline fluid-filled cavity with mixed echogenicity and calcifications adjacent to the anterior abdominal wall. A characteristic CT feature of urachal carcinoma is a midline mass anterosuperior to the dome of the bladder with low-attenuation components, which represent pools of mucin at pathologic examination. As with some other mucinous adenocarcinomas of the abdominal organs, urachal carcinomas may produce typical psammomatous calcifications that are well depicted at CT in 50–70% of cases. Magnetic resonance imaging is an excellent staging tool. Because of the presence of mucin within the tumor, an increased signal intensity that is seen on T2-weighted MR images is usually diagnostic [44]. Both CT and MR imaging are useful for demonstrating both extra- and intravesical extension of the tumor (Figs. 35.39 and 35.40).

Prognosis: The prognosis of urachal carcinoma depends mostly on tumor stage, particularly the presence or absence of metastatic disease. Patients with UraC often present with an advanced disease that cannot be treated with surgery alone. Five-year overall and relative survival was 45–48% [46].

Management: Owing to the lack of evidence-based guidelines, the therapy of UraC remains

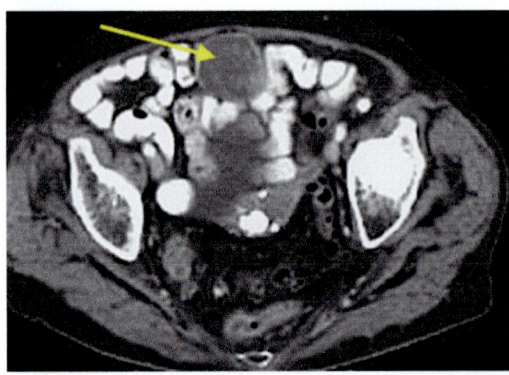

Fig. 35.39 UraC (*arrow*) which is not connected to the bladder and surrounded with bowel loops

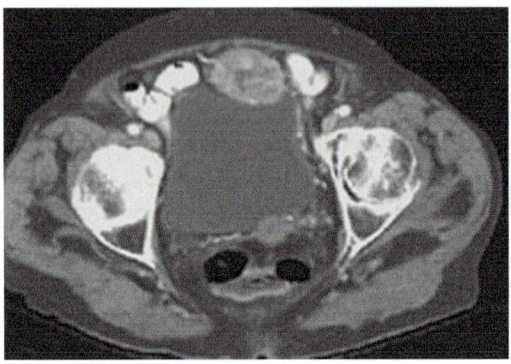

Fig. 35.40 CT features of urachal carcinoma with a midline mass anterosuperior to the bladder with low-attenuation components

challenging. Given the infrequency of UraC, large prospective studies comparing different systemic therapies can hardly be conducted.

Also UraC is rather insensitive to radiotherapy; patients with metastasized UraC are likely to have a poor prognosis. Thus, adequate surgery is crucial in patients with localized disease. Nonetheless, the optimal surgical procedure must be defined. Partial cystectomy provides oncological outcomes similar to those of radical cystectomy. However, it was suggested that umbilectomy and lymphadenectomy should be an integral part of surgery [47].

5-FU-containing chemotherapy regimens are more effective than cisplatin-based treatment modalities, whereas their combination seems to provide the strongest antitumor effect [48].

35.9   Absent Urachus: 'Urachal Agenesis'

Complete absence of urachus along all other umbilical structures is a very rare anomaly, which was discussed with umbilical cord agenesis, but cases of bladder exstrophy, either an open or closed one, may have an absent urachus; this is also quite common with cloacal exstrophy (Fig. 35.41) [49].

We reported herein an interesting case of cloacal exstrophy associated with a ruptured omphalocele with aberrant dilated umbilical vessels, but there is no urachus or median umbilical ligament that could be appreciated in the scene (Fig. 35.42).

In such cases the bladder wall was not developed completely, so the allantois didn't pass to the urachal transition, or the urachus development was disturbed and interfered by the undivided cloaca [50].

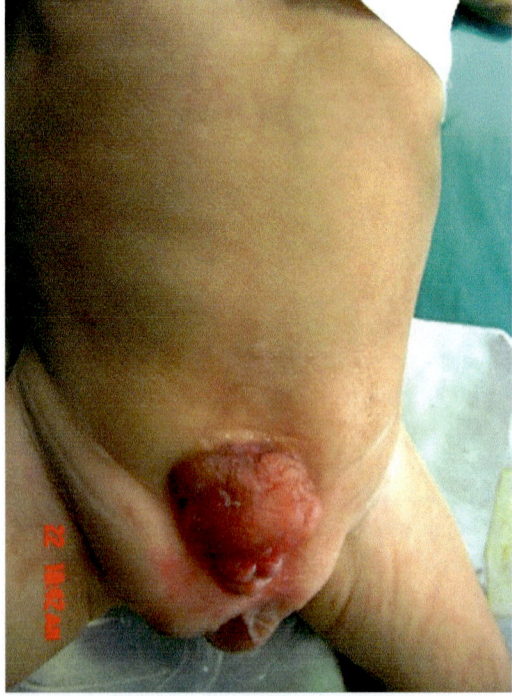

Fig. 35.41 Absent urachus along an absent umbilicus in a case of bladder exstrophy

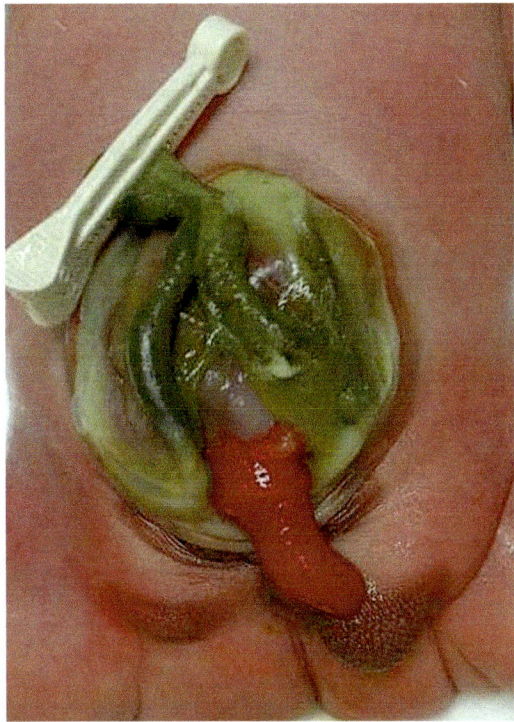

Fig. 35.42 A case of cloacal exstrophy with a ruptured omphalocele; prominent umbilical vessels seen without a median umbilical ligament (urachus)

References

1. Tolaymat LL, Maher JE, Kleinman GE, et al. Persistent patent urachus with allantoic cyst: a case report. Ultrasound Obstet Gynecol. 1997;10(5):366–8. doi:10.1046/j.1469-0705.1997.10050366.x-.
2. Moore KL, Persaud TVN. The developing human: clinically oriented embryology. 5th ed. Philadelphia: Saunders; 1993.
3. Skandalakis JA, Gray SW. Embryology for surgeons. Baltimore: Williams & Wilkins; 1994. p. 675–81.
4. Pazos HMF, Costa WS, Sampaio FJB, Favorito LA. Structural and ontogenetic study of the urachus in human fetuses. Cells Tissues Organs. 2010;191:422–30. doi:10.1159/000258785.
5. Rubin A. A handbook of congenital malformations. Philadelphia: Saunders; 2009.
6. Begg RC. The urachus and umbilical fistulae. Surg Gynecol Obstet. 1927;45:16–78.
7. Bilchert M, Nielsen OV. Congenital patent urachus and acquired variants. Acta Chir Scand. 1971;137:807–14.
8. Yu J, Kim K, Lee H, Lee Y, Yoon C, Kim M. Urachal remnant disease: spectrum of CT and US findings. Radiographics. 2001;21:451–6.
9. Berman SM, Berman BM, Laor E, Freed SZ. Urachal remnants in adults. Urology. 1988;31(1):17–21. doi:10.1016/0090-4295(88)90564-X.
10. Herman TE, Siegel MJ. Prune belly syndrome. J Perinatol. 2009;29:69–71.
11. Bourdelat D, Husson S, Soisic F, Vrsansky P. Embryological study of the mechanism of antenatal lower urinary tract obstruction. Ann Urol (Paris). 1998;32(4):253–68.
12. Sadler TW. Urogenital system. In: Longman's medical embryology. 10th ed. Philadelphia: Lippincott, Williams & Wilkins; 2006. p. 236–8.
13. Bureau M, Bolduc S. Allantoic cysts and posterior urethral valves: a case report. Ultrasound Obstet Gynecol. 2011;38:116–8. doi:10.1002/uog.8910.
14. Gobet R, Bleakley J, Craig A. Peterspremature urachal closure induces hydroureteronephrosis in male fetuses. J Urol. 1998;160(4):1463–7. doi:10.1016/S0022-5347(01)62592-8.
15. Fox JA, McGee SM, Routh JC, Granberg CF, Ashley RA, Hutcheson JC, et al. Vesicoureteral reflux in children with urachal anomalies. J Pediatr Urol. 2011;7:632–5.
16. Atobatele MO, Olalekan IO, Abdulrasheed AN, John OB. Posterior urethral valve with unilateral vesicoureteral reflux and patent urachus: a rare combination of urinary tract anomalies. Urol Ann. 2015;7(2):240–3. doi:10.4103/0974-7796.150496.
17. Razvi S, Murphy R, Shlasko E, Cunningham-Rundles C. Delayed separation of the umbilical cord attributable to urachal anomalie. Pediatrics. 2001;108(2):493–4.
18. Kilicdag EB, et al. Large pseudocyst of the umbilical cord associated with patent urachus. J Obstet Gynaecol Res. 2004;30(6):444–7.
19. Little DC, Shah SR, St Peter SD, et al. Urachal anomalies in children: the vanishing relevance of the preoperative voiding cystourethrogram. J Pediatr Surg. 2005;40:1874–6.
20. Flanagan DA, Mellinger JD. Urachal-sigmoid fistula in an adult male. Am Surg. 1998;64:762–3.
21. Lugo B, McNulty J, Emil S. Bladder prolapse through a patent urachus: fetal and neonatal features. J Pediatr Surg. 2006;41(5):e5–7. doi:10.1016/j.jpedsurg.2005.12.062.
22. Galati V, Donovan B, Ramji F, et al. Management of urachal remnants in early childhood. J Urol. 2008;180(4 Suppl):1824e6. [discussion 1827]
23. Siow SL, Mahendran HA, Hardin M. Laparoscopic management of symptomatic urachal remnants in adulthood. Asian J Surg. 2015;38(2):85–90. doi:10.1016/j.asjsur.2014.04.009.
24. Rivera M, Granberg CF, Tollefson MK. Robotic-assisted laparoscopic surgery of urachal anomalies: a single-center experience. J Laparoendosc Adv Surg Tech A. 2015;25(4):291–4. doi:10.1089/lap.2014.0551.
25. Widni EE, Höllwarth ME, Haxhija QE. The impact of preoperative ultrasound on correct diagnosis

of urachal remnants in children. J Pediatric Surg. 2010;45:1433–7.

26. Pal K, Ashri H, Al-Ghazal FA. Allantoic cyst and ura-chus. Indian J Pediatr. 2009;76:221–3.

27. Ohgaki M, Higuchi A, Chou H, Takashina K, Kawakami S, Fujita Y, Hagiwara A, Yamagishi H. Acute peritonitis caused by intraperitoneal rupture of an infected urachal cyst: report of a case. Surg Today. 2003;33:75–7.

28. Mazzucchelli R, Scarpelli M, Montironi R. Mucinous: adenocarcinoma with superficial stromal invasion and villous adenoma of urachal remnants: a case report. J Clin Pathol. 2003;56:465–7.

29. Blichert-Toft M, Nielson OV. Congenital patent ura-chus and acquired variants: diagnosis and treatment. Review of the literature and report of 5 cases. Acta Chir Scand. 1971;137:807–14.

30. Pesce C, Costa L, Musi L, Campobasso P, Zimbardo L. Relevance of infection in children with urachal cysts. Eur Urol. 2000;38:457–60.

31. Seo IY, Park SC, Oh SJ. Laparoscopic excision of complicated urachal cyst in child. Korean J Urol. 2005;46(3):324–6.

32. Walsh SA, Weiss RM. Case report: persistent dysuria and a suprapubic mass in a 3-year-old boy. Curr Opin Pediatr. 2002;14:647–8.

33. Tiao MM, Ko SF, Huang SC, Shieh CS, Chen CL. Urachal inflammatory mass mimicking an intra-abdominal tumor two years after excision of the ura-chal sinus in a child. Chang Gung Med J. 2003;26(8): 598–601.

34. Yiee JH, Garcia N, Baker LA, Barber R, Snodgrass WT, Wilcox DT. A diagnostic algorithm for urachal anomalies. J Pediatr Urol. 2007;3:500–4.

35. Wang B, Tashiro J, Pelaez L, Rodriguez MM, Perez EA, Neville HL, Sola JE. A unique presentation and rare pathological finding for urachal sinus. J Pediatric Surg. 2013;48(9):1977–80. doi:10.1016/j. jpedsurg.2013.07.002.

36. El Ammari JE, Ahallal Y, El Yazami Adli O, El Fassi MJ, Farih MH. Urachal sinus presenting with abscess formation. ISRN Urol. 2011;2011:820924. doi:10.5402/2011/820924.

37. Mistrya KA, et al. Late presentation of congenital urachal sinus in a middle aged male complicated by an umbilical abscess: a case report. Egypt J Radiol Nuclear Med. 2015;46(3):755–9. doi:10.1016/j.ejrnm.2015.04.010.

38. Blichert-Toft M, Nielsen OV. Diseases of the urachus simulating intra-abdominal disorders. Am J Surg. 1971;122:123–8.

39. Ozbülbül NI, Dagli M, Akdogan G, Olçer T. CT urog-raphy of a vesicourachal diverticulum containing cal-culi. Diagn Interv Radiol. 2010;16:56–8.

40. Ansari MS, Hemal AK. A rare case of urachovesical calculus: a diagnostic dilemma and endo-laparoscopic management. J Laparoendosc Adv Surg Tech A. 2002;12:281–3.

41. Sheldon CA, Clayman RV, Gonzalez R, Williams RD, Fraley EE. Malignant urachal lesions. J Urol. 1984;131:1–8.

42. Ghazizadeh M, Yamamoto S, Kurokawa K. Clinical features of urachal carcinoma in Japan: review of 157 patients. Urol Res. 1983;11(5):235–8.

43. Gopalan A, Sharp DS, Fine SW. Urachal carcinoma: a clinicopathologic analysis of 24 cases with outcome correlation. Am J Surg Pathol. 2009;33:659–68.

44. Szarvas T, et al. Clinical, prognostic, and therapeu-tic aspects of urachal carcinoma—a comprehensive review with meta-analysis of 1,010 cases. Urol Oncol. Semin Orig Invest. 2016;34(9):388–98.

45. Bruins HM, et al. The clinical epidemiology of ura-chal carcinoma: results of a large, population based study. J Urol. 2012;188(4):1102–7. doi:10.1016/j. juro.2012.06.020.

46. Herr HW, Bochner BH, Sharp D, et al. Urachal car-cinoma: contemporary surgical outcomes. J Urol. 2007;178:74.

47. Molina JR, Quevedo JF, Furth AF, et al. Predictors of survival from urachal cancer: a mayo clinicstudy of 49 cases. Cancer. 2007;110:2434.

48. Ashley RA, Inman BA, Sebo TJ, et al. Urachal carcinoma: clinicopathologic features and long-term outcomes of an aggressive malignancy. Cancer. 2006;107:712.

49. Charles HM. Exstrophy of the bladder and its treat-ment. JAMA. 1917;25:2079–81. doi:10.1001/jama.1917.02590520001001.

50. Sakellaris G, Cervellione RM, Dickson AP. An unusual bladder/cloacal exstrophy with urachal exstrophy. Urol Int. 2008;81(1):113–5. doi:10.1159/000137651.

Embryological background: Early in the fourth week of development, the embryo undergoes an elaborate folding process that transforms the flat germ disc into a convex-shaped three-dimensional structure, with the endoderm, mesoderm and ectoderm all meeting and fusing in the midline. The endodermal gut tube initially consists of the blind-ending cranial foregut and caudal hindgut, and the midgut remains open to the yolk sac through the vitelline duct (Fig. 36.1). The boundaries of the foregut, midgut and hindgut are determined by their vascular supply, which originates from derivatives of the vitelline artery: the celiac, superior mesenteric and inferior mesenteric arteries vascularize the foregut, midgut and hindgut, respectively. The intestines normally migrate outside the abdominal cavity through the umbilical ring during a phase of rapid growth in the 6th week of development, and upon returning to the abdominal cavity by the 12th week of development, the bowel normally has rotated 270° counterclockwise before mesenteric fixation occurs in the peritoneal cavity. Meanwhile, the urinary tract is partially derived from the cloaca, which is the distal expansion of the hindgut and gives rise to the urinary bladder, and also from the intermediate mesoderm

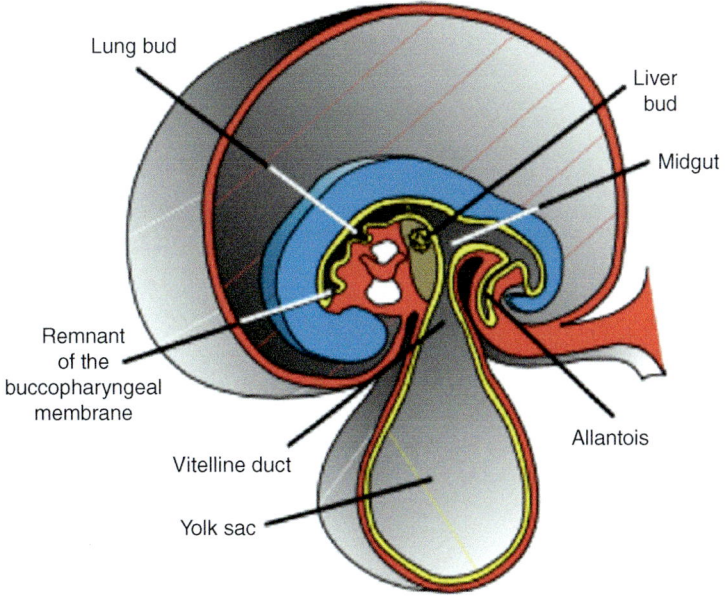

Fig. 36.1 Early development of yolk sac

in the dorsal body wall, which gives rise to the renal parenchyma and collecting systems. As these systems are developing, the abdominal wall is formed by infolding of the cranial, caudal and two lateral embryonic folds (Fig. 36.2) [1].

Persistent vitellointestinal duct is a rare anomaly of the primitive yolk sac. The vitellointestinal duct provides nutrition to the early developing embryo. The duct provides a communication between the primitive yolk sac on the ventral side of the embryo and the midgut loop through the umbilical coelom. The duct lies in the axis of the herniating loop of the midgut and resembles an extension of the superior mesenteric artery towards and beyond the umbilicus. The OMD gradually attenuates and involutes from the terminal part of the ileum by the 5th–9th week of gestational period. Remnants of the duct present as varied anatomical entities. The most common presentation of a persistent duct (67%) is the Meckel's diverticulum, followed by patent OMD; other anomalies are rare and recorded as case reports or cases series [2].

Nomenclatures: Omphalomesenteric ducts (OMD) also known as vitellointestinal duct, yolk stalk and sometimes referred as vitelline duct.

Classifications: Trimingham [3] and Nix and Young [4] classified the failure of closure or persistence of the omphalomesenteric duct into the following categories:

1. Completely patent omphalomesenteric duct (umbilical enteric fistula)
2. Partially patent omphalomesenteric duct
   (a) Peripheral portion (umbilical sinus)
   (b) Intermediate portion (vitelline cyst)
   (c) Enteric portion (Meckel's diverticulum)
3. Mucosa remnant at the umbilicus (umbilical polyp)
4. Congenital band (obliterated omphalomesenteric duct)

This classification ignored different cases reported with bowel prolapse and cases of appendico-umbilical fistula, so we adopt this simple classification of the OMD anomalies, according to the diagram (Fig. 36.3):

- Meckel's diverticulum
- Patent vitellointestinal duct
- Vitellointestinal sinus
- Vitellointestinal cyst
- Vitellointestinal mucosal polyp
- Vitellointestinal fibrous band
- Intestinal prolapse
- Appendico-umbilical fistula

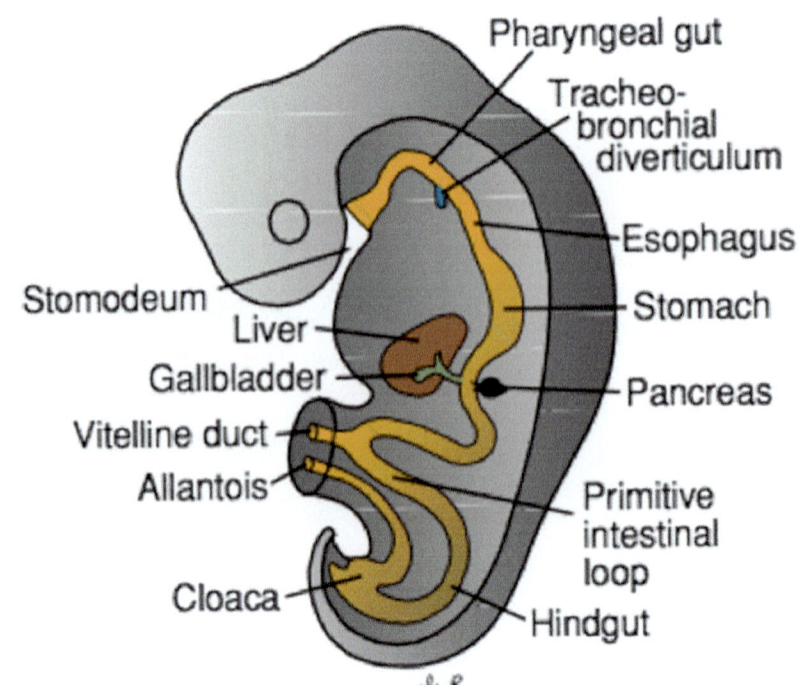

Fig. 36.2 Different parts of the primitive bowel with vitellointestinal duct communicating midgut to the umbilicus

Incidence: Remnants of the vitellointestinal duct are said to be present in 2–4% of all routine postmortem examinations, but presumably many people live their allotted span of life despite their presence and at no time have symptoms referable to them [5].

Six percent of these malformations correspond to persistent omphalomesenteric ducts, and up to 20% of them present with complications [6]. Seventy-three percent of the cases show symptoms within the first 28 days of life and are more frequent in male patients, but other authors believe that these malformations are found with equal frequency between both sexes, and only the incidence of symptoms is significantly greater in males [7].

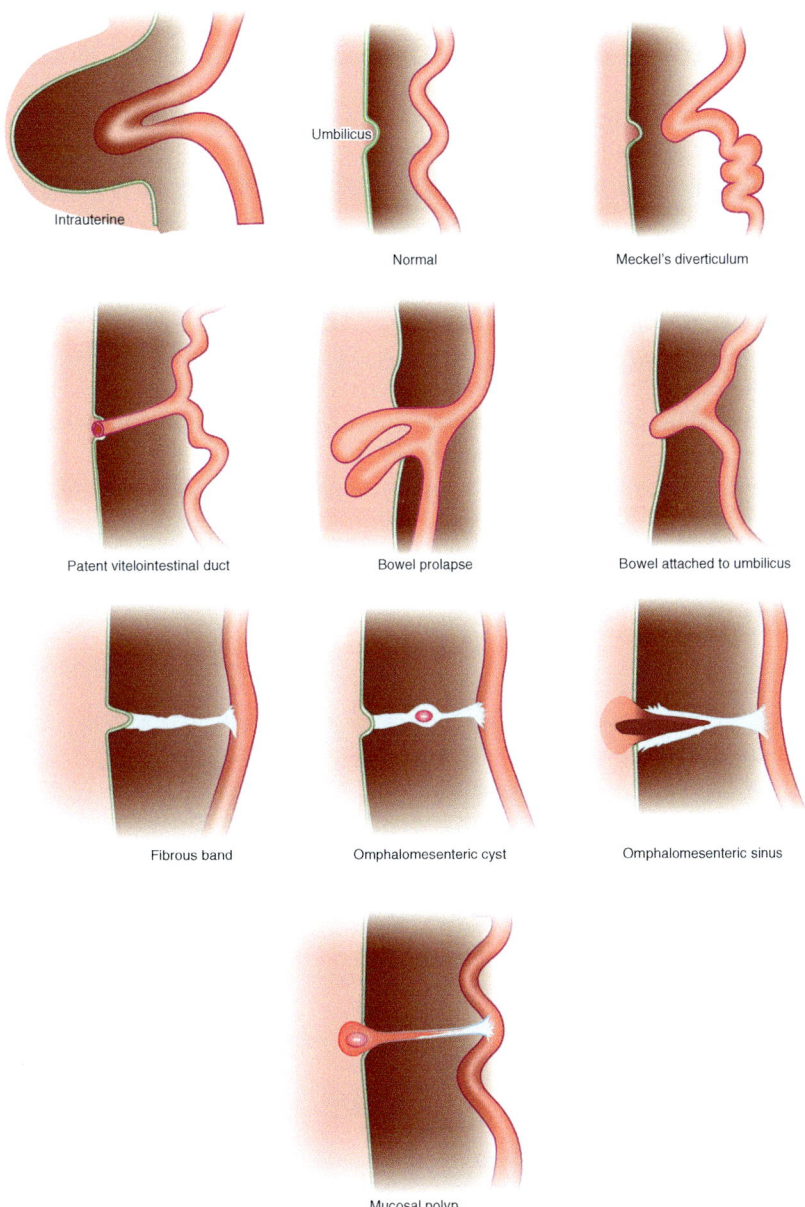

Fig. 36.3 Classifications of different vitellointestinal duct anomalies

Associated anomalies: OMD anomalies may be associated with umbilical and other related embryological remnants anomalies or with systemic malformations.

Umbilical anomalies reported in association with OMD include congenital umbilical hernia, exomphalos, intestinal malrotation, volvulus and bowel atresia [8].

Urachal anomalies are not rare with OMD [9]. Simultaneous coexistence of multiple types of OMD anomalies is not rare; prolapse of the ileum was present in about 50% of cases of patent OMD. Many cases of Meckel's diverticulum with OMD band had been reported and also umbilical polyp and OMD cyst are occasionally diagnosed with Meckel's diverticulum [10].

Systemic anomalies reported are cardiac malformation and cleft lip and palate, and also omphalomesenteric duct may be seen in trisomy 13 [11], Down's syndrome and Ehlers–Danlos syndrome [12].

Clinically: Common symptoms of OMD malformations generally include abdominal pain, rectal bleeding, intestinal obstruction, umbilical drainage and umbilical hernia. All these symptoms appear to be age dependent, usually appearing before the age of 4 years; 85% of infants younger than 1 month and 77% of children aged 1 month to 2 years have a symptomatic presentation, while adult patients are usually asymptomatic [13].

36.1   Meckel's Diverticulum (MD)

The spectrum of MD pathology and management is beyond the scope of this chapter, which is dealing mainly with the umbilical anomalies. The most common presentation of a persistent OMD (67%) is the Meckel's diverticulum, which is found in approximately 2% of the population. Seventeen percent of them might present patches of gastric mucosa and rarely pancreatic islet tissues. This condition causes symptoms in 4–30% of patients [14].

MD was named after Johann Friedrich Meckel, who described the embryological origin of this type of intestinal diverticulum in 1809 [15].

About 10% of the MD may be attached to the umbilicus with a fibrous cord, in several cases, however, the fibrous cord is seen to regress leaving no trace of connection between the MD and the umbilicus. It is well known that MD is more common in males, with a male/female ratio of 1.7:1 [16].

The most common symptoms of Meckel's diverticulum were rectal bleeding, intestinal obstruction and abdominal pain, and other symptoms similar to acute appendicitis are the common presentation.

MD is the most prevalent congenital anomaly of the gastrointestinal tract and often presents a diagnostic challenge. Many tools are available for the diagnosis, including Meckel's technetium scan, US, CT, GI endoscopy and capsule endoscopy [17]. MD may be complicated with bowel perforation and intestinal obstruction, secondary to intussusception or volvulus (Figs. 36.4 and 36.5).

MD is variable in size, mostly seen at the antimesenteric border of the terminal ileum but could be seen nearer to the mesentery or inverted inside the bowel lumen (Fig. 36.6).

A laparoscopic approach is safe and effective in the diagnosis and treatment of Meckel's diverticulum. With the wide use of laparoscopy in almost all specialities during the last two decades, it is expect to have a higher rate of incidentally diagnosed MD [18].

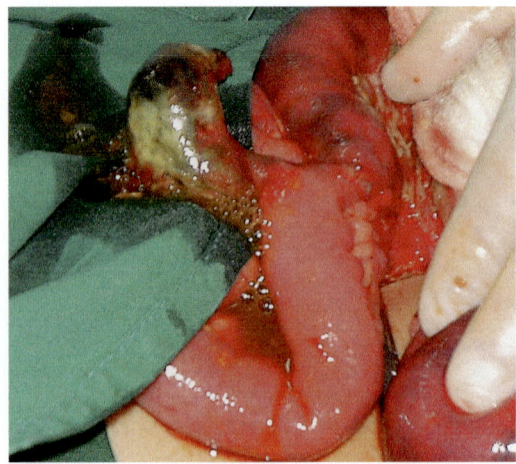

Fig. 36.4 Severely inflamed Meckel's diverticulum with perforation

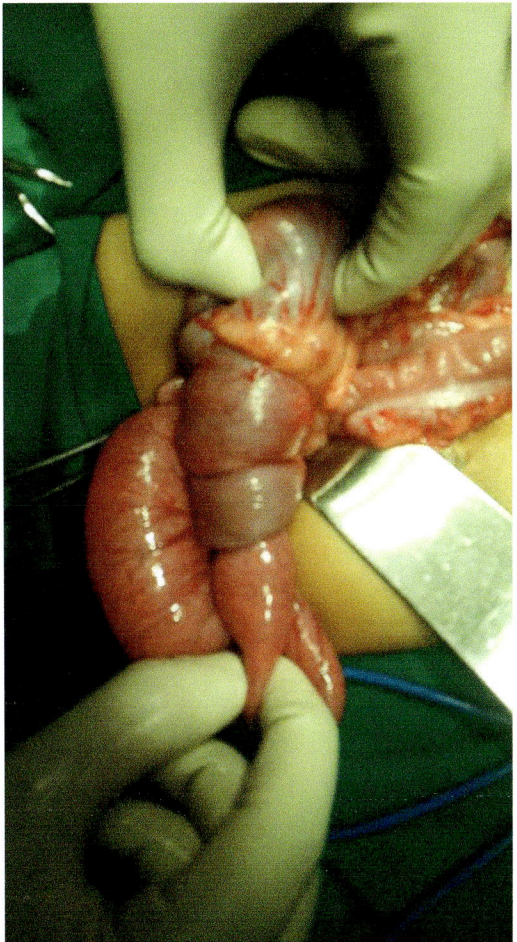

Fig. 36.5 Ileal intussusception secondary to inflamed MD

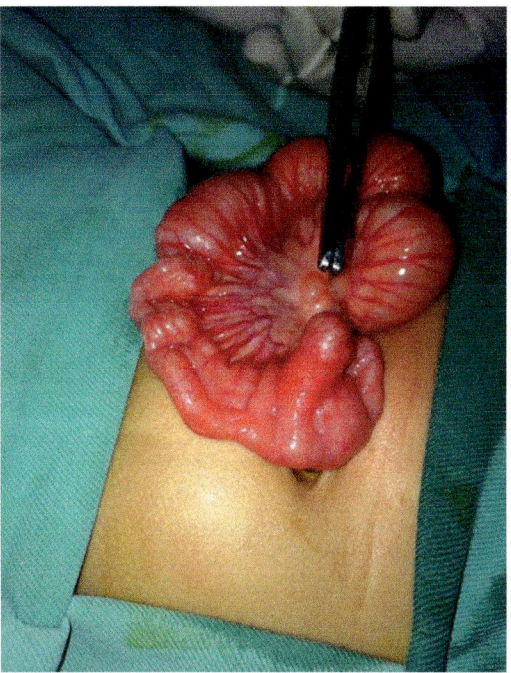

Fig. 36.6 MD near to the mesenteric border of the ileum with ectopic gastric tissue

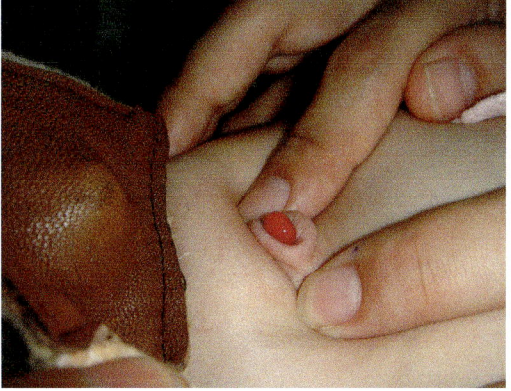

Fig. 36.7 Cherry-like mass at the umbilicus diagnosed wrongly as a granuloma, but latter on a punctum detected at its summit

36.2 Patent Vitellointestinal Duct

Umbilical drainage of gas or intestinal contents in a newborn represents the hallmark finding for a patent OMD; most cases are usually diagnosed after fall down of the umbilical stump, with a resultant cherry-like mass, which may be diagnosed wrongly as a U polyp (Chap. 29) (Fig. 36.7).

Presence of a punctum at the summit of the query polyp with a greenish discharge should arouse suspicion about a patent OMD; passing a fine catheter through this punctum usually confirm the diagnosis, when intestinal contents are retrieved through the catheter (Figs 36.8, 36.9, and 36.10).

The ducts averaged 3.8 cm in length and 1.1 cm in diameter. Ectopic gastric mucosa was found in 10% of the cases [19].

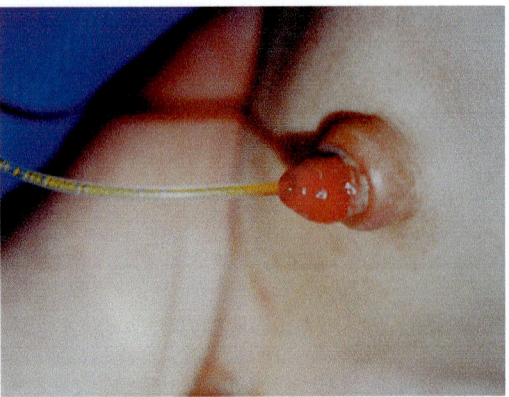

Fig. 36.8 A fleshy umbilical swelling retrieves an intestinal contents after cannulation with a fine catheter

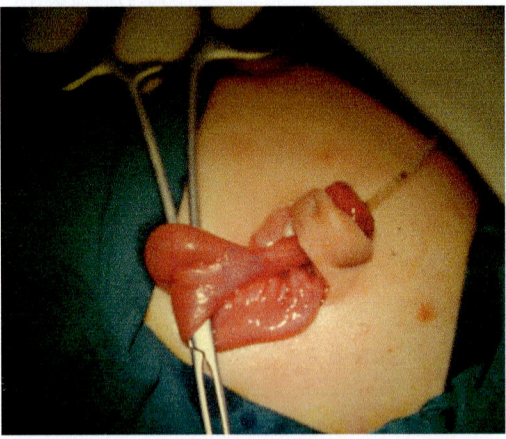

Fig. 36.9 A patent vitellointestinal duct connected to the umbilicus as an ileaoumbilical fistula

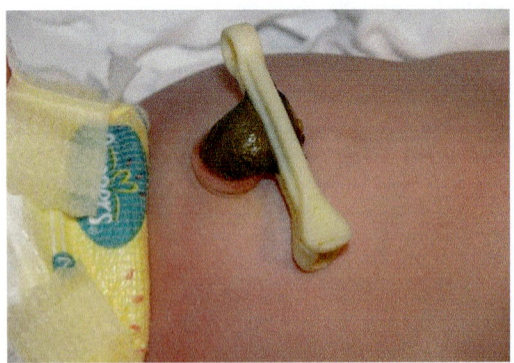

Fig. 36.10 Meconium-stained umbilical stump, an indicator for patent OMD

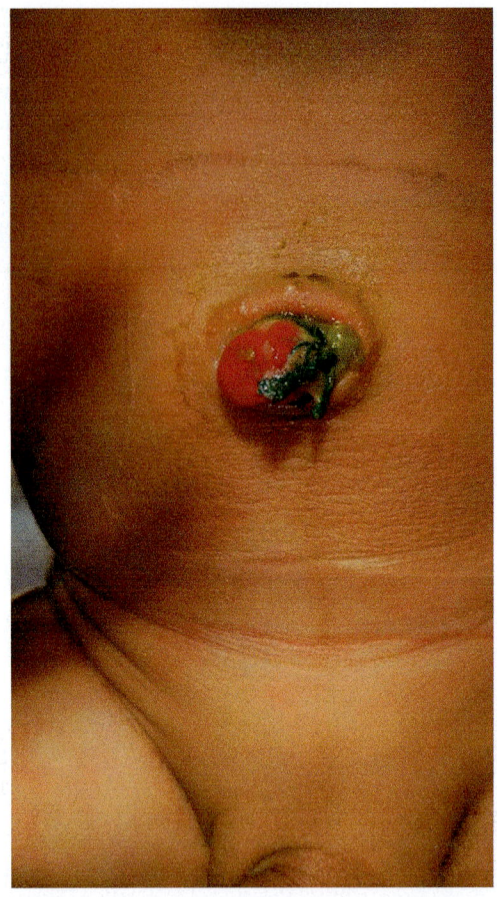

Fig. 36.11 Faecal fistula as a presentation of patent OMD

Recognition of patent vitellointestinal duct by gynaecologist and paediatrician, as early as possible, is crucial for its proper management, so this anomaly may present itself as:

- Meconium staining of the umbilical cord (Fig. 36.10)
- Continuous or intermittent discharge through the umbilicus after fall down of umbilical stump, (enteroumbilical fistula) (Fig. 36.11)
- Prolapsed ileum through the umbilicus with the patent vitellointestinal duct (Fig. 36.12)
- Patent OMD way be associated with cases of exampholas or congenital hernia of umbilical cord (Fig. 36.13)

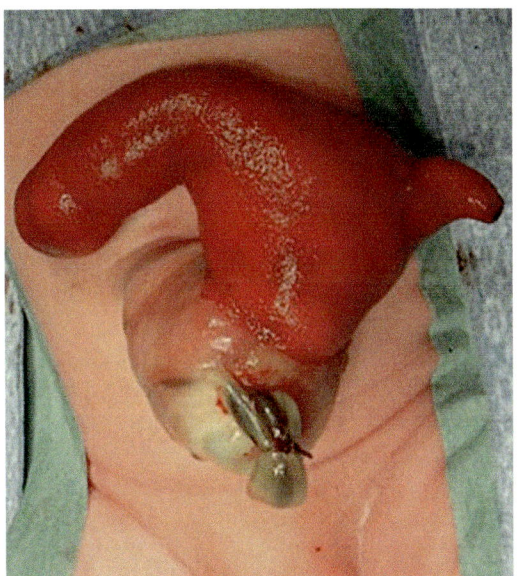

Fig. 36.12 Patent OMD with prolapsed small bowel (Ram's horn-type appearance)

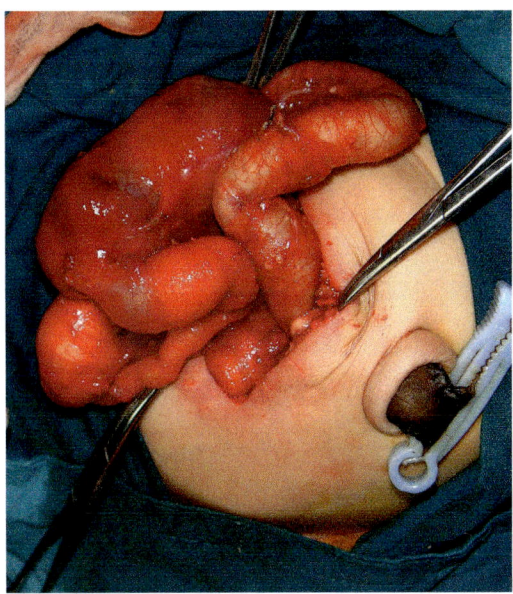

Fig. 36.14 Ileal atresia with the proximal limb ended at the umbilicus as a patent OMD

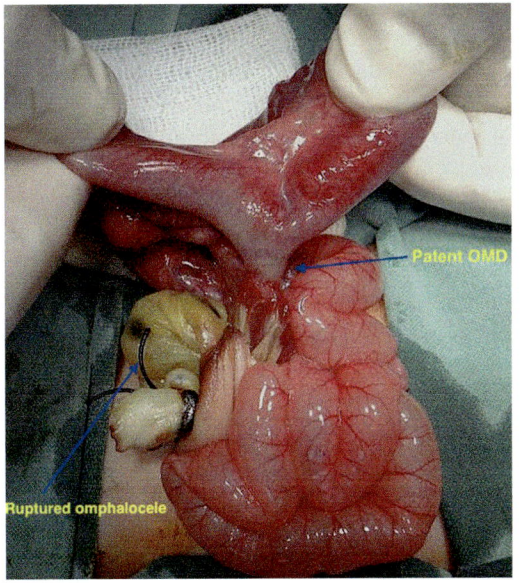

Fig. 36.13 Patent OMD with a ruptured minor omphalocele

In cases of patent OMD, associated with ileal atresis, one bowel end may open in the umbilicus and the other end will be seen as a blind loop (Fig. 36.14).

The defect which is wide enough or the predisposing conditions which increase intra-abdominal pressure leads to partial or total prolapse of the intestine through the patent duct, leading to a T-shaped bowel protrusion through the umbilicus and even Ram's horn-type appearance (Fig. 36.12).

The condition, if not managed promptly by surgical intervention, it may leads to subacute or acute intestinal obstruction, strangulation and gangrene of the prolapsed intestinal loop (Fig. 36.17).

Complications: Intestinal obstruction is reported to be the most serious complication of persistent OMD. Among all neonatal cases of persistent OMDs, about 6% of the babies present as completely patent ducts with complications in the first 28 days of life, characteristically with intussusceptions of the small bowel through the patent vitelline duct in 20% of them [20].

Resection and anastomosis is preferable to wedge resection of patent OMD, because of the associated risk of ectopic gastric or pancreatic mucosa as well as the associated ischaemia secondary to intestinal obstruction and strangulation.

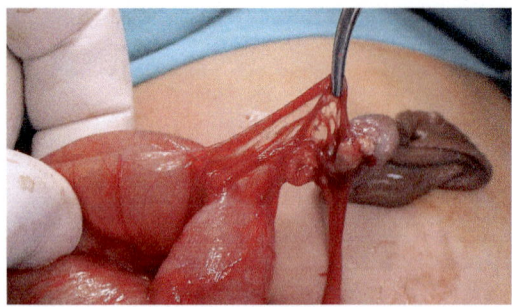

Fig. 36.15 Vitellointestinal band attached to the terminal ileum with a ruptured vitelline cyst at its umbilical end

36.3   Vitellointestinal Sinus

Distal part of the vitellointestinal duct sometimes remains patent to form an umbilical sinus. The mucous membrane of the sinus may evert out to form the 'raspberry tumor' or may be presented as an umbilical polyp, which may had recurrent discharge of mucoid fluid from the umbilicus dating back to the neonatal period. There was no connection to the intestine. Treatment was by excision of the sinus via an infraumbilical incision or minilaparotomy to explore any other associated anomalies [19].

36.4   Vitellointestinal Cyst (Vitelline Duct Cysts)

Remnants of the duct may sometimes show a mucous filled cyst at its centre. The cyst may be attached to the inner aspect of the umbilicus by a fibrous band or to be connected to the terminal ileum (at the site of expected Meckel's diverticulum) [21] (Fig. 36.15).

Omphalomesenteric duct cysts are located at the proximal (fetal) end of the cord and range from 0.4 to 6.0 cm in diameter. They appear as cystically dilated 'miniature' segments of the gastrointestinal tract and are lined by columnar epithelium resembling that of the gastric, small intestinal or colonic mucosa; islands of pancreatic tissue may be associated with the cyst lining. The cysts have peripheral angiomatoid vascularity, and the surface epithelium of the cord at one site tends to be hyperplastic [22]. These lesions occur more often in males than in females and are unrelated to pre-

maturity or to maternal age, race or gravidity. They only rarely cause fetal morbidity or mortality, but evidence is presented to suggest that they may on occasion be associated with potentially dangerous intra-abdominal anomalies of the OM duct [23].

36.5   Vitellointestinal Fibrous band

This remnant presented as a thick cord extending from the umbilicus towards the terminal part of the ileum and beyond. The terminal part of the cord showed a few ramifications that ended in the mesentery. This embryological entity was not found to be associated with any other anomaly, usually related to non-regression of the vitellointestinal duct. Though very rare, the occurrence of such innocuous band of fibrous cord across the abdominal cavity may cause entanglement of intestinal loops around it. Possibility of such a situation should be suspected in an acute abdominal condition [24].

The umbilicus was absolutely normal when observed from the exterior. It is rare to find an asymptomatic vitelline cord unrelated to a Meckel's diverticulum or a cystic dilation of the OMD, in an adult. Sometimes a persistent vitelline artery seen extends along fibrous cord to umbilicus [25] (Fig. 36.15). About 10% of the MD may be attached to the umbilicus with this fibrous band. In several cases, however, the fibrous cord is seen to regress leaving no trace of connection between the Meckel's diverticulum and the umbilicus [26].

36.6   Intestinal Prolapse

Prolapse of different sizes of the mid ileum may be the only manifestation of a vitellointestinal anomalies (Fig. 36.16), but this may be detected with a patent vitelline duct with intussusception of the small bowel (Fig. 36.12).

Ileal intussusception with prolapse of different lengths of bowel is a rarely reported entity [27].

It is the widely patent type of PVID which are more likely to present with either complete or partial prolapse of ileum through the defect. The prolapse itself is probably caused by a sudden increase in intra-abdominal pressure associated with straining in neonates with a widely patent VID. Moreover, since the distance between the ileocecal valve and VID is shorter in neonates, it leads to higher intraluminal pressure causing double intussusception [11, 28].

The prolapsed bowel should be managed early with reduction and exploration for any associated anomalies, mainly Meckel's diverticulum or urachal anomalies; otherwise the exposed bowel may be twisted with impairment of its blood supply and eventually become gangrenous (Fig. 36.17).

Intestinal prolapse through omphalomesenteric fistula is a rare cause of neonatal intestinal obstruction.

36.7 Congenital Umbilical Appendix (Appendico-Umbilical Fistula)

This another congenital anomaly related to OMD presented as an umbilical mass or enteric fistula. Reports of a fistulous connection between appendix and umbilicus are rare. Collins reported only three cases in a review of 50,000 specimens of the human vermiform appendix [29].

From 1922 till now, a total of 11 cases had been reported [30].

In classical patent OMD a connection established between umbilicus with the distal ileum, but very rarely, the bowel connected to the umbilicus is the cecum, ascending colon or the appendix.

Such cases may be presented early as an umbilical mass or later the appendix may perforate in the umbilicus and present as a faecal fistula, appendico-umbilical fistula (Fig. 36.18).

The appendico-umbilical fistula is believed to be a variant of the patent omphalomesenteric duct, one that connected with the appendix instead of the distal ileum or other places like the cecum or the ascending colon.

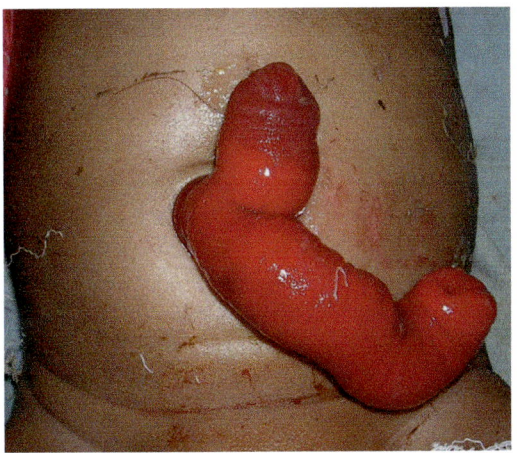

Fig. 36.16 Prolapse of ileum with intussusception

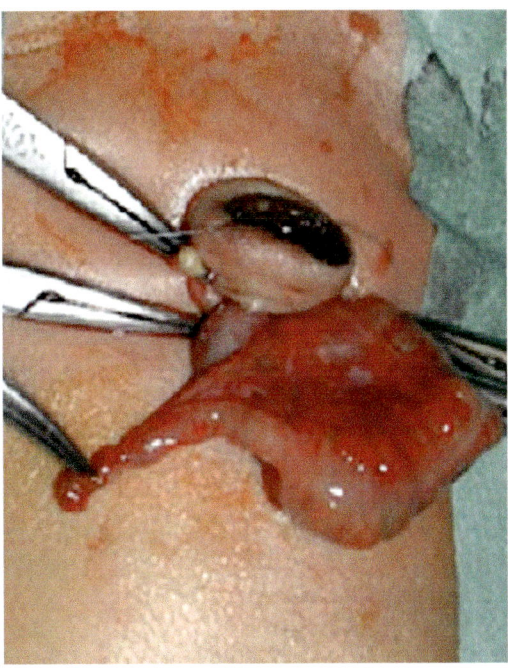

Fig. 36.18 Umbilical appendix; an umbilical mass, with a mobile appendix attached to the umbilicus

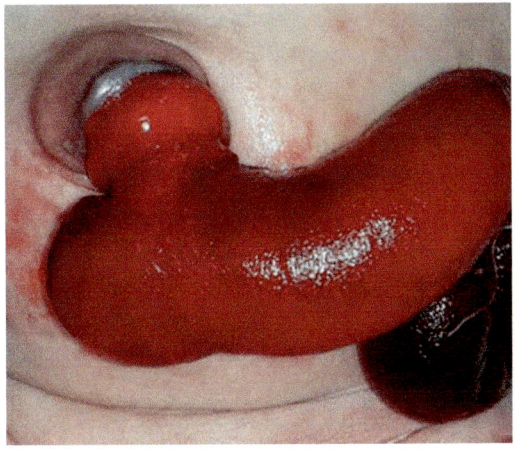

Fig. 36.17 Early bowel gangrene after ileal intussusception

When an umbilical appendix is present, it is known to be associated with various forms of malrotation of the gut [31].

However, these anomalies differ totally from a neonatal appendix protruding in the umbilical cord. This appears to be a different entity of congenital umbilical anomalies.

Recently a theory has been put forward to explain the development of a neonatal umbilical appendix; Borgna-Pignatti et al. [32] postulated that perhaps some of the intestinal loops fail to re-enter the abdominal cavity during the embryological development. In case of failure of a large part of the gut to re-enter the abdomen, a gross omphalocele results, which is often easily diagnosed postpartum. But if the appendix alone fails to re-enter the abdomen, this results only in a small umbilical anomaly, which may not be noticed during neonatal physical examination. When the umbilical cord is cut off straight above the umbilical ring, for example, during the procedure of umbilical vein catherization, this may create an appendico-umbilical fistula (AUF).

It is postulated that the umbilical anomaly reported as AUF in some of the articles in fact are intact neonatal umbilical appendices, which have become a fistula iatrogenically.

Because of the possible association between an umbilical appendix and malrotation of the bowel, it is recommend that in case of a neonatal umbilical appendix, further (radiological) investigation to the anatomical positioning of the bowel needs to be performed following operative procedure.

Investigations: Because more than one omphalomesenteric duct anomaly can be present, radiologic evaluation should be performed in patients with an OMD anomaly. This should include ultrasonography and possibly a Meckel scan (99 m technetium pertechnetate, which has an affinity for gastric mucosa). If the results from ultrasonography are uncertain, computed tomography is performed. CT scan, Meckel's scan and fistulograms are helpful in determining the cause of the symptoms, when the presence of OMD remnants is suspected; moreover, a differential diagnosis from urachal remnants should be made.

Antenatal Diagnosis: Congenital hernia of the umbilical cord or omphalocele associated with a patent omphalomesenteric duct could be diagnosed at midtrimester by ultrasonography, but other OMD anomalies are very rarely diagnosed antenatally in routine examination [33].

Using high-resolution real-time ultrasound in the first trimester of pregnancy is able to demonstrate the yolk sac precisely and the amniotic membrane; high index of suspicion is required to pick up OMD anomalies in the second trimester [34].

Complications: Intestinal obstruction is the most lethal complication of omphalomesenteric duct remnants. The overall lifetime risk of development of complications from Meckel's diverticulum is said to be around 4%, with one-third of cases resulting in small-bowel obstruction [35].

Nearly 20% of patent OMD cases are complicated by intussusception of the small bowel through the patent duct, leading to intestinal obstruction. In view of the high mortality rate of patients with a prolapse of the ileum (18%), and the strong possibility of intestinal obstruction, patent OMD should be resected surgically [36].

Management: Management of this condition requires careful assessment and awareness, while treatment needs to be tailored to the individual case. Surgical resection of remnants of the duct is required for the treatment of bleeding, intussusception and intestinal prolapse causing obstruction.

The principle of surgical management is reduction of the intussuscepted gut along with complete excision of the vitelline duct and restoring the ileal continuity as well as umbilical reconstruction. Three approaches have been described: infraumbilical, supraumbilical or through the umbilicus.

In symptomatic cases the surgical repair could be achieved either by conventional or laparoscopic surgery, while in asymptomatic subjects surgery is not necessary [37].

When haemodynamic conditions are put into question or in the advent of peritoneal sepsis, an initial bowel bypass is needed to avoid the risk of postoperative peritonitis.

For simple fistula, the purpose of surgery is to release the bud by the umbilical route and bowel resection on both sides of the location of the fistula with termino-terminal anastomosis. For some authors, excision of the omphalomesenteric fistula remains justified [27].

Primary closure of the VID following reduction of the prolapse may be possible if the patient arrives early without any gross oedema over the intestinal loops. If the defect is large, one can go for resection of the loop of intestine near the patent duct followed by primary anastomosis [28].

References

1. Kittle CF, Jenkins HP, Dragstedt LR. Patent omphalomesenteric duct and its relation to the diverticulum of Meckel. Arch Surg. 1947;54:10–36.
2. Larsen W. Human embryology. 2nd ed. New York: Churchill Livingstone; 1997. p. 240–2.
3. Trimingham HL, McDonald J. Congenital anomalies in the umbilicus. Surg Gynecol Obstet. 1945;80:152–63.
4. Nix TE Jr, Young JC. Congenital umbilical anomalies. Arch Dermatol. 1964;90:160–5.
5. Aitken J. Remnants of the vitellointestinal duct; a clinical analysis of 88 cases. Arch Dis Child. 1953;28(137):1–7. PMCID: PMC1988648.
6. Markogiannakis H, Theodorou D, Toutouzas KG, Drimousis P. Persistent omphalomesenteric duct causing small bowel obstruction in an adult. World J Gastroenterol. 2007;13(15):2258–60.
7. Ghislain P, Diane C, Christophe A, Xavier C. Intestinal prolapse through a persistent omphalomesenteric duct causing small-bowel obstruction. S Afr J Surg. 2012;50(3):102–3. doi:10.7196/SAJS.1289.
8. Sánchez-Castellanos M, Sandoval-Tress C, Hernández-Torres M. Persistencia del conducto onfalomesentérico. Diagnóstico diferencial de granuloma umbilical en la infancia. Actas Dermosifiliogr. 2006;97:404–5.
9. Griffith GL, et al. Patent urachus associated with completely patent Omphalomesenteric duct. South Med J. 1982;75(2):252. doi:10.1097/00007611-198202000-00041.
10. Ioannidis O, et al. Coexistence of multiple omphalomesenteric duct anomalies. J Coll Physicians Surg Pak. 2012;22(8):524–6. doi: 08.2012/JCPSP.524526.
11. Blair SP, Beasley SW. Intussusception of vitellointestinal tract through an exomphalos in trisomy 13. Pediatr Surg Int. 1989;4:422–3.
12. Bargman H, Stewart WD. A case of Ehlers-Danlos syndrome (type IV) with persisting vitelline duct cyst. Cutis. 1980;25(4):411–4.
13. Miller G, Boman J, Shrier I, et al. Etiology of small bowel obstruction. Am J Surg. 2000;180:33–6.
14. Heider R, Warshauer DM, Behrns KE. Inverted Meckel's diverticulum as a source of chronic gastrointestinal blood loss. Surgery. 2000;128:107–8. [PubMed].
15. Meckel JF. Über die Divertikel am Darmkanal. Arch Physiol. 1809;9:421–53.
16. Coetzee T. Clinical anatomy of the umbilicus. S Afr Med J. 1980;57(12):463–6.
17. Hayashi A, et al. Severe acute abdomen caused by symptomatic Meckel's diverticulum in three children with trisomy 18. Am J Med Genet A. 2015;167A:2447–50.
18. Teitelbaum DH, et al. Laparoscopic diagnosis and excision of Meckel's diverticulum. J Pediatr Surg. 1994;29(4):495–7.
19. Ameh EA, et al. Symptomatic vitelline duct anomalies in children. S Afr J Surg. 2005;43(3):84–5.
20. Yamada T, Seiki Y, Ueda M, Yoshikawa T, Sempuku S, Kurokawa A, Nakata K. Patent omphalomesenteric duct: a case report and review of Japanese literature. Asia Oceania J Obstet Gynaecol. 1989;15(3):229–36.
21. Grosfeld JL, Franken EA. Intestinal obstruction in the neonate due to vitelline duct cysts. Surg Gynecol Obstet. 1974;138(4):527–32.
22. Heifetz SA, Eugenia Rueda-Pedraza M. Omphalomesenteric duct cysts of the umbilical cord. J Pediatr Pathol. 1983;1(3):325–35.
23. Templeton AW, Shebesta E. Communicating vitelline duct cyst. Radiology. 1964;82(3):476–7. doi:10.1148/82.3.476.
24. Schillings GJ. Strangulation ileus caused by a not completely obliterated omphaloenteric duct in a 32-year-old patient. Zentralbl Chir. 1987;112(6):383–6.
25. Kamii Y, Zaki AM, Honna T, Tsuchida Y. Spontaneous regression of patient omphalomesenteric duct: from a fistula to Meckel's diverticulum. J Pediatr Surg. 1992;27(1):115–6.
26. Mahato NK. Obliterated, fibrous omphalomesenteric duct in an adult without Meckel's diverticulum or vitelline cyst. Romanian J Morphol Embryol. 2010;51(1):195–7.
27. Mohite PN, Bhatnagar AM, Hathila VP, Mistry JH. Patent vitellointestinal duct with prolapse of inverted loop of small intestine: a case report. J Med Case Rep. 2007;1:49.
28. Sherer DM, Dar P. Prenatal ultrasonographic diagnosis of congenital umbilical hernia and associated patent omphalomesenteric. Gynecol Obstet Investig. 2001;51(1):66–8. doi:10.1159/000052895.
29. Collins DC. A study of 50,000 specimens of the human vermiform appendix. Surg Gynecol Obstet. 1955;101(4):437–45.
30. Ola Olorun AD, Adesina SA, Adepoju AO, Amole IO. Patent omphalomesenteric duct opening into the vermiform appendix. Int J Case Rep Images. 2015;6(12):743–6.
31. Fuijkschot J, Wijnen RM, Gerrits GP, Dubois SV, Rieu PN. A neonate with an intact congenital umbilical appendix: an alternative theory on the etiology of the appendico-umbilical fistula. Pediatr Surg Int. 2006;22(8):689–93.

32. Borgna Pignatti C, Bergamo Andreis I, Bettili G, Zamboni G. Delayed separation of an appendix containing umbilical stump. J Pediatr Surg. 1995;30:1717–8.

33. Sauerbrei E, et al. Ultrasound demonstration of the normal fetal yolk sac. J Clin Ultrasound. 1980;8(3):217–20. doi:10.1002/jcu.1870080306. Source: PubMed.

34. Srinivas GN, Cullen P. Intestinal obstruction due to Meckel's diverticulum:a rare presentation. Acta Chir Belg. 2007;107:64–6.

35. Vane DW, West KW, Grosfeld JL. Vitelline duct anomalies. Experience with 217 childhood cases. Arch Surg. 1987;122:542.

36. Nursal TZ, et al. Laparoscopic resection of patent omphalomesenteric duct in an adult. Surg Endosc. 2002;16(11):1638. doi:10.1007/s00464-002-4209-2.

37. Dioufa C, Ndoyeb NA, Fayeb AL, Ndourb O, Ngomb G. Intestinal prolapse through omphalomesenteric fistula, a rare cause of neonatal occlusion: a case report. J Pediatr Surg Case Rep. 2016;10:1–2.

Erratum to: Umbilicus and Umbilical Cord

Mohamed Fahmy

Erratum to:
FM (page vi) in: M. Fahmy, *Umbilicus and Umbilical Cord*,
https://doi.org/10.1007/978-3-319-62383-2

This book was inadvertently published missing the following acknowledgement in FM. The original book has been updated accordingly.

Acknowledgement

For additional information and references on the umbilical cord see Silent Risk Issues about the human umbilical cord 2nd Edition Copyright © 2014 by Jason H. Collins, MD, MSCR.

Xlibris Books Library of Congress Control Number: 2014911209.

The online version of the original chapter can be found under
https://doi.org/10.1007/978-3-319-62383-2

© Springer International Publishing AG 2018
M. Fahmy, *Umbilicus and Umbilical Cord*, https://doi.org/10.1007/978-3-319-62383-2_37

Erratum to: Umbilicus in History and Its Religious Background

Mohamed Fahmy

Erratum to:

Chapter 09 (page 29 and 40) in: M. Fahmy, *Umbilicus and Umbilical Cord*, https://doi.org/10.1007/978-3-319-62383-2_9

This Chapter was inadvertently published missing the following reference in the original version. The original chapter has been updated accordingly.

Reference [4] with the following citation in page 29: Jason H. Collins, Silent Risk Issues about the human umbilical cord, 2nd Edition, 2014.

9.2 Umbilicus and Umbilical Cord in Different Cultures

The umbilical cord considered as 'the thread of life' and the placenta are magical doubles of the child and they symbolize the dual union of infant and mother, the tie that unites mother and child.

Umbilical cord in history: One has to wonder what thoughts prehistoric humans had when confronted with the stillbirth of a baby entangled in its umbilical cord. Some insights from more recent times suggest the umbilical cord represented an omen, a sacred talisman, predictor of future fertility. In some popular classes in Europe, Australia, Africa and Hawaii, the umbilical cord was dried and soaked in water for consumption to ensure future fertility. It was eaten, hung from tree branches and stuffed in volcanic rock crevices at sites such as the Birthing Stones in Kukahiioko, Oahu [4]. Chinese literature suggests the cord had many medicinal properties.

The online version of the original chapter can be found under
https://doi.org/10.1007/978-3-319-62383-2_9